Clinical Exercise Science

Clinical Exercise Science is an introduction to core principles and best practice in exercise science for students and practitioners working with clinical populations. Combining the latest scientific research with evidence-based, practitioner-led analysis, the book offers integrated coverage of the full clinical exercise curriculum, including:

- Pathophysiology of exercise and disease
- Exercise as a clinical intervention
- Exercise, nutrition, and lifestyle
- Health behaviour change
- Clinical skills in exercise science.

The book covers a wide range of conditions, including cardiovascular disease, pulmonary disease, metabolic disease, and mental health problems, and includes an array of useful features to guide student learning, such as case studies, study tasks, definitions of key terms and suggestions for further reading. With contributions from leading researchers and health practitioners, this is an invaluable foundation text for any clinical exercise science course, and useful reading for any student or practitioner working in exercise science, exercise rehabilitation, health science, or physical therapy.

Andrew Scott is Course Leader for the MSc in Clinical Exercise Science, and Senior Lecturer in the Department of Sport and Exercise Science at the University of Portsmouth, UK.

Christopher Gidlow is an Associate Professor in the School of Psychology, Sport, and Exercise at Staffordshire University, UK.

Clinical Exercise Science

Edited by
Andrew Scott and
Christopher Gidlow

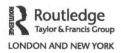

Routledge
Taylor & Francis Group

LONDON AND NEW YORK

First published 2016
by Routledge
2 Park Square, Milton Park, Abingdon, Oxon OX14 4RN

and by Routledge
711 Third Avenue, New York, NY 10017

Routledge is an imprint of the Taylor & Francis Group, an informa business

British Library Cataloguing-in-Publication Data
A catalogue record for this book is available from the British Library

Library of Congress Cataloging in-Publication-Data
Names: Scott, Andrew T., 1979- editor. | Gidlow, Christopher,
    editor.
Title: Clinical exercise science / edited by Andrew Scott and
    Christopher Gidlow.
Description: New York : Routledge, 2016. | Includes bibliographical
    references and index.
Identifiers: LCCN 2015031623| ISBN 9780415708401 (hardback)
    | ISBN 9780415708418 (paperback) | ISBN 9781315885995
    (eBook)
Subjects: LCSH: Clinical psychology. | Exercise—Physiological aspects.
Classification: LCC RC466.8 .C55 2016 | DDC 616.89—dc23
LC record available at http://lccn.loc.gov/2015031623

ISBN: 978-0-415-70840-1 (hbk)
ISBN: 978-0-415-70841-8 (pbk)
ISBN: 978-1-315-88599-5 (ebk)

Typeset in Sabon
by Swales & Willis Ltd, Exeter, Devon, UK.

Printed and bound in the United States of America by
Edwards Brothers Malloy on sustainably sourced paper

Contents

Acknowledgements

Figure 2.1 reproduced with permission from BACPR
Figure 3.1 reproduced with permission from Sage Publications Ltd
Figure 3.2 reproduced with permission from Elsevier
Figure 6.3 reprinted with permission from Betof AS, Dewhirst MW, Jones LW (2013). Effects and potential mechanisms of exercise training on cancer progression: a translational perspective. *Brain Behaviour and Immunity* 30, S75–87. Copyright 2013, Elsevier
Figure 7.3 reproduced with permission from Gallanagh et al. (2011)

Boxes

Figures

Tables

Chapter authors

Chapter 1

Andrew Scott, BSc, MSc, PhD, Course Leader for MSc Clinical Exercise Science and Senior Lecturer
Department of Sport and Exercise Science, University of Portsmouth, United Kingdom.

Chapter 2

Gail Sheppard, BSc, MSc, MPH, Senior Lecturer and Programme Director for BSc Health Studies/Public Health/Health Promotion
School of Public Health, Midwifery and Social Work, Canterbury Christ Church University, United Kingdom.

Steve Meadows, BA, MSc, PhD, Lecturer and Director for BSc Sport and Exercise for Health
School of Sport and Exercise Sciences, University of Kent, United Kingdom.

Chapter 3

Linzy Houchen-Wolloff, PhD, MCSP, Senior Research Associate
Centre for Exercise and Rehabilitation Science, Respiratory Biomedical Research Unit, Glenfield Hospital, University Hospitals of Leicester NHS Trust, United Kingdom.

Lorna Latimer, BSc, Research Exercise Physiologist
Centre for Exercise and Rehabilitation Science, Respiratory Biomedical Research Unit, Glenfield Hospital, University Hospitals of Leicester NHS Trust, United Kingdom.

Michael Steiner, MB BS, BSc, MD, FRCP, Consultant Respiratory Physician[1] and Honorary Clinical Professor[2]
[1]Leicester Respiratory Biomedical Research Unit, Glenfield Hospital, University Hospitals of Leicester NHS Trust, United Kingdom.
[2]School of Sports, Exercise and Health Sciences, Loughborough University, United Kingdom.

Chapter 4

Tom Yates, BSc, MSc, PhD, Senior Lecturer
Diabetes Research Centre, University of Leicester, United Kingdom.
National Institute for Health Research (NIHR) Leicester-Loughborough Diet, Lifestyle, and Physical Activity Biomedical Research Unit, United Kingdom.

Andrew Scott, BSc, MSc, PhD, Course Leader for MSc Clinical Exercise Science and Senior Lecturer
Department of Sport and Exercise Science, University of Portsmouth, United Kingdom.

Chapter 5

Naomi Ellis, BSc, MSc, PhD, Senior Lecturer
School of Psychology, Sport and Exercise, Staffordshire University, United Kingdom.

Leon Meek, BSc, PgCert, Engagement, Activity and Physical Health Lead
Greyfriars PICU, Wotton Lawn Hospital, 2gether NHS Trust for Gloucestershire, United Kingdom.

Chapter 6

Clare Stevinson, BSc, MSc, PhD, Lecturer
School of Sport, Exercise and Health Sciences, University of Loughborough, United Kingdom.

Anna Campbell, BSc, MSc, PhD, Reader
School of Life, Sport and Social Sciences, Edinburgh Napier University, United Kingdom.

Helen Crank, BA, MSc, PhD, Principal Research Fellow
Centre for Sport and Exercise Science, Sheffield Hallam University, United Kingdom.

Chapter 7

Tom Balchin, BA, MSc, PhD
Director, The ARNI Institute, Surrey, United Kingdom.
Honorary Senior Research Fellow, Oxford Brookes University, United Kingdom.

Sarah Valkenborghs, BSc, Research Assistant
Hunter Medical Research Institute, University of Newcastle, Australia.

Chapter 8

Johnathan Collett, BSc, PhD, Senior Clinical Research Fellow
Centre for Rehabilitation, Faculty of Health and Life Sciences, Oxford Brookes University, United Kingdom.

Helen Dawes, BSc, MMedSci, PhD, Elizabeth Casson Trust Chair
Centre for Rehabilitation, Faculty of Health and Life Sciences, Oxford Brookes University, United Kingdom.
Associate Research Fellow, Department of Clinical Neurology, University of Oxford, United Kingdom.
Honorary Professor, Cardiff University, United Kingdom.

James Bateman, MSc, Lecturer
Centre for Rehabilitation, Faculty of Health and Life Sciences, Oxford Brookes University, United Kingdom.

Chapter 9

Gladys Onambélé-Pearson, BSc, MSc, PhD, Reader
Department of Exercise and Sport Science, Manchester Metropolitan University, United Kingdom.

Neil Reeves, BSc, MSc, PhD, Professorial Research Fellow
School of Healthcare Science, Manchester Metropolitan University, United Kingdom.

Chapter 10

Lisa Loughney, BSc, MSc, Clinical Exercise Physiologist [1,2,3]

Sandy Jack, MSc, PhD, Consultant Clinical Scientist, Associate Professor [1,2,3]

Denny Z H Levett, BM BCh, PhD, MRCP, FRCA, Consultant Anaesthesia and Critical Care[1,2,3]
[1]*Integrative Physiology and Critical Illness Group, Clinical and Experimental Sciences, Faculty of Medicine, University of Southampton, United Kingdom.*
[2]*Critical Care Research Area, Southampton NIHR Respiratory Biomedical Research Unit, United Kingdom.*
[3]*Anaesthesia and Critical Care Research Unit, University Hospital Southampton NHS Foundation Trust, United Kingdom.*

Chapter 11

Lynne Johnston, BA, MSc, PhD, DClin Psych, CPsychol, AFBPsS, Principal Clinical Psychologist
South of Tyne Specialist Weight Management Service, Department of Clinical Health Psychology, City Hospitals Sunderland NHS Foundation Trust, United Kingdom.

Andrew Hutchison, PhD, CPsychol
Birmingham and Solihull Mental Health NHS Foundation Trust, United Kingdom.

Chapter 12

Diane Crone, BSc, PhD, Professor of Exercise Science
School of Sport and Exercise, University of Gloucestershire, United Kingdom.

David James, BSc, PhD, Professor of Exercise Science
School of Sport and Exercise, University of Gloucestershire, United Kingdom.

Chapter 13

Christopher Gidlow, BSc, MSc, PhD, Associate Professor
School of Psychology, Sport and Exercise, Staffordshire University, United Kingdom.

Diane Crone, BSc, PhD, Professor of Exercise Science
School of Sport and Exercise, University of Gloucestershire, United Kingdom.

Michelle Huws-Thomas, BSc, MSc, PhD, CPsychol, AFBPsS, CSci, Lecturer in Mental Health
School of Healthcare Sciences, Cardiff University, United Kingdom.

Chapter 14

Samantha Meredith, BSc, MSc, Research Assistant
Department of Sport and Exercise Science, University of Portsmouth, United Kingdom.
Chris Wagstaff, BSc, MSc, PhD, CPsychol, AFBPsS, CSci, Course Leader for MSc Sport and Exercise Psychology and Senior Lecturer
Department of Sport and Exercise Science, University of Portsmouth, United Kingdom.

Glossary

6MWD 6-minute walk distance.

6MWT 6-minute walk test.

AAA abdominal aortic aneurysm.

ACSM American College of Sports Medicine, An organisation which aims to advance and integrate scientific research to provide educational and practical applications of exercise science and sports medicine.

Acute Stroke < 1 month post-stroke.

ADL activities of daily living.

Aerobic exercise in which energy needed is provided by using oxygen inspired to produce ATP.

Ambulatory relates to walking.

Anaemia a marked decrease in haemoglobin in the blood, caused by destruction or decreased production of red blood cells, or blood loss.

Anaerobic exercise in which energy needed exceeds oxidative processes and non-aerobic metabolism is dominant.

Angina Pectoris experience of central retro-sternal chest pain but pain can radiate to upper limbs, back, stomach and jaw.

Angiogenesis the development of new blood vessels.

Angiogram a type of X-ray used following an injection of a dye into the blood vessels to examine the health of blood vessels and location and extent of narrowing.

Anosodiaphoria indifference to the existence of a limitation.

Anosognosia inability or refusal to recognise a defect or disorder that is clinically evident.

Aphasia inability (or impaired ability) to understand or produce speech.

Arrhythmia abnormal heart rhythm (the heart does not beat rhythmically).

AT anaerobic threshold.

Atherosclerosis disease of the arteries characterised by the accumulation of fatty material in arterial wall resulting in narrowing of the vessel lumen.

ATP adenosine triphosphate.

ATS/ACCP The American Thoracic Society/The American College of Chest Physicians.

Autonomic neuropathy affects the nerves that control involuntary bodily processes like digestion and heart rate.

β-blocker β-adrenoceptor antagonist.

BACPR British Association for Cardiovascular Prevention and Rehabilitation.

Basal metabolic rate minimal rate of metabolism of the body in a non-digestive and non-absorptive state.

Behavioural Experiment a technique commonly used in CBT-based therapies to gather information, which leads to either the development of a formulation, an examination of the validity of a person's beliefs, or the development and examination of new beliefs.

Biomechanics the internal and external forces acting on the human body.

BMI body mass index.

BP blood pressure.

BR breathing reserve.

CABG coronary artery bypass graft.

CAG cytosine-adenine-guanine, the codon for the amino acid glutamine. A repeat mutation of this codon on the huntingtin gene is the cause of HD.

Cardiac output volume of blood ejected from heart in litres per minute.

Cardiovascular disease (CVD) disease of the blood vessels (arteries) that can lead to narrowed or blocked blood vessels

Cardiovascular exercise predominantly dynamic exercise using large-muscle groups (e.g. walking or running).

Case Formulation also referred to as case conceptualisation. A process of performing an individualised assessment of a clinical case, which is sensitive to variations in the development, manifestation, and maintaining mechanisms of an individual's difficulties.

Cerebral relating to the cerebrum of the brain.

Cerebrovascular relating to the blood vessels of the brain.

Cerebrovascular accident (CVA) the medical term for a stroke.

CES-D scale Centre for Epidemiologic Studies Depression Scale. A scoring system for depression.

CHD coronary heart disease.

CHF chronic heart failure.

Chronic Stroke > 6 months post-stroke.

Circuit training conditioning exercises designed to improve multiple fitness components (strength, endurance, and aerobic capacity).

Clinical Psychologist an applied practitioner with expertise in the application of psychological theory to practice. Clinical psychologists work in a range of mental and physical health settings and contribute to the assessment and treatment of a range of clinical difficulties.

Cognition the process of acquiring knowledge and understanding through thought, experience, and the senses.

Cognitive Behavioural Therapy (CBT) a classification of psychotherapeutic approaches informed by cognitive and behavioural theory, which typically seek to modify maladaptive thinking, in order to bring about behavioural and emotional change.

Contracture the shortening and hardening of muscles, tendons, or other tissue, often leading to deformity and rigidity of joints.

Contraindication   any factor that makes it unwise to engage in an activity (e.g. exercise) as risks outweigh benefits.

Contralateral   relating to the opposite side of the body to that on which a particular structure or condition occurs.

COPD   chronic obstructive pulmonary disorder.

CPET   cardio-pulmonary exercise test.

CR   cardiac rehabilitation.

Creatine kinase   an enzyme found in the heart which can be leaked into the blood when the myocardium is damaged (e.g. in a myocardial infarction).

CRF   cardio-respiratory fitness.

CT   computerised tomography (scan).

CV   cardiovascular.

Cx   circumflex artery.

Dynamic exercise   muscle contraction producing movement.

ECG   electrocardiagram.

EDSS   Expanded Disability Status Scale, an MS specific scale used to quantify and monitor the level of disability.

Ejection fraction   ratio of left ventricle stroke volume to end-diastolic volume (or percentage of end-diastolic volume ejected with each cardiac contraction); normal range is 60 per cent to 75 per cent.

Electrocardiogram   a graphical record of the electrical changes occurring during the cardiac cycle (heart contraction).

Embolus   solid or fluid material which is carried by the blood from one point in the body to lodge at another point.

Endothelium   cells that forms the inner lining of a blood vessel wall providing a friction-reducing lining.

EuSOS   European Surgical Outcomes Study.

Flexibility activity   activity designed to enhance range of motion of joints.

Gait   a person's manner of walking.

Growth factor   a substance which stimulates growth of cells.

Haemorrhagic stroke   a blood vessel bursts causing bleeding into the brain tissue.

Harris Hip Score (HHS score)   a measure of hip function and symptoms.

HD   Huntington's disease, a genetic neurodegenerative LTNC characterised by striatum dysfunction.

Heart rate variability (HRV)   variation in the time interval between heart beats.

Hemiparesis/ Hemiplegia   paralysis of one side of the body.

Hemispatial neglect   lack of attention or awareness of one side of the body due to inability to process and perceive stimuli, where that inability is not due to a lack of sensation.

High-density lipoprotein (HDL)   a lipoprotein that is often referred to as the 'good cholesterol' as it transfers fat away from artery walls, reducing risk of atherosclerosis.

HIT   high intensity training.

HR   heart rate.

HR$_{max}$ maximum heart rate. The highest number of heart beats per minute an individual can achieve in an all-out effort.

%HR$_{max}$ percentage heart rate maximum.

HRR   heart rate reserve.

%HRR   percentage heart rate reserve.

HRV   heart rate variability.

Hyaline cartilage   the joint capsule. It is shiny, slippery, firm, translucent, and has no nerves or blood vessels.

Hypertonicity   the chronic contraction of a muscle.

ICF   International Classification of Functioning, Disability and Health, a classification system for health and health-related domains.

Ischaemia   restriction of oxygen.

Ischemic stroke   a thrombosis or embolism (a clot) that blocks or narrows a blood vessel that carries oxygenated blood to the brain.

Isometric/static exercise   muscle contraction with no movement.

ISWT   incremental shuttle walk test.

Knee malalignment   Unbalanced set of forces across the patellofemoral joint causing the patella to not be centred within the trochlear groove (see valgus and varus).

KOOS   Knee Injury and Osteoarthritis Outcome Score.

LAD   left anterior descending artery.

LaT   lactate threshold.

Lesion   a region in an organ or tissue that has suffered damage through injury or disease.

LTNC   long-term neurological condition, a neurological condition which results from injury or disease that will affect an individual for the rest of their lives.

Lumen   blood vessel cavity where blood flows through.

Lymphoedema   the accumulation of lymph in soft tissue leading to swelling; caused by damage to, or removal of, lymph channels.

Malignancy   a cluster of cells with the capacity to invade surrounding tissue and spread to other parts of the body.

MCT   moderate intensity continuous training.

MET   metabolic equivalent of task ($3.5 \ mL \cdot kg^{-1} \cdot min^{-1}$ of oxygen uptake).

Meta-analysis   combining the findings from independent studies often used to assess the clinical effectiveness of healthcare interventions.

Metastasis   the spread of cancer cells from the primary site to other parts of the body via the bloodstream or lymph system.

MI   myocardial infarction.

MLWHF   Minnesota Living with Heart Failure questionnaire.

Moment   the muscle force across a joint.

Mortality   the state of being mortal or susceptible to death; mortality rate refers to death rate.

Motivational Interviewing (MI)   a goal-oriented, client-centred counselling style for eliciting behaviour change by helping clients to explore and resolve ambivalence.

Motor control   the process by which humans and animals use their neuromuscular system to activate and coordinate the muscles and limbs involved in the performance of a skill.

MRI   magnetic resonance imagery (scan).

MS   multiple sclerosis, an inflammatory, neurodegenerative LTNC characterised by focal areas of demyelination in the central nervous system.

MSE   muscular strength and endurance (exercise).

MV̇O₂   myocardial oxygen consumption.

MVV maximum voluntary ventilation.

Myelin a fatty material that provides electrical insulation and protection by forming a sheath around a nerve.

Myocardium cardiac muscle cells.

NACR National Audit of Cardiac Rehabilitation.

Neoplasm (tumour) a new growth of tissue characterised by the uncontrolled reproduction of cells.

Neurogenesis the growth and development of nervous tissue.

Neuroplasticity relating to changes in neural pathways and synapses.

Neutropenia a marked decrease in the number of neutrophils (a kind of white blood cell) in the blood.

NICE National Institute for Health and Care Excellence, the executive non-departmental public body of the UK Department of Health providing guidance and advice to improve health and social care.

NO nitric oxide.

NSAID non-steroidal anti-inflammatory drug.

Occlude blockage (normally relates to a blood vessel).

Oedema swelling normally caused by fluid retention.

Osteophyte bone spur.

Parasympathetic part of the autonomic nervous system that creates the internal body conditions found during a resting state.

Pathophysiology the study of the biological and physical manifestations of disease; the study of disease process that results in signs and symptoms of disease.

PCI percutaneous coronary intervention.

Penumbral region the area of hypoxic cells near the location of the original lesion.

Percutaneous coronary intervention a procedure that involves non-surgical widening of the coronary artery, using a balloon catheter to dilate the artery from within (angioplasty); a metallic stent is usually placed in the artery after dilatation.

PETCO$_2$ end tidal carbon dioxide.

PETO$_2$ end tidal oxygen.

Pharmacological drug intervention.

PPI proton pump inhibitor.

Prehab prehabilitation.

Premanifest used to describe the period of someone's life with the mutant HD gene before symptoms become apparent.

Proprioception stimuli that are produced and perceived within the body.

Psycho-education a process of providing education for individuals and/or carers/families on the possible biological, psychological and social determinants of a person's difficulties.

Pulmonary pertaining to the lungs.

PVD peripheral vascular disease.

Pw people with . . . commonly used prefix when referring to people that have a certain disease or condition.

Quality of life a highly subjective measure, but reflects a person's general sense of wellbeing and an ability to enjoy normal life activities.

Rating of perceived exertion (RPE) Borg scale of 6 to 20 or 0 to 10.

RCT randomised controlled trial, a research design that aims to minimise bias, seen as the most robust research design and second to systematic reviews in terms of level of evidence. This approach is often considered the gold standard for a clinical trial.

RER respiratory exchange ratio.

Resistance or strength training muscle contraction with limited movement and against a resistance, which is designed to increase muscle strength.

Risk stratification process of classifying (stratifying) the risk of a further cardiac event (low, moderate, or high risk).

ROS reactive oxygen species.

RPP rate pressure product is an indirect measure of cardiac workload (calculated: SBP × HR / 100); it is a measure of stress placed on the myocardium based on the number of times the heart beats per minute (HR) and the systemic arterial blood pressure that it is pumping against (SBP). It provides an indication of the oxygen demand of the myocardium, and therefore a measure of the oxygen consumption of the heart.

RR respiratory rate.

RT resistance training.

SBP systolic blood pressure.

Sensorimotor function actions involving both sensory and motor pathways.

SF-12 12-Item Short Form Health Survey.

Spasticity altered skeletal muscle performance with a combination of paralysis, increased tendon reflex activity, and hypertonia.

SpO$_2$ oxygen saturation.

Spontaneous recovery the phenomenon of the re-emergence of a previously extinguished conditioned response/ability without professional treatment or formal help.

ST depression horizontal or down-sloping (0.10 mV/ms) segment, measured from isoelectric PR level.

Stenosis narrowing.

Stroke insufficient oxygen supply to the brain due to cerebrovascular stenosis or haemorrhage.

Stroke volume amount of blood ejected from the heart with each contraction; normal range is 80 to 90 mL at rest in a 70kg male.

Sub-acute stroke 1–6 months post-stroke.

Subchondral bone bone that is immediately beneath or below the cartilages.

Subluxation a partial dislocation or misalignment of a joint.

Systematic review a review that aims to evaluate all the possible of the research relevant the question they pose.

Task-specific training breaking down daily skills (e.g. grasping) into part movements that are practiced repeatedly (100–300 reps/day) to stimulate the neural reorganisation that underlies motor learning.

TC total cholesterol.

Thrombolytic drugs used to dissolve blood clots in a procedure termed thrombolysis.

Thrombopenia a reduction in the number of platelets in the blood.

Training physical activity and/or conditioning exercise leading to improved fitness.

Troponin complex protein that is integral to cardiac muscle contraction.

TUG   Timed Up and Go, an often used clinical test of functional mobility, whereby a person is timed to standing from a chair walking around a cone and returning to sitting.

UHDRS   Unified Huntington's Disease Rating Scale; quantifies the clinical features of HD.

Uhthoff phenomenon   an increase in body temperature that leads to a transient intensification of MS symptoms.

Up titration   increase dosage of medication; doctors use the term titration to describe the process of adjusting the standard dosage of a medication up or down based on an individual patient's reactions.

Valgus knee angle   this is when the line joining the centre of the hip joint passes through the knee (i.e. the mechanical axis of the knee), in a bent position causing the knee to face outwardly.

Varus knee angle   this is when the line joining the centre of the hip joint passes through the knee (i.e. the mechanical axis of the knee), in a bent position causing the knee to face inwardly.

VAS score   the Visual Analogue Scale (VAS) is commonly used to scale pain.

Vascular   relating to vessels, particularly those carrying blood.

Vasoconstriction   a physiological response in the vascular system where the lumen of the vessel narrows.

Vasodilation   a physiological response in the vascular system where the lumen of the vessel expand.

$\dot{V}_E$ minute expired ventilation.

$\dot{V}_E/\dot{V}O_2$ ventilatory equivalents for oxygen.

$\dot{V}_E/\dot{V}CO_2$ ventilatory equivalents for carbon dioxide.

$\dot{V}O_2$ oxygen uptake.

$\dot{V}CO_2$ carbon dioxide production.

$\dot{V}O_{2max}$ maximum oxygen uptake. A factor that can determine a person's capacity to perform a sustained aerobic effort.

$\dot{V}O_{2peak}$ peak oxygen uptake.

$\dot{V}O_2R$ oxygen uptake reserve.

$\%\dot{V}O_{2max}$ percentage maximum oxygen uptake.

$\%\dot{V}O_2R$ percentage oxygen uptake reserve. A method of exercise intensity monitoring or prescription that utilises the fraction of the difference between resating and maximal $\dot{V}O_2$.

$\dot{V}O_2/HR$ oxygen pulse. The volume of oxygen consumed relative to each heart beat; an indicator of cardiovascular efficiency.

V_T tidal volume.

WHO   World Health Organization, agency of the United Nations concerned with health.

WOMAC index   Western Ontario and McMaster Universities' index. It is a disability functional scale using 24 parameters.

Chapter 1

Introduction to clinical exercise science

Andrew Scott

Introduction

This book has been developed to complement other similar books in the area of clinical exercise science by bringing together expert exercise practitioners in the UK who also have an academic background, to provide evidence-based exercise guidance that academic texts in clinical exercise do not provide. This textbook aims to discuss information on exercise considerations for medical conditions in Chapters 2–10, and also discusses methods of facilitating exercise referral and long-term physical activity behaviour change in Chapters 11–14.

This chapter and the subsequent chapters in the book follow a general pattern including:

- A brief discussion of the pathophysiology of the condition
- Specific exercise guidelines and a discussion of the evidence that underpins these
- A case study
- Suggestions for future research
- A chapter summary
- Study tasks
- Further reading/resources.

A key theme in this book is the promotion of physical activity, not just the study of exercise physiology, as is the case with many such textbooks and, especially, journal articles. There is often a disconnection between working in an ideal physiological scenario, yet forgetting that those who can benefit from being more physically active will not necessarily have the contacts, intrinsic motivation, or confidence to become more physically active by themselves. Therefore, the remit of this book was to bring together a team of authors who are not only exercise scientists, but are also experienced practitioners in the study of physical activity, and are themselves exercise practitioners. This has led to a practitioner focus to the chapters rather than them just reporting data from laboratory studies. Importantly, there are four chapters that are focused on the soft skills of engaging sedentary individuals in becoming more physically active using evidence-based research and the professional experiences of the authors.

Chapters 2–9 in this book are largely defined by the range of specialist exercise instructor awards for the management of chronic diseases or disorders that are available in the UK, while Chapter 10 presents information on well-established techniques being applied in a relatively new context that have not been presented in other such textbooks. Exercise services in cardiac rehabilitation, pulmonary rehabilitation, stroke rehabilitation, neurological rehabilitation, and physiotherapy for musculoskeletal conditions are well-established in hospitals in the UK; however, referral pathways for patients following outpatient care can be variable. Referral for exercise for individuals recovering from cancer treatment is increasing, although it is still not widely available, while dedicated physical activity counselling for diabetes and mental health needs to be prioritised in care pathways, since increasing numbers of patients are suffering from such disorders, which have a strong and inverse relationship with physical activity and fitness levels. Chapter 10 is not related to exercise leadership *per se*, but is concerned with the increasing utilisation of pre-operative exercise testing to objectively assess a patient's fitness for surgery rather than clinical judgement alone. Such tests can be used to indicate to a patient how much they might struggle during the peri-operative period (during and after surgery). In previous years, these tests would screen out patients who would be unable to receive surgical treatment – usually for cancer resection – however, increasing research has demonstrated that, as with apparently healthy individuals, it is possible to significantly and clinically improve fitness for surgery through structured exercise training. The remaining challenge is to optimise the exercise prescription for improving fitness for surgery and post-surgical prognosis with the minimum of frequency, intensity, and time of exercise.

The final four chapters in the book present the authors' experience of promoting health behaviours in a physical activity context, particularly relating to exercise referral services in the UK. The use of physical activity counselling underpinned by psychological principles is under-utilised in the UK, with behavioural medicine still not as available as traditional medicine in the prevention and treatment of chronic diseases and disorders. This is further exacerbated by sport and exercise psychology, and, indeed, often sport and exercise in general, being largely focused on sport and less on exercise. There is often a token nod to physical activity in most respects, rather than the promotion of health-enhancing physical activity being the primary focus that is needed to help the National Health Service (NHS) and regional and central governments in their challenge to engage individuals in physical activity across the lifespan of diverse groups of individuals. Chapter 11 outlines the theory and application of psychological principles to enhancing health behaviours and parallels this with physical activity, where there is less evidence. Chapters 12 and 13 discuss the promotion of physical activity through an evaluation of research interventions, and those applied specifically in exercise referral services. Finally, Chapter 14 discusses the relatively new advent of 'stealth physical activity interventions' to enhance physical activity participation in hard-to-reach groups, i.e. those who do not wish to take part in structured physical activity or do not personally take responsibility for their health. The message is to perform a particular activity, such as gardening, as the primary driver to deliver an end result, i.e. a tidy garden, but at the same time increase incidental energy expenditure too.

Physical activity in healthcare

During the last fifty years there has been considerable growth in the appreciation of physical activity in preventive medicine and in the secondary treatment of a range of communicable and non-communicable disorders, based on a range of anecdotal, epidemiological, and interventional reports (Blair and Morris, 2009; Fiuza-Luces et al., 2013; Sallis, 2009). The evidence is so broad that physical inactivity is increasingly being seen as a key public health issue, equal to smoking and obesity (Kohl et al., 2012; Lee et al., 2012). In the general population, it has long been recognised that engaging adults in regular exercise could achieve important health benefits at relatively low cost (Morris, 1994). Physical activity reduces the risk of developing chronic diseases including type 2 diabetes (Hopper et al., 2011), cancer of the breast (Friedenreich, 2011), kidney (Behrens and Leitzmann, 2013) and colon (Thompson et al., 2003), osteoporosis (Howe et al., 2011), obesity (Tate et al., 2007) and depression (Mammen and Faulkner, 2013). Further benefits may include increased employment rates and decreased mental health problems for both patients and carers.

Fitter patients have been shown to have better outcomes in a wide variety of conditions, including diabetes (Hayashino et al., 2012; Thomas et al., 2006), coronary artery disease (Thompson et al., 2003; Thompson et al., 2007), heart failure (Belardinelli et al., 1999; Mandic et al., 2012; O'Connor et al., 2009), hypertension (Cornelissen and Smart, 2013), COPD (Waschki et al., 2011), chronic kidney disease (Heiwe and Jacobson, 2011), cancer (Brunelli et al. 2014; Des Guetz et al., 2013), stroke (Austin et al., 2014; Saunders et al., 2013), depression (Cooney et al., 2013) and dementia (Forbes et al., 2013).

Although there is a transiently-increased risk of mortality during physical activity or training (De Backer et al., 2003; Thompson et al., 2007), this is outweighed by the cumulative benefit of regular physical activity (Thompson et al., 2003). Supervised and unsupervised training programmes have been shown to be beneficial in a variety of conditions, including COPD, stroke, heart failure, and intermittent claudication (Carson et al., 2013; Lane et al., 2014; Mehrholz et al., 2014; Puhan et al., 2011; Taylor et al., 2014). Furthermore, exercise has been shown to improve the quality of life and the ability to perform activities of daily living in the frail elderly (Chou et al., 2012). Likewise, the public health promotion of physical activity is generally effective (Heath et al., 2012).

Exercise referral services

The evidence for physical activity in the management of long-term health conditions is now beginning to be implemented through the development of condition-specific community exercise programmes in the UK. The referral pathways for various medical conditions are analogous to the well-established rehabilitation services for patients with cardiac disease, where patients graduate from outpatient rehabilitation programmes and are referred to community-based exercise programmes that are sometimes part of broader exercise referral services. These collaborations between NHS Trusts and council-run leisure centres provide a range of exercise programmes delivered in either small group or one-to-one sessions (Nicholson et al., 2013). Additionally, some UK charities, such as Breathe Easy, Action from Rehabilitation for Neurological Injury (ARNI), MacMillan and Mind offer free or minimal-cost group exercise classes.

As with all health interventions the cost-effectiveness of exercise referral has been scrutinised. The available evidence suggests that structured exercise is one of the most cost-effective interventions available, using chronic obstructive pulmonary disease (COPD) as an example. A recent summary of the relative value of treatments for COPD suggested that pulmonary rehabilitation (PR) was one of the highest value interventions to improve health outcomes in this patient group (British Thoracic Society, 2012). However, even in the optimal environment of an outpatient unit, the time dedicated to each patient's therapy is restricted by economic constraints, such as limited resources and personnel (Gallanagh et al., 2011). Individual therapy is labour intensive (Studenski et al. 2005), whereas reduced self-esteem and low mood in patients can contribute to decreased motivation to participate in group-based physical activity (Gallanagh et al., 2011). However, circuit class therapy (CCT) can be as effective as individual physiotherapy sessions for inpatient rehabilitation and in reducing the length of hospital stay (English and Hillier, 2011; English et al., 2007). Thus, the provision of CCT over individual therapy is more cost-effective, and also facilitates socialisation and the reduction of perceptions of isolation. An age-old yet persistent challenge is increasing the 'graduation' of patients receiving acute hospital-based exercise therapy, such as cardiac rehabilitation, pulmonary rehabilitation, stroke rehabilitation or cancer treatment, into community-based physical activity programmes to maintain lifelong physical activity to help in secondary prevention. The main challenge here, besides funding, is ensuring that exercise practitioners engage in appropriate training, gain experience, and maintain their continuing professional development in planning, instructing, and adapting physical activities for a range of referred conditions. This is important since such individuals are increasingly presenting with multiple morbidities besides their primary referral condition.

Physical activity and health training pathways

Professionals involved in the delivery of hospital- and community-based clinical exercise services require condition-specific training and experience in prescribing and supervising exercise for such patient groups, along with up to date cardiopulmonary resuscitation (CPR) training. Referral pathways may include input from professionals in several disciplines, including: general physicians, consultants, physiotherapists, occupational therapists, nurses, dieticians, exercise physiologists, and health psychologists. The balance of the contribution of these healthcare professionals depends on the particular patient group and the level of service that has been commissioned. A number of training pathways are available for individuals to train to deliver clinical exercise programmes, and those in the UK and USA will be discussed here.

UK accredited certifications

During the previous two decades a number of training organisations have begun to deliver specialist exercise instructor training for defined medical conditions, mapped to National Occupational Standards on the Register of Exercise Professionals (REPs). The most well-established courses address the conditions in the third column of Figure 1.1. The prerequisite for these courses is a level 2 qualification in fitness instruction, such as exercise to music or gym-based exercise. The entry-level award is followed by a level 3 exercise referral instructor award relating to low/moderate-risk referred

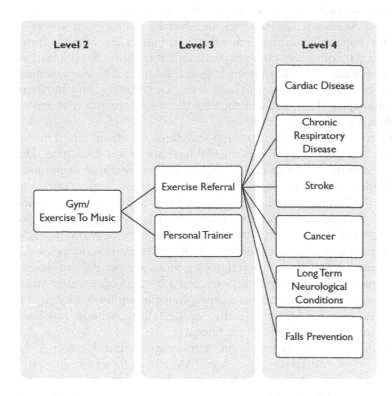

Figure 1.1 SkillsActive specialist exercise instructor pathway.

conditions to serve as an introductory grounding in planning and instructing adapted exercise for conditions such as:

- Hypertension
- Hypercholesterolaemia
- Chronic obstructive pulmonary disease
- Asthma
- Obesity
- Type 1 and 2 diabetes
- Osteoarthritis
- Rheumatoid arthritis
- Osteoporosis
- Depression
- Stress
- Anxiety
- Simple mechanical back pain
- Joint replacement.

After completing the exercise referral course and 150 hours of experience in providing exercise guidance at this level, exercise professionals wishing to deliver exercise for patients with known diseases/disorders are eligible to train in exercise for higher risk medical conditions. As Figure 1.1 indicates, the exercise courses that are most well-established are for patients in cardiac rehabilitation, pulmonary rehabilitation, stroke rehabilitation, as part of cancer rehabilitation, falls prevention for the frail or elderly and exercise for the management of neurological conditions. These are medical conditions that cannot be ameliorated by exercise, but exercise training can contribute towards successfully managing them, and can decrease the risk of secondary events or complications arising as a result of the condition.

There are currently nine National Occupational Standards for Health and Fitness, with the remainder being obesity and diabetes, mental health, and low back pain. The conditions demonstrated in the level 4 column of Figure 1.1 are led by, or in conjunction with, academic leaders in these fields, and there is potential for further courses to be developed in Metabolic Disorders, Mental Health, and Musculoskeletal Conditions that are led by Higher Education Institutions (HEI). The level 4 specialist exercise instructor courses are generally studied in block delivery, for instance two weekends, combined with home study and gaining experience of clinical exercise services for the relevant medical condition(s) that the course relates to, and a further day for assessment is a common format. The assessments can vary, but a common assessment strategy includes a written exam and a case study of a client, sometimes followed by an oral exam. A practical exam is required for exercise after stroke, falls prevention, low back pain and exercise for long-term neurological conditions.

In terms of HEI involvement in the provision of training in clinical exercise, the British Association of Sport and Exercise Sciences (BASES) endorses graduates in sport and exercise subjects who have completed a course of studies that includes sufficient notional hours in biomechanics, physiology, psychology, inter-disciplinary studies, laboratory experience, research methods and independent study, in addition to having completed at least one qualification at level 4 for referred clients (Figure 1.2). Furthermore, there are an increasing number of clinical exercise science degree programmes across the UK. These include both undergraduate and postgraduate pathways, and invariably provide professional experience in clinical exercise embedded as part of them and also qualifications mapped to REPs level 2 for the entry level fitness instructor course, which include the practical component of exercise delivery that is often missing from degrees. Increasingly, level 3 personal trainer awards and exercise referral diplomas are also being provided. This, then, enables practitioners-in-training to progress directly to level 4 qualifications to work with individuals with medical conditions. This is the UK's way of professionalising clinical exercise as a graduate profession; however, possessing a degree is not yet mandatory for working with higher-risk clients.

The usual employment route following level 4 qualifications is to work for a local authority leisure service or to become self-employed, and there is a wealth of opportunities in the UK to become employed in either of these capacities, providing that effective communication pathways are developed to ensure that there are referrals from acute care providers of exercise rehabilitation in hospitals. A good example of an exercise referral service is the Wales National Exercise Referral Scheme, which provides a national service for preventing and managing a range of referred conditions. This is a nationally-coordinated service, where any staff involved are provided with similar continuing professional development (CPD) opportunities, and service users

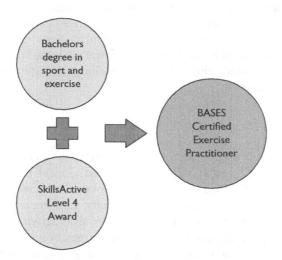

Figure 1.2 The BASES pathway for certified exercise practitioner status.

can expect a similar service irrespective of location. When this service was evaluated, the benefits were largely correlated with adherence, where it was particularly effective in increasing the physical activity of individuals referred with coronary heart disease (CHD) risk factors, but not in individuals referred with mental health conditions (Murphy et al., 2012). The analysis of the increase in quality adjusted life years (QALY) experienced in the scheme is likely to be cost-effective at under £12,000 per QALY relative to the £20,000–£30,000 per QALY. QALY is a measure of cost effectiveness of healthcare interventions, with £20–£30,000 being reasonable. If the rest of the UK follows this current gold standard for exercise referral then there is great potential to improve professionalism and achieve improved patient outcomes.

In addition to community employment, the aim of BASES is to advocate the employment of sport and exercise scientists as clinical exercise physiologists in healthcare settings, through the BASES Certified Exercise Practitioner pathway. Traditionally, physiotherapists and nurses provide hospital-based exercise therapy; however, Hospital and Community Trusts are increasingly employing sport and exercise graduates as clinical exercise physiologists to provide such services, particularly in the area of health and fitness assessments, including cardiopulmonary exercise stress testing. As an alternative to the NHS, private healthcare providers, such as BUPA and Nuffield Health, also employ exercise physiologists as either health advisors or health and wellbeing physiologists, respectively. Nuffield Health have a defined career route from 'academy health and wellbeing physiologist' through to 'physiology leadership' positions. This programme begins with a five-week training course; the first four weeks are an intense theory-based residential training programme including intermediate life support and venepuncture courses, and conducting sub-maximal electrocardiography (ECG) exercise testing, and the fifth week is shadowing an experienced health and wellbeing physiologist. After approximately 2,400 hours of working as a health and wellbeing physiologist, promotion to senior health and wellbeing physiologist is possible, potentially leading to opportunities to work as a regional clinical lead physiologist.

Without entering the Nuffield pathway or taking an MSc in clinical exercise science, practical exercise and health techniques are still not covered in depth on every sport and exercise degree, hence the relative lack of awareness of the potential of such graduates. However, it is still possible for students to gain such experience post-graduation, and the ACSM qualifications aim to provide this training in fulfilling the experience requirement of their clinical certifications.

USA accredited certifications

The ACSM clinical certifications have been provided for many years and include the ACSM certified clinical exercise physiologist (CEP) and registered clinical exercise physiologist® (RCEP) awards. The CEP is trained to deliver physical activity programmes with individuals presenting cardiovascular, pulmonary and metabolic, diseases and disorders, whereas the RCEP is trained to deliver physical activity programmes with individuals presenting cardiovascular, pulmonary, metabolic, orthopaedic, musculoskeletal, neuromuscular, neoplastic, immunologic or haematologic diseases or disorders. The CEP requires a minimum of a bachelor's degree in exercise science, basic life support certification, and 500 hours of practical experience in health education, exercise delivery, and/or exercise testing, whereas the RCEP requires a minimum of a master's degree in exercise science, basic life support and 600 hours of documented experience of exercise consultation and delivery in the following areas: cardiovascular (200 hours), pulmonary (100 hours), metabolic (120 hours), orthopaedic/musculoskeletal (100 hours), neuromuscular (40 hours), and immunological/haematological (40 hours). The taught aspect of these courses is via distance learning, using learning materials such as the ACSM's own texts, and the courses are assessed via a written examination. To remain in good standing, CEPs and RCEPs must log sixty continuing education credits (CECs) as evidence of their CPD every three years. Other certifications are also available, such as the 'Exercise is Medicine® Credential', the 'ACSM/ACS Certified Cancer Exercise Trainer'™ 'ACSM/NCHPAD Certified Inclusive Fitness Trainer' and the 'ACSM/NPAS Physical Activity in Public Health Specialist' awards (Figure 1.3).

In the UK the CEP is most likely to be used by an exercise practitioner, since there are not many common community-based exercise referral pathways available to individuals presenting neuromuscular, neoplastic, immunologic or haematologic diseases or disorders. However, the UK pathways for the level 4 specialist exercise instructor courses (column 3 of Figure 1.1) can act as precursors to the ACSM certifications, since these provide a good background to allow an exercise professional to gain experience in all areas highlighted for RCEP certification. Generally, in training and education it is difficult to gain experience without already being skilled in some way. The practical experience that is gained in the process of producing the case study for each level 4 course can be used to evidence the practical hours required, while gaining a range of specialist exercise instruction would provide a gateway to then fulfilling the requisite experience hours for ACSM certification through employment without the need to search for volunteer experience, which is not so easy to find.

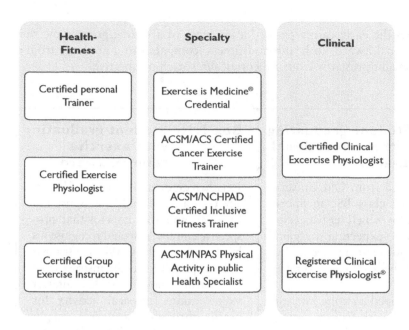

Health-Fitness	Specialty	Clinical
Certified personal Trainer	Exercise is Medicine® Credential	
	ACSM/ACS Certified Cancer Exercise Trainer	Certified Clinical Excercise Physiologist
Certified Exercise Physiologist	ACSM/NCHPAD Certified Inclusive Fitness Trainer	
Certified Group Exercise Instructor	ACSM/NPAS Physical Activity in public Health Specialist	Registered Clinical Excercise Physiologist®

Figure 1.3 ACSM certifications.

Exercise is Medicine® and special interest groups

The 'exercise is medicine' movement started by the ACSM in 2008 now has a worldwide following, with universities and communities promoting physical activity as a means of preventing and managing chronic diseases and disorders in local areas rather than just in the USA. The main thrust of the movement is to encourage general physicians to consult with patients on their physical activity levels and to treat this as a vital sign to utilise the doctor's position as a beacon of health promotion to increase their patients' physical activity levels too. This is highly dependent on the doctors' knowledge of physical activity and confidence in consulting on a matter outside of their training. It has already been proposed that exercise physiology be taught on medical degrees, but, generally, unless student doctors intercalate with a sport and exercise degree, or even if they study for a degree in sport and exercise medicine, they are not exposed to the merits of exercise for health.

A number of special interest groups have been set up for students, researchers and exercise practitioners to join, learn, or share experiences of professional practice in clinical exercise, disseminate research opportunities and foster effective working collaborations between professionals with shared interests. In the UK such groups include the Clinical Exercise Physiology and Exercise for Health Practitioners specialist interest groups allied to BASES and exercise instructor networks (EIN), such as the British Association for Cardiovascular Prevention and Rehabilitation (BACPR) EIN. The ACSM also hosts interest groups in 'Aging', 'Bone and Osteoporosis Network Exchange', and 'Cancer'.

Case study

Box 1.1 illustrates the early career path of a graduate of a degree programme that mapped to vocational awards in health and fitness, compared to a graduate from a degree that was taught primarily from a theoretical/research perspective.

Box 1.1a Student graduating without vocational awards

Joseph graduated from Old University with a first class BSc in Sport and Exercise, for which he was very proud and was expecting to gain full-time employment immediately. He wanted to be a clinical exercise physiologist.

Joseph developed a strong interest in exercise and health science during his exercise physiology lectures and, due to his institution's focus on generating research funding, he was able to work with MSc and PhD students on a funded project as part of his own undergraduate project, for which he attained a very high grade. However, most of the focus of his degree was towards sport research, rather than professional practice in exercise, and thus he had only developed vocational skills in research with healthy individuals.

Following a holiday to celebrate his graduation, he began looking online for positions in clinical exercise physiology and noticed that he did not have any of the qualifications and experience required for such positions. He sent his CV in anyway, but after three months he had still not received any replies. Rather than aimlessly apply for jobs, he decided to work backwards from the experiences and qualifications that such employers required and realised that he almost needed to start again.

Box 1.1b Student graduating with exercise referral award

Jonathan graduated from New University with a 2.1 class BSc in Sport and Exercise, and was hopeful that prospective employers would recognise his hard work to achieve this. He wanted to be a specialist exercise instructor.

Jonathan developed his interest in promoting physical activity for health through his varied taught units in exercise science, but particularly developed his personal and technical skills by studying a series of vocational awards on his degree, including gym instructor, personal trainer, and also exercise referral certifications that had been embedded into his taught units. He also studied a professional development unit to further develop the skills that he had gained from these courses in an exercise referral service.

Immediately following graduation he began working as an exercise referral specialist at the fitness centre where he gained his work experience during his studies, based on the good impression he had made and his qualifications. He was soon enrolled on specialist exercise instructor courses, such as cardiac rehabilitation, since the service was becoming more popular with higher-risk clients. Within one year he was a full-time employee and managing the scheme's referral pathway for high-risk medical conditions.

This led to him looking for a gym instructor training course. He noticed the cost and realised that he must work to pay for it and started working as a barman in various bars. Within six months he had saved enough for a gym course and exercise referral course soon afterwards. On completion, he thought he would now be in a good place to gain related employment; however, on applying for jobs, other individuals were preferred due to their work experience, and he could only be employed as a gym instructor at first. Due to his persistence in asking the fitness manager, he was allowed to shadow other exercise referral specialists in their consultations, inductions and reviews with clients, and within eighteen months was able to gain casual hours each week assisting with the exercise referral service.

He then realised that he was missing his studies and saved up sufficiently to study for an MSc in clinical exercise, hoping to later study for a PhD, where he realised his interests lay.

His employer is now paying for him to study an MSc in clinical exercise so that he can improve his research skills in order to fully evaluate their service provision.

Future research

The recent proliferation of training providers in clinical exercise, and the development of postgraduate courses in clinical exercise science in the UK, highlights the increasing demand for such courses, particularly from learners, but also from the wider community. Therefore, it is essential that such training is underpinned by research and professional practice is evidence-based. A key theme throughout this book is that the health effects of exercise have been understood for centuries; however, a remaining issue in clinical exercise is how to effectively encourage individuals who can benefit from exercise, but who have been largely sedentary, to engage in exercise as a part of improvements to their lifestyle. Much research should focus on facilitating exercise for the prevention of chronic diseases and disorders in general, but also for individuals with specific conditions, since barriers can vary. Although the chapters included within this book are presented according to each specific condition, patients very rarely only present in such a way, and comorbidities are a common concern. This often means that patients are referred to an exercise specialist to deal with the most serious concern, who then has to deal with the comorbidities too, without necessarily having received full training or having had prior experience of such comorbidities. Future work should be performed to determine the effect of comorbidities on the exercise responses and adaptations experienced relating to the primary condition, and training providers should also work together to develop training routes for adapting exercise according to common comorbidities.

Summary

Clinical exercise science is a growing field in the UK, with more sport and exercise graduates being trained in the application of exercise to healthcare, and growing connections between exercise professionals and medical professionals and physiotherapists. These relationships can only start up and flourish with appropriately-trained and experienced clinical exercise specialists whom such professionals trust with their patients. The UK qualifications may not be as well-established as the ACSM's clinical certification track, but they serve an increasing need for trained exercise professionals to be able to provide 'exercise as medicine' to an increasingly ageing UK population. There is a range of professional organisations that individuals can engage with to become trained, gain experience, be employed and to receive CPD, particularly through those referred to in the main discussion in this chapter and the 'further reading/resources' section. However, there is still much work to be done to research effective means of facilitating physical activity for those in need, and to enhance the professional standing of clinical exercise specialists.

Study tasks

1   Perform a checklist of the exercise qualifications that you have to help you to become a specialist exercise instructor:

    a   Fitness instructor award
    b   Exercise referral diploma
    c   Experience in delivering exercise at level 3
    d   At least one level 4 specialist exercise instructor certification
    e   Preferably a degree in an exercise science-related area.

2   Using any means you wish, identify the higher education institutions that provide exercise referral and/or level 4 specialist exercise instructor awards as part of their degrees.

3   Based on consulting the recommended sources below and reading the chapters in this book, contact your local leisure services or NHS Trust to determine whether exercise services for these conditions are provided. If so, try to get some experience working with their exercise practitioners. If not, work towards setting up a referral pathway from outpatient rehabilitation by leading some exercise classes yourself. Do this by consulting with your local council, leisure providers, and the healthcare team to determine feasibility.

Further reading/resources

For further information regarding commissioning and managing exercise referral services in general, consult:

National Institute for Health and Care Excellence (2014). Exercise referral schemes to promote physical activity: NICE guidelines [PH54]. London, UK: NICE: https://www.nice.org.uk/guidance/ph54

Wales National Exercise Referral Scheme: http://www.wlga.gov.uk/ners

For information on continuing professional development in exercise training for referred medical conditions, consult the following sources:

Register of Exercise Professionals

http://www.exerciseregister.org/

BASES Certified Exercise Practitioner

http://www.bases.org.uk/Certified-Exercise-Practitioner

Cardiac rehabilitation

British Association for Cardiovascular Prevention and Rehabilitation www.bacpr.com/pages/default.asp

Pulmonary rehabilitation

British Lung Foundation www.blf.org.uk/Page/Become-an-instructor

Cancer and exercise rehabilitation

CanRehab http://canrehab.co.uk/

Exercise for long-term neurological conditions

Oxford Brookes University http://www.shs.brookes.ac.uk/clear/course

Exercise after stroke

Later Life Training www.laterlifetraining.co.uk/courses/exercise-for-stroke-instructor/

The ARNI Institute www.arni.uk.com/BRIDGINGper cent20THEper cent20GAPper cent20INITIATIVE.htm

Falls prevention in the frail and elderly

Later Life Training www.laterlifetraining.co.uk/courses/postural-stability-instructor/

American College of Sports Medicine clinical certifications

* ACSM Certified Clinical Exercise Physiologist (ACSM CEP) http://certification.acsm.org/acsm-certified-clinical-exercise-physiologist
* ACSM Registered Clinical Exercise Physiologist® (ACSM RCEP) http://certification.acsm.org/acsm-registered-clinical-exercise-physiologist

References

Austin, M. W., Ploughman, M., Glynn, L. and Corbett, D. (2014). Aerobic exercise effects on neuroprotection and brain repair following stroke: a systematic review and perspective. *Neurosci Res*, doi: 10.1016/j.neures.2014.06.007.

Behrens, G. and Leitzmann, M. F. (2013). The association between physical activity and renal cancer: systematic review and meta-analysis. *Br J Cancer*, 108(4), 798–811. doi: 10.1038/bjc.2013.37.

Belardinelli, R., Georgiou, D., Cianci, G. and Purcaro, A. (1999). Randomized, controlled trial of long-term moderate exercise training in chronic heart failure: effects on functional capacity, quality of life, and clinical outcome. *Circulation*, 99(9), 1173–82.

Blair, S. N. and Morris, J. N. (2009). Healthy hearts – and the universal benefits of being physically active: physical activity and health. *Annals of Epidemiology*, 19(4), 253–6.

British Thoracic Society (2012). IMPRESS guide to the relative value of COPD interventions – executive summary. www.impressresp.com/index.php?option=com_docmanand task=doc_viewand gid=52and Itemid=82.

Brunelli, A., Pompili, C., Salati, M., Refai, M., Berardi, R., Mazzanti, P. and Tiberi, M. (2014). Preoperative maximum oxygen consumption is associated with prognosis after pulmonary resection in stage I non-small cell lung cancer. *Ann Thorac Surg*, 98(1), 238–42. doi: 10.1016/j.athoracsur.2014.04.029.

Carson, K. V., Chandratilleke, M. G., Picot, J., Brinn, M. P., Esterman, A. J. and Smith, B. J. (2013). Physical training for asthma. *Cochrane Database Syst Rev*, (9), CD001116. doi: 10.1002/14651858.CD001116.pub4.

Chou, C. H., Hwang, C. L. and Wu, Y. T. (2012). Effect of exercise on physical function, daily living activities, and quality of life in the frail older adults: a meta-analysis. *Arch Phys Med Rehabil*, 93(2), 237–44. doi: 10.1016/j.apmr.2011.08.042.

Cooney, G. M., Dwan, K., Greig, C. A., Lawlor, D. A., Rimer, J., Waugh, F. R., McMurdo, M. and Mead, G. E. (2013). Exercise for depression. *Cochrane Database Syst Rev*, (9), CD004366. doi: 10.1002/14651858.CD004366.pub6.

Cornelissen, V. A. and Smart, N. A. (2013). Exercise training for blood pressure: a systematic review and meta-analysis. *J Am Heart Assoc*, 2(1), e004473. doi: 10.1161/jaha.112.004473.

De Backer, G., Ambrosioni, E., Borch-Johnsen, K., Brotons, C., Cifkova, R., Dallongeville, J., Ebrahim, S., Faergeman, O., Graham, I., Mancia, G., Manger Cats, V., Orth-Gomér, K., Perk, J., Pyörälä, K., Rodicio, J. L., Sans, S., Sansoy, V., Sechtem, U., Silber, S., Thomsen, T. and Wood, D. (2003). European guidelines on cardiovascular disease prevention in clinical practice: third joint task force of European and other societies on cardiovascular disease prevention in clinical practice (constituted by representatives of eight societies and by invited experts). *Eur J Cardiovasc Prev Rehabil*, 10(4), S1-S10. doi: 10.1097/01.hjr.0000087913.96265.e2.

Des Guetz, G., Uzzan, B., Bouillet, T., Nicolas, P., Chouahnia, K., Zelek, L. and Morere, J. F. (2013). Impact of physical activity on cancer-specific and overall survival of patients with colorectal cancer. *Gastroenterol Res Pract*, 2013, 340851. doi: 10.1155/2013/340851.

English, C. and Hillier, S. (2011). Circuit class therapy for improving mobility after stroke: a systematic review. *Journal of Rehabilitation Medicine*, 43(7), 565–73.

English, C. K., Hillier, S. L., Stiller, K. R. and Warden-Flood, A. (2007). Circuit class therapy versus individual physiotherapy sessions during inpatient stroke rehabilitation: a controlled trial. *Archives of Physical Medicine and Rehabilitation*, 88(8), 955–63.

Fiuza-Luces, C., Garatachea, N., Berger, N. A. and Lucia, A. (2013). Exercise is the real polypill. *Physiology (Bethesda)*, 28(5), 330–58. doi: 10.1152/physiol.00019.2013.

Forbes, D., Thiessen, E. J., Blake, C. M., Forbes, S. C. and Forbes, S. (2013). Exercise programs for people with dementia. *Cochrane Database Syst Rev*, (12), CD006489. doi: 10.1002/14651858.CD006489.pub3.

Friedenreich, C. M. (2011). Physical activity and breast cancer: review of the epidemiologic evidence and biologic mechanisms. *Recent Results Cancer Res*, 188, 125–39. doi: 10.1007/978-3-642-10858-7_11.

Gallanagh, S., Quinn, T. J., Alexander, J. and Walters, M. R. (2011). Physical activity in the prevention and treatment of stroke. *International Scholarly Research Notices*. doi: 10.5402/2011/953818.

Hayashino, Y., Jackson, J. L., Fukumori, N., Nakamura, F. and Fukuhara, S. (2012). Effects of supervised exercise on lipid profiles and blood pressure control in people with type 2 diabetes mellitus: a meta-analysis of randomized controlled trials. *Diabetes Res Clin Pract*, 98(3), 349–60. doi: 10.1016/j.diabres.2012.10.004.

Heath, G. W., Parra, D. C., Sarmiento, O. L., Andersen, L. B., Owen, N., Goenka, S., Montes, F. and Brownson, R. C. (2012). Evidence-based intervention in physical activity: lessons from around the world. *Lancet*, 380(9838), 272–81. doi: 10.1016/s0140-6736(12)60816-2.

Heiwe, S. and Jacobson, S. H. (2011). Exercise training for adults with chronic kidney disease. *Cochrane Database Syst Rev*, (10), CD003236. doi: 10.1002/14651858.CD003236.pub2.

Hopper, I., Billah, B., Skiba, M. and Krum, H. (2011). Prevention of diabetes and reduction in major cardiovascular events in studies of subjects with prediabetes: meta-analysis of randomised controlled clinical trials. *Eur J Cardiovasc Prev Rehabil*, 18(6), 813–23. doi: 10.1177/1741826711421687.

Howe, T. E., Shea, B., Dawson, L. J., Downie, F., Murray, A., Ross, C., Harbour, R. T., Caldwell, L. M. and Creed, G. (2011). Exercise for preventing and treating osteoporosis in postmenopausal women. *Cochrane Database Syst Rev*, (7), CD000333. doi: 10.1002/14651858.CD000333.pub2.

Kohl, H. W., 3rd, Craig, C. L., Lambert, E. V., Inoue, S., Alkandari, J. R., Leetongin, G. and Kahlmeier, S. (2012). The pandemic of physical inactivity: global action for public health. *Lancet*, 380(9838), 294–305. doi: 10.1016/s0140-6736(12)60898-8.

Lane, R., Ellis, B., Watson, L. and Leng, G. C. (2014). Exercise for intermittent claudication. *Cochrane Database Syst Rev*, (7), CD000990. doi: 10.1002/14651858.CD000990.pub3.

Lee, I. M., Shiroma, E. J., Lobelo, F., Puska, P., Blair, S. N. and Katzmarzyk, P. T. (2012). Effect of physical inactivity on major non-communicable diseases worldwide: an analysis of burden of disease and life expectancy. *Lancet*, 380(9838), 219–29. doi: 10.1016/s0140-6736(12)61031-9.

Mammen, G. and Faulkner, G. (2013). Physical activity and the prevention of depression: a systematic review of prospective studies. *Am J Prev Med*, 45(5), 649–57. doi: 10.1016/j.amepre.2013.08.001.

Mandic, S., Myers, J., Selig, S. E. and Levinger, I. (2012). Resistance versus aerobic exercise training in chronic heart failure. *Curr Heart Fail Rep*, 9(1), 57–64. doi: 10.1007/s11897-011-0078-0.

Mehrholz, J., Pohl, M. and Elsner, B. (2014). Treadmill training and body weight support for walking after stroke. *Cochrane Database Syst Rev*, (1), CD002840. doi: 10.1002/14651858.CD002840.pub3.

Morris, J. N. (1994). Exercise in the prevention of coronary heart disease: today's best buy in public health. *Medicine and Science in Sports and Exercise*, 26(7), 807–14.

Murphy, S. M., Tudor Edwards, R., Williams, N., Raisanen, L., Moore, G., Linck, P., Hounsome, N., Ud Din, N. and Moore, L. (2012). An evaluation of the effectiveness and cost effectiveness of the National Exercise Referral Scheme in Wales, UK: a randomised controlled trial of a public health policy initiative. *J Epidemiol Community Health*, 66(8), 745–53. doi: 10.1136/jech-2011-200689.

Nicholson, S., Sniehotta, F. F., Wijck, F., Greig, C. A., Johnston, M., McMurdo, M. E., Dennis, M. and Mead, G. E. (2013). A systematic review of perceived barriers and motivators to physical activity after stroke. *International Journal of Stroke*, 8(5), 357–64.

O'Connor, C. M., Whellan, D. J., Lee, K. L., Keteyian, S. J., Cooper, L. S., Ellis, S. J., Leifer, E. S., Kraus, W. E., Kitzman, D. W., Blumenthal, J. A., Rendall, D. S., Miller, N. H., Fleg, J. L., Schulman, K. A., McKelvie, R. S., Zannad, F. and Piña, I. L. (2009). Efficacy and safety of exercise training in patients with chronic heart failure: HF-ACTION randomized controlled trial. *JAMA*, 301(14), 1439–50. doi: 10.1001/jama.2009.454.

Puhan, M. A., Gimeno-Santos, E., Scharplatz, M., Troosters, T., Walters, E. H. and Steurer, J. (2011). Pulmonary rehabilitation following exacerbations of chronic obstructive pulmonary disease. *Cochrane Database Syst Rev*, (10), CD005305. doi: 10.1002/14651858.CD00 5305.pub3.

Sallis, R. E. (2009). Exercise is medicine and physicians need to prescribe it! *Br J Sports Med*, 43(1), 3–4. doi: 10.1136/bjsm.2008.054825.

Saunders, D. H., Sanderson, M., Brazzelli, M., Greig, C. A. and Mead, G. E. (2013). Physical fitness training for stroke patients. *Cochrane Database Syst Rev*, (10), CD003316. doi: 10.1002/14651858.CD003316.pub5.

Studenski, S., Duncan, P. W., Perera, S., Reker, D., Lai, S. M. and Richards, L. (2005). Daily functioning and quality of life in a randomized controlled trial of therapeutic exercise for subacute stroke survivors. *Stroke*, 36(8), 1764–70.

Tate, D. F., Jeffery, R. W., Sherwood, N. E. and Wing, R. R. (2007). Long-term weight losses associated with prescription of higher physical activity goals. Are higher levels of physical activity protective against weight regain? *Am J Clin Nutr*, 85(4), 954–59.

Taylor, R. S., Sagar, V. A., Davies, E. J., Briscoe, S., Coats, A. J., Dalal, H., Lough, F., Rees, K. and Singh, S. (2014). Exercise-based rehabilitation for heart failure. *Cochrane Database Syst Rev*, (4), CD003331. doi: 10.1002/14651858.CD003331.pub4.

Thomas, D. E., Elliott, E. J. and Naughton, G. A. (2006). Exercise for type 2 diabetes mellitus. *Cochrane Database Syst Rev*, (3), CD002968. doi: 10.1002/14651858.CD002968.pub2.

Thompson, P. D., Buchner, D., Piña, I. L., Balady, G. J., Williams, M. A., Marcus, B. H., Berra, K., Blair, S. N., Costa, F., Franklin, B., Fletcher, G. F., Gordon, N. F., Pate, R. R., Rodriguez, B. L., Yancey, A. K. and Wenger, N. K. (2003). Exercise and physical activity in the prevention and treatment of atherosclerotic cardiovascular disease: a statement from the Council on Clinical Cardiology (Subcommittee on Exercise, Rehabilitation, and Prevention) and the Council on Nutrition, Physical Activity, and Metabolism (Subcommittee on Physical Activity). *Circulation*, 107(24), 3109–16. doi: 10.1161/01.cir.0000075572.40158.77.

Thompson, P. D., Franklin, B. A., Balady, G. J., Blair, S. N., Corrado, D., Estes, N. A. 3rd, Fulton, J. E., Gordon, N. F., Haskell, W. L., Link, M. S., Maron, B. J., Mittleman, M. A., Pelliccia, A., Wenger, N. K., Willich, S. N. and Costa, F. (2007). Exercise and acute cardiovascular events placing the risks into perspective: a scientific statement from the American Heart Association Council on Nutrition, Physical Activity, and Metabolism and the Council on Clinical Cardiology. *Circulation*, 115(17), 2358–68. doi: 10.1161/circulationaha.107.181485.

Waschki, B., Kirsten, A., Holz, O., Muller, K. C., Meyer, T., Watz, H. and Magnussen, H. (2011). Physical activity is the strongest predictor of all-cause mortality in patients with COPD: a prospective cohort study. *Chest*, 140(2), 331–42. doi: 10.1378/chest.10-2521.

Chapter 2

Physical activity for cardiac rehabilitation

Gail Sheppard and Steve Meadows

The cardiovascular system

The heart consists of four chambers, the 'upper' right and left atrium, and the 'lower' right and left ventricles. Valves between the upper and lower chambers ensure the one directional flow of blood. Both atria contract at approximately the same time, as do both ventricles, ejecting blood out of the heart, ensuring effective blood flow to the pulmonary (right side of the heart) and systemic circulation (left side of the heart). The heart muscle, the myocardium, receives its supply of blood and nutrients via the coronary arteries, which form part of the coronary circulation. The coronary circulation emerges at the root of the aorta, distributing blood and oxygen to the myocardium, with deoxygenated blood returned to the right atrium via coronary veins. The two main coronary arteries are the left (otherwise known as the left main stem) and right coronary arteries, each serving the left and right side of the heart respectively. The left artery further divides into the left anterior descending artery (LAD) and the circumflex artery (Cx), supplying blood to different regions of the myocardium. For a more in depth discussion of cardiovascular physiology, consult Levick (2009).

Pathophysiology of cardiovascular disease

Atherosclerosis

Atherosclerosis is the term used to describe the changing physiology and structure of the arterial wall that results in endothelial dysfunction and causes the narrowing of the arterial lumen. The complex process of atherosclerosis is slow and progressive, and symptoms do not usually present until the artery is more than two-thirds blocked. Two mechanisms can occur that clinically exacerbate the process: either the narrowing (stenosis) is such that blood flow to that area of the myocardium is reduced and the flow cannot meet the demands for oxygen; and/or the plaque can rupture, leading to thrombosis, which, subsequently, can then either further occlude the artery, or break off (embolus), travel downstream and impede blood supply.

Risk factors that may contribute to the development of atherosclerosis are uncontrolled type 2 diabetes, physical inactivity, smoking, stress, hypertension, and dyslipidaemia. The initial stages of the process have been found in children and can potentially occur in any of the arteries of the body, but it is commonly found in the coronary arteries (coronary heart disease, CHD), the arteries of the head and neck (cerebrovascular disease or stroke) and the peripheral (leg) arteries (peripheral vascular disease,

PVD), the latter causing leg pain when exercising. It is possible for one artery to have multiple atherosclerotic lesions.

Acute coronary syndromes

Angina pectoris is the pain sensation caused by ischaemia to the myocardium due to a partially-blocked artery. These symptoms disappear with rest (oxygen demand decreases) or use of a prescribed nitrate spray (inducing dilation of coronary blood vessels). Stable angina refers to symptoms that are predictable, for example during exercise at a known intensity or after a heavy meal. Unstable angina has no pattern and can occur at any time, even at rest, and is an absolute contraindication for exercise.

A myocardial infarction (MI) is caused by the same atherosclerotic process as angina, but refers to the death of the myocardium caused by complete restriction of oxygen due to plaque rupture. The term 'acute MI' is given to a sudden episode of complete stenosis that precipitates myocardial damage. MI can be further classified according to which coronary artery has been occluded; for example, an anterior MI (the anterior site of the left ventricle) will result from occlusion of the left anterior descending artery (LAD) and an occlusion in the right coronary artery will result in an inferior MI (the inferior heart wall).

Symptoms of ischaemia may include pain, shortness of breath, sweating, confusion, and nausea, although patients can experience a 'silent MI' where no signs or symptoms are present; this is common in those with diabetes due to neuropathy. The range of symptoms differs widely between individuals, however, with an MI, symptoms do not resolve with rest. If an MI is suspected, medical attention should be sought immediately, with the aim of restoring blood flow to the myocardium by removing the blockage and re-establishing blood supply with thrombolytic medication or surgical procedure (percutaneous coronary angioplasty [PCI] or coronary artery bypass graft [CABG]).

Diagnostic testing following a coronary event may include:

- Testing of biochemical (enzyme) markers, for example troponin and creatinine kinase. Levels of these biomarkers will typically rise following MI and remain raised for several days;
- ECG (electrocardiogram) monitoring. In the days or weeks following MI, some patients may be required to undergo an ECG stress test that usually involves an incremental exercise test (e.g. walking on a treadmill) while attached to an ECG monitor. This procedure examines how the heart responds to exertion and identifies areas of the heart experiencing ischaemia, indicated by changes in the ECG trace (ST elevation or depression);
- Coronary angiogram, which is an X-ray procedure using intravenous dye into the coronary arteries to determine the extent of atherosclerosis and stenosis;
- CT (computerised tomography) or MRI (magnetic resonance imaging) to determine the extent of myocardial damage.

Chronic heart failure

The term chronic heart failure (CHF) refers to the inability of the heart to effectively deliver blood around the body, often due to valvular disease, a large MI, or multiple smaller MIs having damaged extensive areas of the myocardium. When the heart is unable to maintain its ability to pump, cardiac output decreases and congestion can develop within the circulatory system. Symptoms of heart failure include peripheral and pulmonary oedema and shortness of breath.

For a more comprehensive discussion of cardiovascular pathophysiology, consult Sheppard (2011).

Cardiac rehabilitation

Cardiac rehabilitation (CR) is a multi-disciplinary, professionally-supervised intervention that aims to improve the health and wellbeing of cardiac patients. CR usually consists of a six to twelve-week programme of exercise, education, psychological support, behavioural change, and medical risk factor management. In the UK there are currently over 300 CR programmes that are audited by the National Audit of Cardiac Rehabilitation (NACR) (Doherty and Lewin, 2013).

The multi-disciplinary team may include the following health professionals:

- Cardiologist
- Cardiac specialist nurse
- Exercise physiologists/specialist
- Dietician
- Psychologist or other mental health specialist
- Pharmacist
- Physiotherapist
- Occupational therapist.

Benefits of exercise-based cardiac rehabilitation:

- 13–26 per cent reduction in all-cause mortality
- 26–46 per cent reduction in cardiac mortality
- 23–56 per cent reduction in hospital re-admission
- Cost-effective intervention
- Improved quality of life
- Improved functional capacity
- Supports early return to work
- Empowers the development of self-management skills.
              (Davies et al., 2010; Heran et al., 2011; Lawler et al., 2011;
                    NICE, 2008; Papadakis et al., 2005; Taylor et al., 2004;
                                              Yohannes et al., 2010).

The British Association for Cardiovascular Prevention and Rehabilitation (BACPR) suggest seven core components that should be included within CR in order to ensure a competent, cost-effective, and clinically-effective service (BACPR, 2012). These include health behaviour change and education, lifestyle risk factor management, psychosocial health, cardioprotective therapies, medical risk factor management, long-term management and audit and evaluation.

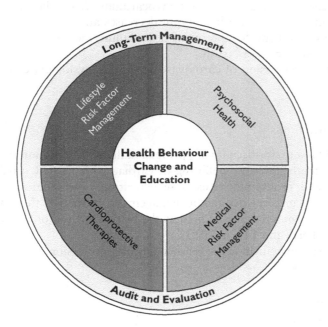

Figure 2.1 Components of cardiac rehabilitation. Reproduced with permission from BACPR, 2012.

With the four-stage structure of cardiac rehabilitation in the UK, patients do not graduate to the next phase until it is deemed medically safe to do so (Table 2.1). In the context of exercise, there are a variety of approaches to encouraging physical activity on a Trust by Trust basis.

Ideally, patients will be encouraged to perform bed-based activities using therabands and squeezing sponge balls as well as performing ambulatory activities, such as walking in the ward and to the toilet by themselves during Phase I. Patients may even be required to walk one flight of stairs in hospital to demonstrate that they are fit for discharge. Patients are not able to be bed-bound anymore, and this approach decreases the length of hospitalisation and improves prognosis. Phase II commences on discharge. In this phase, structured exercise is available to patients in the USA, but in the UK patients have to wait to be enrolled onto the next phase, which could be up to twelve weeks post-discharge. The heart manual may be provided to patients to provide information on managing their condition and modifying their lifestyle, such as being physically active for thirty minutes five times per week. In some Trusts nurses/physiotherapists may make home visits to provide personal physical activity advice, amongst other guidance that is provided relating to medication use and diet. Formal structured exercise begins in Phase III and is led by cardiac nurses/physiotherapists up to twice per week in an outpatient setting, and takes the form of circuit training with simple equipment that could also be used at home. Community centres and leisure centres are the usual venues used, as this reduces the clinical appearance of the service and generates confidence in exercising away from the hospital. Education sessions on diet, medication, smoking cessation, CVD risk factors and relaxation are also provided alongside exercise.

Table 2.1 The UK phases of cardiac rehabilitation

Phase	Service provision
Phase I	**Before discharge from hospital**
	• Assessment of physical, psychological and social needs for cardiac rehabilitation, including a written individual plan for meeting these identified needs
	• Advice on lifestyle e.g. smoking cessation, physical activity, diet, alcohol consumption and employment
	• Prescription of medication and education about its use
	• Provision of written information about cardiac support groups and cardiac rehabilitation.
Phase II	**Early post-discharge period**
	• Comprehensive assessment of cardiac risk, including physical, psychological, and social needs for cardiac rehabilitation, and a review of the initial plan for meeting these needs
	• Provision of lifestyle advice and psychological interventions according to the agreed plan from relevant trained therapists who have access to support from a cardiologist.
Phase III	**As early post-discharge period plus:**
	• Structured exercise sessions to meet the assessed needs of individual patients
	• Maintain access to relevant advice and support from people trained to offer advice about exercise, relaxation, psychological interventions, health promotion, and vocational advice.
Phase IV	**Long-term maintenance of changed behaviour**
	• Long-term follow-up in primary care
	• Offer involvement with local cardiac support groups
	• Referral to specialist cardiac, behavioural (e.g. exercise, smoking cessation), or psychological services as clinically indicated.

Adapted from Department of Health (2000)

Following eight to twelve weeks of Phase III, depending on the commissioned service, patients graduate to Phase IV, which is led by fitness instructors who provide services in the community. These are generally the only places where cardiac patients may perform structured exercise under appropriate supervision. Such instructors are trained to Level 4 standard in providing safe and effective exercise for patients with various heart conditions. A problem with Phase IV exercise is that there are limited spaces in leisure centre schedules for such sessions and they take place during the day. As a result, working age adults, i.e. those who would benefit most from this service, are effectively barred from taking part, and only older adults use these services. The graduation rate from Phase III to Phase IV is therefore limited.

Cardiac exercise physiology

Cardiorespiratory fitness

Cardiorespiratory fitness (CRF) is an independent risk factor of cardiac mortality in men and women with CVD. Patients possessing low CRF are two to five times more likely to die than those patients with higher CRF (Franklin and McCullough, 2009). Furthermore, every one metabolic equivalent of task (MET) increase in patients' CRF after a twelve-week training programme is associated with a 13 per cent reduction in mortality and a 30 per cent reduction in those who started with lower CRF (Martin et al., 2013). The clinical effectiveness of CR can be clearly reflected by increases in peak oxygen consumption ($\dot{V}O_{2peak}$), as CRF is not influenced by pharmacological intervention, unlike blood lipid profiles or blood pressure measurements (Hansen et al., 2010). Generally, most studies report increases in $\dot{V}O_{2peak}$ following training, with increases ranging from 2 per cent to 78 per cent (Hansen et al., 2005). Gender, age or β-adrenoceptor antagonist (β-blocker) use do not seem to influence potential increases in $\dot{V}O_{2peak}$ (Balady et al., 1996; Pavia et al., 1995). However, some patients cannot increase their $\dot{V}O_{2peak}$ through exercise, with possible explanations including a high baseline $\dot{V}O_{2peak}$, the presence of a hibernating myocardium, or that the exercise stimulus was insufficient to stimulate a training response (Hansen et al., 2005). Research evidence suggests that the exercise dose in some UK CR programmes is too limited to significantly influence key patient outcomes, such as CRF and mortality, and challenges the efficacy of contemporary exercise CR interventions (Sandercock et al., 2013a). This should provide the stimulus for CR programmes to review their exercise component and ensure that it delivers an effective intervention according to recommended guidelines, particularly in terms of exercise intensity and enhancing activities of daily living away from structured CR. Due to changes in service commissioning, it may become necessary to evaluate and provide evidence of measurable patient outcomes; exercise capacity is an outcome with potential global benefits to a range of cardiac patients, and a metric that can be easily captured. CR programmes should also aim to encourage broader engagement in domestic, occupational and recreational physical activities outside formally-delivered CR exercise sessions. This should reinforce the need to engage in a physically active lifestyle, not just one to two structured exercise sessions per week, and should minimise sedentary behaviour.

Patients with CVD who were randomised to long-term moderate exercise training (n = 48) significantly increased $\dot{V}O_{2peak}$ by 18 per cent (P ≤ 0.001) and decreased resting heart rate (P ≤ 0.01) compared to a sedentary control group (n = 46) (Bellardinelli et al., 1999). Other studies have found 17 per cent (Giannuzzi et al., 2003) and 29 per cent (Gielen et al., 2003) improvement in $\dot{V}O_{2peak}$ compared to control groups, with either no detrimental effect on left ventricular re-modelling, or attenuating abnormal re-modelling. Physiological adaptations have resulted in improved exercise tolerance, reflected in a 20 per cent increased walking distance in the 6-minute walk test, increased quality of life measures, and fewer hospital re-admissions (Giannuzzi et al., 2003).

More recent studies have also found improvement in $\dot{V}O_{2peak}$ of 2.06 mL·kg⁻¹·min⁻¹ (Van Tol et al., 2006) and 2.70 mL·kg⁻¹·min⁻¹ (Chien et al., 2008), which are clinically significant since $\dot{V}O_{2peak}$ decreases by ~ 0.14 ml·kg·min⁻¹ yearly in patients with CHF after the age of forty (Forman et al., 2009). Furthermore, those with a

$\dot{V}O_{2peak}$ < 15 mL·kg⁻¹·min⁻¹ are at the greatest risk of mortality but an increase of 1 mL·kg⁻¹·min⁻¹ in an individual's $\dot{V}O_{2peak}$ is associated with a 15 per cent decrease in the risk of mortality, indicating how important even marginal improvements in CRF can be (Keteyian et al., 2008).

Besides improvements in maximal exercise capacity, favourable adaptations in sub-maximal measures can be gained following exercise, such as increased exercise time, ventilatory threshold, and quality of life in patients with CHF (Wielenga et al., 1999a). The potential improvements in functional capacity in older adults with CHF can be under-estimated, given the age-related decline in physiological function experienced with advancing age. Although patients with CHF aged > 65 years old do not increase their $\dot{V}O_{2peak}$ to the same extent as those aged < 65 years old, clinically significant improvements can still occur (Wielenga et al., 1999b). Older patients with CHF aged seventy five to ninety years improved their 6 minute walk test distance (6MWD) significantly – by over 40m – representing a 20 per cent increase in the distance walked, following a twelve-week tailored exercise programme (Owen and Croucher (2000). Whilst many research studies have indicated favourable outcomes following exercise interventions, more research is needed in exercise interventions across a diverse demographic of the cardiac population (Lloyd-Williams et al., 2002).

Cardiac function

CRF should improve following an exercise regime; a number of physiological adaptations occur to achieve this, especially in cardiac functional capacity. This is reflected in an increased cardiac output during maximal symptom-limited exercise (Hansen et al., 2010; Hambrecht et al., 1995). Haykowsky et al. (2007) found significant improvements in left-ventricular ejection fraction, end diastolic volume and end systolic volume when aerobic training was performed. These cardiac adaptations may contribute to the reduction in secondary cardiac events and mortality rates associated with exercise participation.

Although many arrhythmias of the heart are not life-threatening; some can lead to cardiac arrest. Heart rate variability (HRV), the variation in time between R-R intervals (the time interval between ventricular contractions), can be used as a key predictor of secondary events (Tsuji et al., 1994). Exercise training within CR has been shown to enhance patients' HRV, thus lowering resting and exercising heart rate (HR). When HR is high, there is an increased risk of arrhythmia due to shortening of the diastolic phase, where myocardial oxygenation occurs (Rennie et al., 2003). A reduction in patients' resting and exercise HR is associated with arterial re-modelling and adaptation in the cardiorespiratory centre, providing cardio-protective mechanisms to reduce sympathetic drive and enhance parasympathetic outflow (Nelson et al., 2005).

Vascular function

A decrease in vasoconstriction of blood vessels, both at rest and during exercise, can reduce hypertension, a key risk factor for CVD (Graham et al., 2007). The endothelium produces numerous vasoactive substances, including nitric oxide (NO), which are crucial anti-atherogenic mediators, but may precipitate CVD when they become dysfunctional (Green et al., 2008). The benefit of exercise-based CR upon endothelial function appears to be a crucial factor in secondary prevention and management of risk factors, as impaired endothelial function inhibits redistribution of blood flow, thus potentially limiting oxygen delivery to the exercising muscles (Maxwell et al., 1998). Improvement in endothelial function increases the ability of the cells to respond to varying vascular conditions and exercise training seems to confer a degree of vascular conditioning, providing a cardioprotective benefit (Green et al., 2004; Green et al., 2008). Exercise-based CR has been shown to directly benefit the coronary vasculature through improved endothelial function to meet $M\dot{V}O_2$ more effectively (Green et al., 2004). CR exercise provides the potential to induce a training adaptation in endothelial function and thus preferential redistribution of blood flow to the working muscles during exercise. This may help the cardiac patient improve their exercise tolerance (Demopoulos et al., 1997; Maxwell et al., 1998).

Exercise-based CR, incorporating both large and small muscle groups (cardiovascular and muscular strength endurance exercises) decreases vasoconstriction in response to a vasoconstrictor stimulus (Hambrecht et al., 2000). This leads to an improvement in NO vasodilatory function, increasing blood flow to exercising limbs, which in turn enhances the peak vasodilatory capacity of the vasculature (Green, et al., 1996).

Exercise and secondary cardiac events

Cardiac mortality

Cardiovascular disease is progressive and there is a strong likelihood of a secondary cardiac event through weakening of the structure and function of the heart (Van Stel et al., 2012; Leon et al., 2005). Vigorous physical activity in individuals unaccustomed to such exertion may disrupt unstable atherosclerotic plaques, causing vasospasm rather than vasodilation, triggering the onset of an MI (Mittleman et al. 1993). However, exercise can significantly reduce the occurrence and severity of a secondary cardiac event (Artham et al., 2008; Lavie and Milani, 1997). A Cochrane review of forty seven studies determined that exercise reduces the mortality rates of cardiac patients, yet found no significant relationship between the overall physical activity dose of the exercise programme (session intensity, frequency, and duration of individual sessions), and mortality rates (Heran et al., 2011). Secondary MIs were reduced by 25 per cent in a sample group of 4554 participants (O'Connor et al., 1989), and secondary cardiac events were reduced by 27 per cent in 8440 participants following CR (Jolliffe et al., 2001). Furthermore, after fourteen years of follow-up, those who attended CR had a 58 per cent lower mortality risk than those who did not attend (Beauchamp et al., 2012). This demonstrates the value of attending a CR programme, and also that lifestyle change can potentially contribute to quality of life and survival.

Not only do mortality rates among patients with CVD decrease with exercise training; the number of hospitalisations also decreases (Davies et al., 2010). Following the completion of sixteen exercise sessions over the course of eight weeks, 10.6 per cent of the exercise group was admitted to hospital compared to 20.2 per cent of the non-exercising control group within twenty four weeks after completion of training (Austin et al., 2005). Furthermore, those in the non-exercise group had more multiple admissions and remained in hospital longer. A meta-analysis of the effects of the exercise component of CR found significant reductions in hospital admissions when a study with poor adherence was excluded from the analysis (Davies et al., 2010). In contrast, a multi-centre trial of 2331 patients with CVD found that 759 patients in the exercise group were hospitalised, or died, compared to 796 patients in the control group (O'Connor et al., 2009). However, these findings need to be treated with caution since only 30 per cent of the exercise group completed all of the prescribed exercise, whilst 8 per cent of the control group increased their physical activity levels.

Psychological health and quality of life

Health problems associated with CVD are not just physical; anxiety and depression have a negative inter-relationship with patient cardiovascular health and patient outcomes such as quality of life, and they potentially increase mortality risk (Carney et al., 1999; Rozanski et al., 2005; Stein et al., 1995). Anxiety and/or depression can also adversely affect patient recovery (Lavie et al., 2009). Patients who attend CR have a 40–70 per cent decrease in anxiety and depression, along with a 70 per cent decrease in mortality risk (Lavie et al., 2009). Since CR can potentially provide a supportive social setting for exercise, some of the psychological benefits may accrue from exposure to this environment, not just the physicality element of exercise. Attending CR sessions does place patients within an 'exercise and health-promoting environment', and increases their opportunities to increase physical activity levels. Although patients gain functional improvements through exercise, they often report that the most noticeable benefits of CR are psychosocial in nature. This has implications for CR delivery, as individualised exercise programmes may be insufficient to improve psychological health, and potentially quality of life (Ades, 2001; Chien et al., 2008).

Multidisciplinary CR, including education, individual therapy and group workshops, has been shown to decrease both anxiety and depression; however, this is not routinely provided by all CR programmes (Child et al., 2010; Doherty and Lewin, 2013). Exercise can still prevent depression, and is therefore valued as an important psychosocial support mechanism compared to other interventions (Rozanski et al., 2005). Exercise for post-MI patients can increase their wellbeing, confidence, and happiness, as well as decreasing depression and anxiety (Taylor et al., 1986).

A meta-analysis of 3647 participants from nineteen studies of exercise-based CR reported that all studies found an improvement in quality of life (Davies et al., 2010), with one study in particular finding an average improvement of 9.7 points, using the Minnesota Living With Heart Failure questionnaire (MLWHF) (Van Tol et al., 2006). Such improvements are also experienced relatively consistently across sex, age, race, and other sub-groups, with 54 per cent of those in exercise-based CR demonstrating clinically noticeable improvements in quality of life compared to only 29 per cent of a non-exercise control group (Flynn et al., 2009). Improvements in quality of life scores have been closely correlated with improvements in 6MWD following high-intensity training, which may reflect improved endurance capability during active daily living (Nilsson et al., 2008). Physical attributes associated with improved quality of life following CR include improved physical function, energy availability, body pain, and exercise tolerance (Lavie and Milani, 1995; Saeidi and Mostafavi, 2013; Marchionni et al., 2003).

Physical activity in cardiac rehabilitation

Is exercise in cardiac rehabilitation safe?

There are potential risks with vigorous physical activity. It is known to trigger cardiac complications, as up to a fifth of all MIs are induced after physical exertion (Fletcher et al., 2001). However, in a CR context, these risks are relatively low due to the emphasis on moderate intensity effort. Cardiac mortality has been reported at a rate of only 0.61 deaths per 100,000 hours of exercise in CR programmes (Fletcher et al., 1996). Similarly low incident rates have been reported elsewhere, with figures ranging from one cardiac event in 50,000 to one in 120,000 patient exercise hours, with a reported two fatalities within 1.5 million hours of exercise (Franklin et al., 1998; Thompson et al., 2003). As the benefits of exercise are widely reported, it is understandable that doctors and health care professionals consider the benefits to outweigh the risks. Of the relatively small numbers of MIs that are experienced during or after vigorous exercise, the majority are seen in those who are unaccustomed to this type of activity and whose cardiac profile is undiagnosed (Hambrecht et al., 2000).

Referred cardiac patients are initially risk stratified and then supervised during CR exercise sessions. In various risk stratification criteria, risk is ascribed based on the possibility of an adverse event during exercise, i.e. a cardiac event or musculoskeletal injury, and the degree of supervision required. The majority of cardiac patients are less physically active than similar individuals without a cardiac history and have significantly impaired cardiac function, which increases the supervision that they require during exercise. This places cardiac patients in the high risk of suffering a cardiac event category compared to other exercisers, which necessitates supervision by specialist cardiac rehabilitation exercise instructors. Within this high risk category, there is a further subset of low, moderate, and high risk classifications for patients with known CVD, based on cardiac function rather than CVD risk factors. The classifications of cardiac function can be based on multiple measures, but the two most commonly applied are aerobic capacity (METs) and ejection fraction. The recommended hierarchy of MET thresholds for risk stratification in cardiac rehabilitation are: low risk (> 7 METs capacity three or more weeks following clinical event), moderate risk (5–6 METs three or more weeks following clinical event) and high risk patients (< 5 METs) (American Association for Cardiovascular and Pulmonary Rehabilitation [AACVPR], 2013; Association of Chartered Physiotherapists in Cardiac Rehabilitation [ACPICR], 2015). Most cardiac rehabilitation exercise is likely to be pitched at a moderate intensity (3–6 MET range) to conform to recommended guidelines (Sandercock et al., 2013b), so the risk of a fatal cardiac related event is significantly reduced. MET capacity is determined from an incremental exercise test on a treadmill, usually the modified Bruce protocol, prior to exercise training; however, increasingly fewer exercise tests are performed in cardiac rehabilitation, and thus the MET method is now rarely available for risk stratification. Alternatively, the left ventricular ejection fraction can be used to indicate the severity of cardiac dysfunction (AACVPR, 2013). The ejection fraction is the proportion of blood that is ejected during each cardiac cycle from the left ventricle relative to end-diastolic volume. The greater the ejection fraction the greater the left ventricle function and the lower risk to the patient during exercise, since there would be a lower risk of exercise-induced ischaemia. The levels of risk determined by left ventricular ejection fraction are: < 40 per cent (high risk), 40–50 per cent (moderate risk) and > 50 per cent (low risk). The ejection fraction of the patient is most likely to be used by Phase III professionals to indicate the risk stratification of the patient on their Phase IV transfer form. See the AACVPR Stratification Algorithm for Risk of Event for further modifying variables for cardiac patients (AACVPR, 2013).

Warm-ups and cool-downs

Warm-ups should be gentle and prolonged in cardiac patients due to impaired coronary circulation. The oxygen extraction rate of the coronary circulation is 80 per cent at rest; therefore, the only means of increasing $M\dot{V}O_2$ is through increased blood supply. If the warm-up is too brisk then $M\dot{V}O_2$ would increase disproportionately to myocardial oxygen supply – the ability of the heart to supply itself with oxygenated blood – which is likely to result in ischaemia. Ischaemia can initiate the ischaemic cascade (Figure 2.2). Each stage is further exacerbated by ischaemia, where O_2 supply to the myocardium is further diminished with diminishing cardiac function. Therefore, gentle increases in intensity are required, using progressively larger or faster movements to decrease the risk of reaching the ischaemic threshold before the appropriate training intensity has been attained. Warming-up for a longer duration may appear counter-intuitive, but it allows for steady increases in intensity and will allow a higher training intensity to be achieved more safely. Fifteen to twenty minutes is advised as an appropriate duration including mobility, pulse raising, and dynamic stretching activities.

A sufficiently long cool-down is required to prevent the risk of blood pooling, postural hypotension, and elevated catecholamine activity. An ineffective cool-down (<10 minutes), particularly in cardiac patients, predisposes to cardiovascular dysfunction. The previous exercise session encourages blood flow to the extremities and significantly elevates cardiac output to achieve this, by increasing adrenaline in the circulation and norepinephrine in the sympathetic nervous system. Following exercise,

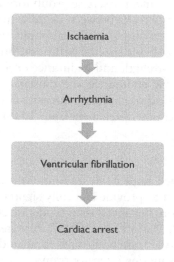

Figure 2.2 Ischaemic cascade.

this can create difficulties that are exacerbated by anti-hypertensive medications. If exercise ceases immediately or too abruptly, heart rate, and thus cardiac output, slows rapidly. This causes impaired circulation and lack of pressure to return blood in the veins of the extremities back to the heart, and, through lack of the 'muscle pump', to enhance venous return. This process reduces blood supply to the myocardium, which may still be working at an increased rate, and predisposes ischaemia to the heart and brain, resulting in syncope. The interaction of anti-hypertensive medication and exercise-induced vasodilation exacerbate this effect. Furthermore, many cardiac events occur in the period following exercise while sympathetic nervous system activity remains elevated; therefore, the prolonged cool-down and social chat afterwards allows instructors and peers to check that pulse rates have returned to resting before leaving the session.

Aerobic exercise training

Physical activity has been known as a therapeutic intervention for disease since ancient times, but was neglected until 1772 when William Heberden reported wood sawing as a cure for angina pain. However, the incorporation of exercise rehabilitation into contemporary CR programmes is a more recent phenomenon, and structured physical activity is regarded as the cornerstone component of CR, not only to help re-establish function, but also to address low physical fitness as a precursor for CVD (Balady et al., 1994; BACPR, 2012; Fletcher et al., 1996; Piepoli, et al., 2010). The British Association for Cardiovascular Prevention and Rehabilitation (BACPR, 2012) describes the aim of cardiac rehabilitation (CR) as a means to encourage patients to regain full physical, psychological, and social status and ultimately slow, or even reverse the progression of, CVD to encourage exercise independence and to return the patient to occupational or recreational activities (Fletcher et al., 2001; Pescatello et al., 2014).

Exercise in CR tends to be delivered in a circuit training format, which allows for easy adaptation, the potential for a more social environment (exercise group format), and, due to its intermittent nature, facilitates recovery breaks between exercise intervals (ACPICR, 2015). This provides a format that suits an older clinical population, allowing them to recover their breath and not over-work one specific part of the body, by alternating aerobic exercise bouts with muscular strength and endurance exercise (MSE) as an active recovery. Improvements in aerobic endurance and musculoskeletal strength have been demonstrated following a period of moderate intensity circuit training, without causing any cardiovascular complications (Kelemen et al., 1986).

Interval vs. continuous aerobic training

Interval training prescribed in isolation, or combined with MSE training (which is often the typical CR exercise format) has been shown to provide clinically significant adaptations in cardiac patients, and is potentially more beneficial than moderate continuous intensity CV training (Cornish et al., 2011). Wisløff et al. (2007) reported a 46 per cent improvement in VO_{2peak} among an interval training group, compared to a substantially smaller 14 per cent increase in a continuous intensity training group, with less tedium reported. More recently Moholdt et al. (2012) completed a similar study finding a larger improvement in VO_{2peak} in an interval training group against a continuous training group. When comparing four interval training protocols, a period of thirty seconds of exercise followed by a passive recovery, was found to be safest, and enabled exercisers to operate above 85 per cent of their $\dot{V}O_{2peak}$ with no adverse effects reported (Meyer et al., 2012). Normal operating CR procedures encourage an active recovery period to reduce the risk of a sudden drop in blood pressure, which could occur due to blood pooling in the legs during inactive periods, and as a side-effect of anti-hypertensive medications.

Resistance training

Besides the obvious strength gains, the benefits of resistance training (RT) go further by also improving muscular endurance, metabolism, and CVD risk factors, such as reduced blood pressure, as well as enhancing cardiovascular function and exercise capacity (Pollock et al., 2000). RT has been shown to increase other aspects of health, including functional independence, self-efficacy, and quality of life (Bjarnason-Wehrens, et al., 2004; Cornelissen and Fagard, 2005; Fletcher, 2001; McCartney, 1998; Williams et al., 2007). There appears to be no increased risk of cardiovascular events with resistance training compared to aerobic training (Bjarnason-Wehrens et al., 2004). The physical adaptations seem to benefit the heart directly; the rate pressure product (RPP) has been shown to decrease when muscle strength has improved (Parker et al., 1996). This is important to the cardiac patient, as RPP is an indirect measurement of myocardial workload ($M\dot{V}O_2$), combining heart rate (HR) and systolic blood pressure (SBP), calculated using the following formula: $RPP = HR \times SBP$. This measurement takes into account not only the rate of myocardial contraction but also the force of contraction (afterload). RT adaptations could therefore lead to a decrease in $M\dot{V}O_2$ during the activities of daily life. For example, carrying groceries or completing DIY jobs will be easier and there will be less risk of exceeding the ischaemic threshold of CVD patients (Pollock et al., 2000).

Heavy RT is not advised immediately after cardiac surgery as it may lead to further complications, such as re-opening of surgical wounds and osteomyelitis (Williams et al., 2007; Pollock et al., 2000). Consequently, the implementation of RT should be delayed until a patient's condition permits safe engagement (usually four to eight weeks post-surgery, or until able to exercise > 5 METs), but should be incorporated as a core component of physical conditioning (Williams et al. 2007). Bjarnason-Wehrens et al., (2004) acknowledge the risks of increasing blood pressure during resistance exercise with cardiac patients. Blood pressure increases depending on load intensity, the muscle mass engaged, and the nature of the repetitions performed. Therefore, correct technique and supervision is necessary, as well as appropriate screening of cardiac patients, their cardiac stress tolerance, and clinical status to ensure safety during RT (Bjarnason-Wehrens et al., 2004). Breath holding, or the Valsalva manoeuvre (attempting to exhale against a closed glottis), should be avoided (Wise and Patrick, 2011).

One of the main concerns with RT is with elevations in blood pressure, which may relate to the nature of the muscle contraction. Dynamic exercises tend to be favoured over static (isometric) contractions (Bethell, 1999). Isometric exercises are not normally recommended due to the adverse blood pressure response associated with them (Fletcher et al., 1996; Wenger, 2008). However, performing isometric muscular work is unavoidable when lifting or carrying, for example, children or shopping bags, and when performing many active daily living tasks, such as DIY or gardening. Some researchers have found beneficial effects from isometric exercise; however, it is safer to teach patients to regulate their breathing if isometric actions cannot be avoided (McCartney et al., 1991).

Combining aerobic and resistance-based training in exercise programmes appears to be optimum, and current guidelines recommend that an exercise regime for cardiac patients should incorporate both aerobic and resistance exercises (ACPICR, 2015; Fletcher et al., 2001). Smart and Marwick (2004) systematically reviewed studies on patients with CHF. These indicated positive trends of survival rates, along with improved functional capacity and reduced cardiorespiratory symptoms, after a combination of supervised aerobic and resistance training. This approach has been shown to attenuate the loss of skeletal muscle, which could otherwise lead to reductions in basal metabolic rate, and therefore contribute to long-term weight management and improved quality of life, which is particularly important in an older patient demographic (Bryner et al., 1999). Improvements in muscular strength and overall functional capacity occur due to a combination of these exercise modalities, supporting a more active lifestyle and potentially improved quality of life (Hansen et al., 2010).

Case study task

As a cardiac rehabilitation exercise specialist, consider the patient below. She was referred for Phase III outpatient exercise following a PCI of the LAD, which was performed after suffering an anterior MI, resulting in significantly impaired left ventricle function.

On presentation at the cardiac rehabilitation programme (eight weeks post cardiac event), the following information was collected:

Name:	Carol
Age:	61
Cardiac event:	Anterior MI – primary PCI (LAD)
Ejection fraction:	48 per cent
BP:	120/80 mmHg
Resting pulse:	66 bpm and regular
Past medical history:	Hypertension, palpitations
Medication:	Aspirin 75 mg, Clopidogrel 75 mg, Citalopram 20 mg, Bisoprolol 2.5 mg, Atorvastatin 80 mg, Ramipril 5 mg, nitrate spray.

The Phase III cardiac rehabilitation intervention:

- Twelve week programme of exercise
- 2 × one hour sessions per week of interval- (circuit)-based exercise prescribed according to evidence-based guidelines
- Daily walking programme commenced (home)
- Referral to cardiac counsellor
- Goal setting
- Twelve weekly lifestyle education sessions
- Up titration of medications.

Table 2.2 Health behaviours at diagnosis

	Present	Risk details, level, and action plan
Physical inactivity	✓	None reported
Ex-smoker	✓	Stopped 1½ years ago
Stress	✓	Husband recently diagnosed with lymphoma
Alcohol		< 2 units per week

Carol has now graduated from Phase III cardiac rehabilitation and has been referred to you as a Phase IV specialist exercise instructor. You may wish to consider the following:

1   What is the difference between CVD risk factor analysis and risk stratification for a cardiac event?
2   List which data are most important to you as an exercise specialist and discuss why.
3   Describe how you would help Carol to maintain a physically active lifestyle.

Future research in cardiac exercise rehabilitation

High-intensity training

There is a growing interest amongst health professionals in the role of high-intensity exercise training (HIT) in CR, both in terms of catering for younger cardiac patients, and also striving to achieve optimal health benefit (Sandercock et al., 2013b). HIT involves exercise bouts of usually < 300 seconds at > 70 per cent VO_{2peak} or > 90 per cent peak heart rate (or RPE > 15), interspersed with bouts of lower intensity exercise, or active recovery. This mixture of work and recovery periods allows more intense exercise to be tolerated before fatigue; in time it potentially also allows efficiency and greater cardiac adaptations in the patient, due to the higher-intensity workloads. The intensity of exercise matters in terms of outcomes and, whilst there are many variations of HIT, early research indications suggest it is safe for a CR population with stable CVD to engage in this training, performing it under controlled conditions. Rognmo, et al. (2004) found significantly superior improvements

Table 2.3 Carol's anthropometric, cardiovascular and functional capacity scores in Phase III

Outcome measure	Pre-rehabilitation	Post-rehabilitation
Weight (kg)	86.4	82.3
BMI (kg·m^2)	32.5	31.0
Waist circumference (cm)	101	95
Cholesterol (TC; mmol·L^{-1})	6.1	4.2
TC/HDL ratio	4.4	2.9
Ejection fraction (%)	48	55
ISWT score (metres)	260	340

in $\dot{V}O_{2peak}$ following HIT (17.9 per cent) compared to a moderate-intensity approach (7.9 per cent); however, there were no significant changes in other health outcomes, for example resting heart rate, blood pressure, or body mass. An exercise-based CR programme, consisting of repeated fifteen-second phases of exercise at 100 per cent peak power output, improved health outcomes in stable CVD patients. However, 35 per cent of the group reported exercise-induced ischemia (Guiraud et al., 2009), although it was not prolonged.

It is difficult to compare the relative risk of different forms of exercise training; however, the rates of cardiac complications to the number of patient-exercise hours were one fatal cardiac arrest per 129,456 hours of moderate intensity exercise and one non-fatal cardiac arrest per 23,182 hours of HIT, with no MIs being reported for either exercise modality (Rognmo et al., 2012). Due to the shorter nature (36 per cent) of the HIT sessions compared to moderate intensity training, the rate appears to be further elevated for HIT. Both statistics suggest that exercise, at moderate to high intensity, presents a small and manageable risk of an adverse event occurring.

Cardiac patients are a heterogeneous population; therefore, although these patients may 'tolerate' the HIT, other patients may experience difficulties maintaining high workloads, or may have poor exercise adherence due to low tolerance of the exercise regime. This highlights the need for further investigation to gain a better understanding of the nature, scope, and tolerability of HIT for cardiac patients.

Exercise adherence

The potential benefits of exercise will only be realised through continued participation, so adherence to exercise programmes is fundamental to improved health outcomes. Due to the low uptake of CR both in the UK and the USA (UK ~ 44 per cent [Doherty and Lewin, 2013]; USA < 40 per cent [Keteyian et al., 2012]), research needs to focus on increasing the number of eligible patients being referred for CR and promoting long-term exercise adherence. Of the 30 per cent of eligible patients referred to CR, only one-third still attend CR after six months (10 per cent overall) (Daly et al., 2002). The main factors that were reported for lack of adherence included a lack of social support, motivation, and commitment (Daly et al., 2002). Tracking physical activity levels beyond Phase III CR is not currently catered for in the NACR. This should be considered a priority, in order to determine the longer-term impact of CR on physical activity behaviours and patient outcomes. Methods of promoting 'graduation' from Phase III to Phase IV CR exercise programmes should also be explored, including patient-exercise instructor relationships and effective referral pathways.

Summary

Substantial evidence supports the incorporation of exercise within CR programmes to promote the recovery of physical and psychological health. The evidence presented highlights the positive effect of exercise intervention on secondary cardiac events, mortality rates, cardiac function, and the physical fitness of cardiac patients to supplement contemporary clinical care. However, further research is needed on a greater variety of cardiac patient groups to fully verify the effectiveness of different exercise regimes. Many of the studies cited were performed with CHF patients, who potentially may experience greater improvements in physical function and quality of life, due to the debilitating nature of this condition. Though CHF patients are incorporated into contemporary CR delivery, they are not representative of the wider patient demographic that access CR. Finally, combined aerobic and resistance training provides the greatest potential improvements to physical fitness; however, further research is needed to validate the delivery of contemporary CR services across a heterogeneous patient demographic to ensure that the exercise component meets an appropriate dose to elicit favourable adaptations that impact positively on patient outcomes.

Further reading

American Association for Cardiovascular and Pulmonary Rehabilitation (2013). *Guidelines for cardiac rehabilitation and secondary prevention programs*. 5th ed. Champaign, Illinois: Human Kinetics.

Association of Chartered Physiotherapists in Cardiac Rehabilitation (ACPICR) (2015). *Standards of physical activity and exercise in the cardiovascular population*. 3rd ed. Retrieved from: http://acpicr.com/sites/default/files/ACPICR%20Standards%202015.pdf on 17th March 2015.

British Association for Cardiovascular Prevention and Rehabilitation (BACPR) (2012) *BACPR standards and core components for cardiovascular disease prevention and rehabilitation*. 2nd ed. London: BACPR.

Dalal, H. M., Zawada, A., Jolly, K., Moxham, T. and Taylor, R. S. (2010) Home-based versus centre-based cardiac rehabilitation: Cochrane Systematic Review and Meta-Analysis. *British Medical Journal*, 340. doi: http://dx.doi.org/10.1136/bmj.b5631.

Hamm, L. F., Sanderson, B. K., Ades, P. A., Berra, K., Kaminsky, L. A., Roitman, J. L., and Williams, M. A. (2011). Core competencies for cardiac rehabilitation/secondary prevention professionals: 2010 update: position statement of the American Association of Cardiovascular and Pulmonary Rehabilitation. *Journal of Cardiopulmonary Rehabilitation and Prevention*, 31(1), 2–10. doi: 10.1097/HCR.0b013e318203999d.

Leon, S., Franklin, B. A., Costa, F, Balady, G. J., Berra, K. A., Stewart, K. J., Thompson, P. D., Williams, M. A. and Lauer, M. S. (2005) Cardiac rehabilitation and secondary prevention of coronary heart disease: an American Heart Association scientific statement from the Council on Clinical Cardiology (Subcommittee on Exercise, Cardiac Rehabilitation, and Prevention) and the Council on Nutrition, Physical Activity, and Metabolism (Subcommittee on Physical Activity), in collaboration with the American Association of Cardiovascular and Pulmonary Rehabilitation. *Circulation*, 111, 369–76.

Piepoli, M. F., Corrà, U., Benzer, W., Bjarnason-Wehrens, B., Dendale, P., Gaita, D., McGee H., Mendes, M., Niebauer, J., Zwisler, O. A. and Schmid J. (2010) Secondary prevention through cardiac rehabilitation: from knowledge to implementation. A position paper from the Cardiac Rehabilitation Section of the European Association of Cardiovascular Prevention and Rehabilitation. *European Journal of Cardiovascular Prevention and Rehabilitation*, 17, 1–17.

References

Ades, P. A. (2001). Cardiac rehabilitation and secondary prevention of coronary heart disease. *The New England Journal of Medicine*, 345(12), 892–902.

American Association for Cardiovascular and Pulmonary Rehabilitation (2013). *Guidelines for cardiac rehabilitation and secondary prevention programs*. 5th ed. Champaign, Illinois: Human Kinetics.

Artham, S. M., Lavie, C. J., Milani, R. V., Chi, Y., and Goldman, C.K. (2008). Benefits of exercise training in secondary prevention of coronary and peripheral arterial disease. *Vascular Disease Prevention*, 5(3), 156–68.

Association of Chartered Physiotherapists in Cardiac Rehabilitation (ACPICR) (2015). *Standards of Physical Activity and Exercise in the Cardiovascular Population*. 3rd ed. Retrieved from: http://acpicr.com/sites/default/files/ACPICR%20Standards%202015.pdf on 17th March 2015.

Austin, J., Williams, R., Ross, L., Moseley, L., and Hutchison, S. (2005). Randomised controlled trial of cardiac rehabilitation in patients with heart failure. *European Journal of Heart Failure*, 7(3), 411–17.

Balady, G. J., Fletcher, B. J., Froelicher, E. S., Hartley, L. H., Krauss, R. M., Oberman, A. Pollock, M. L., and Taylor, C. B. (1994). Cardiac rehabilitation programs: a statement for healthcare professionals from the American Heart Association. *Circulation*, 90, 1602–10.

Balady, G., Jette, D., Scheer, J., and Downing, J. (1996) Changes in exercise capacity following cardiac rehabilitation in patients stratified according to age and gender: results of the Massachusetts Association of Cardiovascular and Pulmonary Rehabilitation Multicenter Database. *Journal of Cardiopulmonary Rehabilitation*, 16(1), 38–46.

Beauchamp, A., Worcester, M., Ng, A., Murphy, B., Tatoulis, J., Grigg, L., Newman, R., and Goble, A. (2012). Attendance at cardiac rehabilitation is associated with lower all-cause mortality after 14 years of follow-up. *Heart*, 99(9), 620–5.

Belardinelli, R., Georgiou, D., Cianci, G., and Purcaro, A. (1999). Randomized, controlled trial of long-term moderate exercise training in chronic heart failure. *Circulation*, 99, 1173–82.

Bethell, H. J. (1999). Exercise in cardiac rehabilitation, *British Journal of Sports Medicine*, 33(2), 79–86.

Bjarnason-Wehrens, B., Mayer-Berger, W., Meister, E., Baum, K., Hambrecht, R., and Gielen, S. (2004). Recommendations for resistance exercise in cardiac rehabilitation. Recommendations of the German Federation for Cardiovascular Prevention and Rehabilitation. *European Journal of Preventive Cardiology*, 11(4), 352–61.

British Association for Cardiovascular Prevention and Rehabilitation (BACPR) (2012) *BACPR Standards and Core Components for Cardiovascular Disease Prevention and Rehabilitation*. 2nd ed. London: BACPR.

Bryner, R. W., Ullrich, I. H., Sauers, J., Donley, D., Hornsby, G, Kolar, M., and Yeater, R. (1999). Effect of resistance vs. aerobic training combined with an 800 calorie liquid diet on lean body mass and resting metabolic rate. *Journal of American College of Nutrition*, 18(2), 115–21.

Carney, R. M., Freedland, K. E., Veith, R. C., and Jaffe, A. S. (1999). Can treating depression reduce mortality after an acute myocardial infarction? *Psychosomatic Medicine*, 61, 666–75.

Chien, C. L., Lee, C. M., Wu, Y. W., Chen, T. A., and Wu, Y. T. (2008). Home-based exercise increases exercise capacity but not quality of life in people with chronic heart failure: a systematic review. *Australian Journal of Physiotherapy*, 54(2), 87–93.

Child, A., Sanders, J., Sigel, P., and Hunter, M. S. (2010). Meeting the psychological needs of cardiac patients: an integrated stepped-care approach within a cardiac rehabilitation setting. *The British Journal of Cardiology*, 17(4), 175–9.

Cornelissen, V. A., and Fagard, R. H. (2005). Effect of resistance training on resting blood pressure: a meta-analysis of randomized control trials. *Journal of Hypertension*, 23(2), 251–9.

Cornish, A. K., Broadbent, S., and Cheema, B. S. (2011). Interval training for patients with coronary artery disease: a systematic review. *European Journal of Applied Physiology*, 111, 579–89.

Department of Health (2000). *National service framework for coronary heart disease: modern standards and service models*. London: Crown Copyright.

Daly, J., Sindone, A.P., Thompson, D. R., Hancock, K., and Chang, E. (2002). Barriers to participation in and adherence to cardiac rehabilitation programs: a critical literature review. *Progress in Cardiovascular Nursing*, 17(1), 8–17.

Davies, E. J., Moxham, T., Rees, K., Singh, S., Coats, A. J. S., Ebrahim, S., Lough F., and Taylor, R. S. (2010). Exercise training for systolic heart failure: Cochrane systematic review and meta-analysis. *European Journal of Heart Failure*, 12(7), 706–15.

Demopoulos, L., Bijou, R., Fergus, I., Jones, M., Strom, J., and Le Jemtel, T.H. (1997). Exercise training in patients with severe congestive heart failure: enhancing peak aerobic capacity while minimising the increase in ventricular wall stress, *Heart Failure*, 29, 597–603.

Doherty, P., and Lewin, R. (2013). *The national audit of cardiac rehabilitation annual statistical report 2013*. Birmingham, UK: British Heart Foundation.

Fletcher, G. F., Balady, G., Blair, S. N., Blumenthal, J., Caspersen, C., Chaitman, B., Epstein, S., Sivarajan Froelicher, E. S., Froelicher, V. F., Piña, I. L., and Pollock, M. L. (1996). Statement on exercise: benefits and recommendations for physical activity programs for all Americans. *Circulation*, 94, 857–62.

Fletcher, G. F., Balady, G. J., Amsterdam, E. A., Chaitman, B., Eckel, R., Fleg J., Froelicher, V. F., Leon, A. S., Piña, I. L., Rodney, R., Simons-Morton, D. A., Williams, M. A., and Bazzarre, T. (2001). Exercise standards for testing and training: a statement for healthcare professionals from the American Heart Association. *Circulation*, 104. 1694–1740.

Flynn, K. E., Piña, I. L., Whellan, D. J., Lin, L., Blumenthal, J. A., Ellis, S. J., Fine, L. J., Howlett, J. G., Keteyian, S. J., Kitzman, D. W., Kraus, W. E., Miller, N. H., Schulman, K. A., Spertus, J. A., O'Connor, C. M. and Weinfurt, K. P. (2009). Effects of exercise training on health status in patients with chronic heart failure. HF-action randomised controlled trial. *Journal of the American Medical Association*, 301(14), 1451–9.

Forman, D. E., Cannon, C. P., Hernandez, A. F., Liang, L., Yancy, C. and Fonarow, G. C. (2009). Influence of age on the management of heart failure: findings from Get With the Guidelines-Heart Failure (GWTG-HF). *American Heart Journal*, 157(6), 1010–17.

Franklin, B. A., Bonzheim, K., Gordon, S. and Timmis, G. C. (1998) Safety of medically supervised cardiac rehabilitation exercise therapy: a 16-year follow-up. *Chest*, 114, 902–6.

Franklin, B. A., and McCullough, P. A. (2009). Cardiorespiratory fitness: an independent and additive marker of risk stratification and health outcomes. *Mayo Clinic Proceedings*, 84(9), 776–9.

Giannuzzi, P., Temporelli, P. L., Corrà, U., and Tavazzi, L. (2003). Antiremodelling effect of long term exercise training in patients with stable chronic heart failure. *Circulation*, 108, 554–9.

Gielen, S., Adams, V., Möbius-Winkler, S., Linke, A., Erbs, S., Yu, J., Kempf, W., Schubert, A., Schuler, G., and Hambrecht, R. (2003). Anti-inflammatory effects of exercise training in the skeletal muscle of patients with chronic heart failure, *Journal of the American College of Cardiology*, 4(5), 861–8.

Graham, I., Atar, D., Borch-Johnsen, K., Boysen, G., Burell, G., Cifkova, R., Dallongeville, J., De Backer, G., Ebrahim, S., Gjelsvik, B., Herrmann-Lingen, C., Hoes, A., Humphries, S., Knapton, M., Perk, J., Priori, S. G., Pyorala, K., Reiner, Z., Ruilope, L., Sans-Menendez, S., Scholte op Reimer, W., Weissberg, P., Wood, D., Yarnell, J., Zamorano, J. L., Walma, E., Fitzgerald, T., Cooney, M. T., and Dudina, A.; (2007). European guidelines on cardiovascular disease prevention in clinical practice. *European Heart Journal*, 28, 2375–2414.

Green, D. J., Fowler, D. T., O'Driscoll, J. G., Blanksby, B. A., and Taylor, R. R. (1996). Endothelium-derived nitric oxide activity in forearm vessels of tennis players. *Journal of Applied Physiology*, 81, 943–8.

Green, D. J., Maiorana, A., O'Driscoll, G., and Taylor, R. (2004). Effects of exercise training on endothelium-derived nitric oxide function in humans. *Journal of Physiology*, 561, 1–25.

Green, D. J., O'Driscoll, G., Joyner, M. J., and Cable, N. T. (2008). Exercise and cardiovascular risk reduction: time to update the rationale for exercise? *Journal of Applied Physiology*, 105, 766–8.

Guiraud, T., Nigam, A., Juneau., Meyer, P., Gayda, M., and Bosquet, L. (2009). Acute responses to high-intensity intermittent exercise in CHD patients. *Medicine* and *Science in Sports and Exercise*, 43, 211–17.

Hambrecht, R., Niebauer, J., Fiehn, E., Kälberer, B., Offner, B., Hauer, K., Riede, U., Schlierf, G., Kübler, W., and Schuler, G. (1995). Physical training in patients with stable chronic heart failure: effects on cardiorespiratory fitness and ultrastructural abnormalities of leg muscles. *Journal of American College of Cardiology*, 25(6), 1239–49.

Hambrecht, R., Wolf, A., Gielen, S., Linke, A., Hofer, J., Erbs, S., Schoene, N., and Schuler, G. (2000). Effect of exercise on coronary endothelial function in patients with coronary artery disease. *The New England Journal of Medicine*, 342, 454–60.

Hansen, D., Dendale, P., Berger, J., and Meeusen, R. (2005). Rehabilitation in cardiac patients: what do we know about training modalities? *Sports Medicine*, 35(12), 1063–84.

Hansen, D., Dendale, P., Van Loon, L., and Meeusen, R. (2010). The impact of training modalities on the clinical benefits of exercise intervention in patients with cardiovascular disease risk or type 2 diabetes mellitus. *Sports Medicine*, 40(11), 921–40.

Haykowsky, M. J., Liang, Y., Pechter, D., Jones, L. W., McAlister, F. A., Clark, A. M. (2007). A meta-analysis of the effects of exercise training on left ventricular remodeling in heart failure patients. *Journal of the American College of Cardiology*, 49(24), 2329–36.

Heran, B. S., Chen, J. M. H., Ebrahim, S., Moxham, T., Oldridge, N., Rees, K., Thompson, D. R., and Taylor, R. S. (2011). Exercise-based cardiac rehabilitation for coronary heart disease. *Cochrane Database of Systematic Reviews*, 7, CD001800.

Jolliffe, J., Rees, K., Taylor, R. R. S., Thompson, D. R., Oldridge, N., and Ebrahim, S. (2001). Exercise-based rehabilitation for coronary heart disease. *Cochrane Database of Systematic Reviews*, 1, CD001800.

Kelemen, M. H., Stewart, K. J., Gillilan, R. E., Ewart, C. K., Valenti, S. A., Manley, J. D, Kelemen, M. D. (1986). Circuit weight training in cardiac patients. *Journal of the American College of Cardiology*, 7(1), 38–42.

Keteyian, S. J., Brawner, C. A., Savage, P. D., Ehrman, J. K., Schairer, J., Divine, G., Aldred, H., Ophaug, K., and Ades, P. A. (2008). Peak Aerobic Capacity Predict Prognosis in Patients with Coronary Heart Disease. *American Heart Journal*, 156(2), 292–300.

Keteyian, S. J., Leifer, E. S., Houston-Miller, N., Kraus, W. E., Brawner, C. A., O'Connor, C. M., Whellan, D. J., Cooper, L. S., Fleg, J. L., Kitzman, D. W., Cohen-Solal, A., Blumenthal, J. A., Rendall, D. S. And Piña, I. L. (2012). Relation between volume of exercise and clinical outcomes in patients with heart failure. *Journal of the American College of Cardiology*, 60(19), 1899–1905.

Lavie, C. J. and Milani, R. V. (1995). Effects of cardiac rehabilitation and exercise training on exercise capacity, coronary risk factors, behavioural characteristics, and quality of life in women. *The American Journal of Cardiology*, 75(5), 340–3.

Lavie, C. J., and Milani, R. V. (1997). Effects of cardiac rehabilitation, exercise training, and weight reduction on exercise capacity, coronary risk factors, behavioural characteristics, and quality of life in obese coronary patients. *The American Journal of Cardiology*, 79(4), 397–401.

Lavie, C. J., Thomas, R. J., Squires, R. W., Allison, T. G., Milani, R. V. (2009). Exercise training and cardiac rehabilitation in primary and secondary prevention of coronary heart disease. *Mayo Clinic Proceedings*, 84(4), 373–83.

Lawler, P. R., Filion, K. B., and Eisenberg, M. J. (2011). Efficacy of exercise-based cardiac rehabilitation post-myocardial infarction: a systematic review and meta-analysis of randomized controlled trials. *American Heart Journal*, 162, 571–84.

Leon, S., Franklin, B. A., Costa, F, Balady, G. J., Berra, K. A., Stewart, K. J., Thompson, P. D., Williams, M. A., and Lauer, M. S. (2005). Cardiac rehabilitation and secondary prevention of coronary heart disease: an American Heart Association scientific statement from the Council on Clinical Cardiology (Subcommittee on Exercise, Cardiac Rehabilitation, and Prevention) and the Council on Nutrition, Physical Activity, and Metabolism (Subcommittee on Physical Activity), in collaboration with the American Association of Cardiovascular and Pulmonary Rehabilitation. *Circulation*, 111, 369–76.

Levick, R. J (2009). *An introduction to cardiovascular physiology*. 5th ed. Boca Raton, Florida: CRC Press.

Lloyd-Williams, F., Mair, F. S., and Leitner, M. (2002). Exercise training and heart failure: a systematic review of current evidence. *British Journal of General Practice*, 52(474), 47–55.

Marchionni, N., Fattirolli, F., Fumagalli, S., Oldridge, N., Del Lungo F., Morosi L., Burgisser, C., and Masotti, G. (2003). Improved exercise tolerance and quality of life with cardiac rehabilitation of older patients after myocardial infarction. *Circulation*,107, 2201–06.

Martin, B. J., Arena, R., Haykowsky, M., Hauer, T., Austford, L. D., Knudtson, M., Aggarwal, S., and Stone, J. A. (2013). Cardiovascular fitness and mortality after contemporary cardiac rehabilitation. *Mayo Clinic Proceedings*, 88(5), 455–63.

Maxwell, A. J., Schauble, E., Bernstein, D., and Cooke, J. P. (1998). Limb blood flow during exercise is dependent on nitric oxide. *Circulation*, 98, 369–74.

McCartney, N. (1998). Role of resistance training in heart disease. *Medicine and Science in Sports and Exercise*, 30(10 suppl.), S396–S402.

McCartney, N., McKelvie, R. S., Haslam, D. R., and Jones, N. L. (1991). Usefulness of weight-lifting training in improving strength and maximal power output in coronary artery disease. *The American Journal of Cardiology*, 67(11), 939–45.

Meyer P., Normandin, E., Gayda, M., Billon, G., Guiraud, T., Bosquet, L., Fortier, A., Juneau, M., White, M., and Nigam, A. (2012). High-intensity interval exercise in chronic heart failure: protocol optimisation. *Journal of Cardiac Failure*, 18(2), 126–33.

Mittleman, M. A., Maclure, M., Tofler, G. H., Sherwood, J. B., Goldberg, R. J., and Muller, J. E. (1993) Triggering of acute myocardial infarction by heavy physical exertion – protection against triggering by regular exertion. *The New England Journal of Medicine*, 329, 1677–83.

Moholdt, T., Aamot, I. L., Granøien, I, Gjerde, L., Myklebust, G., Walderhaug, L., Brattbakk, L., Hole, T., Graven, T., Stølen, T. O., Amundsen, B. H., Mølmen-Hansen, H. E., Støylen, A., Wisløff, U., and Slørdahl, S.A. (2012). Aerobic interval training increases peak oxygen uptake more than usual care exercise training in myocardial infarction patients: a randomised controlled study. *Clinical Rehabilitation*, 26(1), 33–44.

National Institute for Health and Clinical Excellence (NICE) (2008). *Cardiac rehabilitation service*. Commissioning guide: Implementing NICE guidance.

Nelson, A. J., Juraska, J. M., Musch, T. I., and Iwamoto, G. A. (2005). Neuroplastic adaptations to exercise: neuronal remodelling in cardiorespiratory and locomotor areas. *Journal of Applied Physiology*, 99, 2312–22.

Nilsson, B. B., Westheim, A., and Risberg, M. A. (2008). Effects of group-based high-intensity aerobic interval training in patients with chronic heart failure. *American Journal of Cardiology*, 102(10), 1361–5.

O'Connor, C. M., Whellan, D. J., Lee, K. L., Keteyian, S. J., Cooper, L. S., Ellis, S. J., Leifer, E. S., Kraus, W. E., Kitzman, D. W., Blumenthal, J. A., Rendall, D. S., Miller, N. H., and Fleg, J. L. (2009). Efficacy and safety of Exercise Training in Patients with Chronic Heart Failure: HF-Action Randomised Controlled Trial. *Journal of the American Medical Association*, 301(14), 1439–50.

O'Connor, G. T., Buring, J. E., Yusuf, S., Goldhaber, S. Z., Olmstead, E. M., Paffenbarger, R., and S. Hennekens, C. H. (1989). An overview of randomized trials of rehabilitation with exercise after myocardial infarction. *Circulation*, 80(2), 234–44.

Owen, A., and Croucher, I. (2000). Effect of an exercise programme for elderly patients with heart failure. *European Journal of Heart Failure*, 2, 65–70.

Papadakis, S., Oldridge, N. B., Coyle, D., Mayhew, A., Reid, R. D., and Beaton, L. (2005). Economic evaluation of cardiac rehabilitation: a systematic review. *European Journal of Cardiovascular Prevention and Rehabilitation*, 12(6), 513–20.

Parker, N. D., Hunter, G. R., Treuth, M. S., Kekes-Szabo, T., Kell, S. H., Weinsier, R. and White, M. (1996) Effects of strength training on cardiovascular responses during a submaximal walk and a weight-loaded walking test in older females. *Journal of Cardiopulmonary Rehabilitation*, 16(1), 56–62.

Pavia, L, Orlando, G., Myers, J., and Maestri, M. (1995). The effect of beta-blockade therapy on the response to exercise training in postmyocardial infarction patients. *Clinical Cardiology*, 18, 716–20.

Pescatello, L. S., Arena, R., Riebe, D., and Thompson, P. D. (2014). *ACSM's Guide for Exercise Testing and Prescription*. 9th ed. Baltimore, MD: Wolters Kluwer Health/Lippincott, Williams and Wilkins.

Piepoli, M. F., Corrà, U., Benzer, W., Bjarnason-Wehrens, B., Dendale, P., Gaita, D., McGee H., Mendes, M., Niebauer, J., Zwisler, O. A., and Schmid J. (2010). Secondary prevention through cardiac rehabilitation: from knowledge to implementation. A position paper from the Cardiac Rehabilitation Section of the European Association of Cardiovascular Prevention and Rehabilitation. *European Journal of Cardiovascular Prevention and Rehabilitation*, 17, 1–17.

Pollock, M. L., Franklin, B. A., Balady, G. J., Chaitman, B. L., Fleg, J. L., Fletcher, B., Limacher, M., Piña, I. L., Stein, R. A., Williams, M. and Bazzarre, T. (2000). Resistance exercise in individuals with and without cardiovascular disease: benefits, rationale, safety, prescription. An advisory from the Committee on Exercise, Rehabilitation, and Prevention, Council on Clinical Cardiology, American Heart Association. *Circulation*, 101, 828–33.

Rennie, K. L., Hemingway, H., Kumari, M., Brunner, E., Malik, M., and Marmot, M. (2003). Effects of moderate and vigorous physical activity on heart rate variability in a British study of civil servants. *American Journal of Epidemiology*, 158, 135–43.

Rognmo, Ø., Hetland, E., Helgerud, J., Hoff, J., Slørdahl, S. (2004). High intensity aerobic interval exercise is superior to moderate intensity exercise for increasing aerobic capacity in patients with coronary artery disease. *European Journal of Preventive Cardiology*, 11, 216–22.

Rognmo, Ø., Moholdt, T., Bakken, H., Hole, T., Mølstad, P., Myhr, N., Grimsmo, J., and Wisløff, U. (2012). Cardiovascular risk of high-versus moderate-intensity aerobic exercise in coronary heart disease patients. *Circulation*, 126, 1436–40.

Rozanski, A., Blumenthal, J. A., Davidson, K. W., Saab, P. G., Kubzansky, L. (2005). The epidemiology, pathophysiology, and management of psychosocial risk factors in cardiac practice. The emerging field of behavioural cardiology. *Journal of the American College of Cardiology*, 45(5), 637–51.

Saeidi, M., and Mostafavi, M. (2013). Effects of a comprehensive cardiac rehabilitation program on quality of life in patients with coronary artery disease. *Heart*, 99(3), A140-A141.

Sandercock, G., Hurtado, V., and Cardoso, F. (2013b). Changes in cardiorespiratory fitness in cardiac rehabilitation patients: a meta-analysis. *International Journal of Cardiology*, 167(3), 894–902.

Sandercock, G. R. H., Cardoso, F., Almodhy, M., and Pepera, G. (2013a). Cardiorespiratory fitness changes in patients receiving comprehensive outpatient cardiac rehabilitation in the UK: a multicentre study. *Heart*, 99, 785–90.

Sheppard, M. (2011). *Practical cardiovascular pathology (Second edition)*. Boca Raton, Florida: CRC Press.

Smart, N., and Marwick, T. H. (2004). Exercise training for patients with heart failure: a systematic review of factors that improve mortality and morbidity. *American Journal of Medicine*, 116, 693–706.

Stein, P. K., Carney, R. M., Freedland, K. E., Skala, J. A., Jaffe, A. S., Kleiger, R. E., and Rottman, J. N. (1995). Severe depression is associated with markedly reduced heart rate variability in patients with stable coronary heart disease. *Journal of Psychosomatic Research*, 46(4–5), 493–500.

Taylor, C. B., Houston-Miller, N., Ahn, D. K., Haskell, W., and DeBusk, R. F. (1986). The effects of exercise training programs on psychosocial improvement in uncomplicated post-myocardial infarction patients. *Journal of Psychosomatic Research*, 30(5), 581–7.

Taylor, R. S., Brown, A., Ebrahim, S., Jolliffe, J., Noorani, H., Rees, K., Skidmore, B., Stone, J. A., Thompson, D. R., and Oldridge, N. (2004). Exercise-based rehabilitation for patients with coronary heart disease: systematic review and meta-analysis of randomized controlled trials. *The American Journal of Medicine*, 116(10), 682–92.

Thompson, P. D., Buchner, D., Piña, I. L., Balady, G. J., Williams, M. A., Marcus, B. H., Berra, K., Blair, S. N., Costa, F., Franklin, B., Fletcher, G. F., Gordon, N. F., Pate, R. R., Rodriguez, B. L., Yancey, A. K., and Wenger, N. K. (2003). Exercise and physical activity in the prevention and treatment of atherosclerotic cardiovascular disease: a statement from the Council on Clinical Cardiology (Subcommittee on Exercise, Rehabilitation, and Prevention) and the Council on Nutrition, Physical Activity, and Metabolism (Subcommittee on Physical Activity). *Circulation*, 107, 3109–16.

Tsuji, H., Venditti, F. J., Manders, E. S., Evans, J. C., Larson, M. G., Feldman, C. L., and Levy, D. (1994). Reduced heart rate variability and mortality risk in the elderly cohort. The Framingham Heart Study. *Circulation*, 90, 878–83.

Van Stel, H. F., Busschbach, J. J. V., Hunink, M. M. G., and Buskens, E. (2012). Impact of secondary cardiovascular events on health status. *Value in Health*, 15(1), 175–82.

Van Tol, B.A. F., Huijsmans, R. J., Kroon, D. W., Schothorst, and M., Kwakkel, G. (2006). Effects of exercise training on cardiac performance, exercise capacity and quality of life in patients with heart failure: a meta-analysis. *European Journal of Heart Failure*, 8, 841–50.

Wenger, N. K. (2008). Current status of cardiac rehabilitation. *Journal of the American College of Cardiology*, 51(17), 1619–31.

Wielenga, R. P., Huisveld, L. A., Bol, E., Dunselman, P. H. J. M., Erdman, R. A. M., Baselier, M. R. P., Mosterd, W. L. (1999a). Safety and effects of physical training in chronic heart failure and graded exercise study (CHANGE). *European Heart Journal*, 20(12), 872–9.

Wielenga, R. P., Huisveld, L. A., Bol, E., Dunselman, P. H. J. M., Erdman, R. A. M., Baselier, M. R. P., Mosterd, W. L. (1999b). Exercise training in elderly patients with chronic heart failure. *Coronary Artery Disease*, 9, 765–70.

Wise, F. M., Patrick, J. M. (2011). Resistance exercise in cardiac rehabilitation. *Clinical Rehabilitation*, 25, 1058.

Wisløff, U., Støylen, A., Loennechen, J. P., Bruvold, M., Rognmo, Ø., Haram, P. M., Tjønna, A. E., Helgerud, J., Slørdahl, S. A., Lee, S. J., Videm, V., Bye, A., Smith, G. L., Najjar, S. M., Ellingsen, Ø. and Skjærpe, T. (2007) Superior cardiovascular effect of aerobic interval training versus moderate continuous training in heart failure. *Circulation*, 115, 3086–94.

Williams, M. A., Haskell, W. L., Ades, P. A., Amsterdam, E. A., Bittner, V., Franklin, B. A., Gulanick, M., Laing, S. T., and Stewart, K. (2007). Resistance exercise in individuals with and without cardiovascular disease: 2007 update. A scientific statement from the American Heart Association Council on Clinical Cardiology and Council on Nutrition, Physical Activity and Metabolism. *Circulation*, 116, 572–84.

Yohannes, A. M., Doherty, P., Bundy, C., Yalfani, A. (2010). The long-term benefits of cardiac rehabilitation on depression, anxiety, physical activity and quality of life. *Journal of Clinical Nursing*, 19(19–20), 2806–13.

Chapter 3

Physical activity for chronic respiratory disease

Linzy Houchen-Wolloff, Lorna Latimer, and Michael Steiner

Introduction

Chronic respiratory disease (CRD) can be considered an umbrella term for a number of long-term conditions caused by a variety of underlying lung pathologies. Collectively, these conditions are an important and prevalent cause of morbidity and mortality, and impose a substantial burden to health services in the developed and developing world. Globally chronic obstructive pulmonary disease (COPD), the most prevalent form of chronic respiratory disease, is the fourth most common cause of death, but also imposes a substantial burden of disability for those living with the disease (WHO, 2014). The prevalence and health burden of CRDs are expected to increase worldwide in line with trends in global tobacco consumption, population ageing, and environmental pollution. A common feature of most CRDs is the tendency to exacerbate acutely, often in response to respiratory infection. These events can have major implications for patients and health services, particularly those with more severe diseases. For example, in the UK, COPD is the second most common cause of unscheduled acute hospital admission, with estimated annual costs to the National Health Service (NHS) in excess of £1 billion.

Chronic respiratory diseases have complex and diverse causes such as smoking, respiratory infections, and environmental/occupational exposures, which interact with the host's genetic susceptibility to cause disease. Anatomically, CRD can predominantly affect the airways (asthma and bronchiectasis), the lung parenchyma (interstitial lung diseases) or both (COPD). Indeed, current thinking about the classification of these diseases recognises the limitations of these terms in describing discrete disease entities, given that each may encompass several underlying lung pathologies and that there may be considerable overlap between them in an individual patient. The diagnosis of specific CRDs relies on the recognition of a compatible clinical syndrome in association with confirmatory diagnostic tests. In the case of COPD, for example, the diagnosis is suggested by typical clinical features and is confirmed by the finding of obstructive spirometry that is not completely reversible (see Box 3.1).

It is not the intention of this chapter to provide a detailed review of the aetiology, pathology, diagnosis, and treatment of the range of common CRDs. However, impaired physical performance and activity are common and key features of all these diseases, and in the following sections we review the pathophysiology of performance and activity limitation in CRD, and discuss the role of exercise therapies in managing this clinical problem. It is now appreciated that CRD is associated with systemic, extra-pulmonary manifestations, which in themselves are responsible for considerable morbidity.

Box 3.1 Diagnosis of COPD

Clinical syndrome

- Breathlessness
- Exercise limitation
- Sputum production
- Winter bronchitis and respiratory infections
- Smoking history.

Diagnostic

Post bronchodilator spirometry showing:

- Forced expiratory volume in 1 second (FEV_1)/Forced vital capacity (FVC) ratio < 0.7
- Reduced FEV_1 (< 80 per cent predicted).

Examples include increased risk of cardiovascular disease, osteoporosis, anaemia, and psychological morbidity (anxiety and depression). Some, such as skeletal muscle dysfunction, directly affect activity limitation and are amenable to exercise-based therapies. Most of the scientific evidence in this area has been derived from populations of patients with COPD, and we will focus in the following section on the key issues in the COPD population with reference to other respiratory diseases where relevant.

Impaired physical activity and performance in COPD

Exercise limitation is a hallmark feature of most chronic respiratory diseases (CRDs) including COPD. The inability to be physically active due to breathlessness is one of the key complaints expressed by patients with COPD, which may extend to the restriction to perform simple physical tasks required for day-to-day living. This is best considered as an 'exercise problem' because it is the quantitative restriction to physical capacity more than the sensation of breathlessness or fatigue during exercise (something we all experience) that is the abnormal symptom. Lung damage leading to impaired lung function is the initiating event in the development of exercise limitation, but the longer-term impact on the patient is the result of a complex interaction of pulmonary and extra-pulmonary pathophysiology that may develop over many years in relation to changes in the individual's habitual levels of physical activity. The development of breathlessness during activity almost universally results in the avoidance of the circumstances which cause the symptom (in this case exercise), resulting in the adoption of a less physically active lifestyle. The consequence is progressive physical deconditioning, which in itself exacerbates the symptom, and thereby compounds the behavioural adaption, a process that has been described as the 'spiral of disability' (Figure 3.1). This may be compounded by additional factors such as drug therapy (beta-agonists, corticosteroids), hypoxia, or inflammation in some individuals. Moreover, the propensity for the condition to exacerbate secondary to recurrent respiratory infection may result in periods of enforced inactivity either in the home or in hospital, which in some

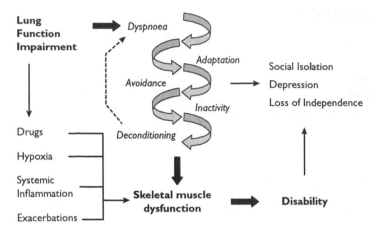

Figure 3.1 The spiral of disability in chronic respiratory disease. Reproduced with permission from Sage Publications Ltd.

patients may be an important driver of progressive deconditioning. In turn, deconditioning is a key driver of skeletal muscle dysfunction, which in itself contributes to impaired performance (see below). In addition, adaptations to activity behaviours may have major adverse consequences for the wider well-being of the patient through changes in mood, loss of social participation, and dependence on others.

Ventilatory limitation to exercise in lung disease

In healthy humans, ventilatory function is not a physiological limit to maximum exercise performance, but in patients with respiratory disease, particularly when it is severe, exercise may be constrained by a limit to maximum ventilation that is imposed by the disease. This may take a variety of forms depending on the underlying pathology. In COPD, expiratory airflow obstruction is the hallmark pathophysiological feature, and the key diagnostic test for the disease (see Box 3.1). The impact of abnormal lung mechanics on exercise performance in COPD has been extensively studied (detailed accounts can be found in Cooper, 2009, Decramer and O'Donnell, 2013, and O'Donnell, 2006). Briefly, when airflow obstruction becomes severe it may limit expiratory flow during tidal breathing. Under these circumstances, expiratory flow cannot rise as exercise intensity increases, and, as a result, incomplete lung emptying occurs during expiration, leading to an increase in lung volume. This 'dynamic hyperinflation' is compounded by increased lung compliance in COPD caused by emphysema, which increases operating lung volumes through an imbalance between 'outward' chest wall and 'inward' lung elastic forces. Dynamic hyperinflation has been shown to increase respiratory muscle work during exercise and is a major cause of premature exercise limitation in COPD. In other CRDs, lung mechanics may be different; for example, in interstitial lung diseases, lung compliance is reduced rather than increased (as in COPD), which also leads to an increase in respiratory muscle work. However, in addition, impaired diffusion of oxygen across the alveolar-capillary barrier may lead to marked haemoglobin desaturation during exercise, which may limit exercise in interstitial lung disease.

Skeletal muscle dysfunction in lung disease

There is now a wealth of evidence indicating that skeletal muscle function (particularly of the locomotor musculature) is impaired in patients with COPD, and that this impairment is an important determinant of impaired physical performance. The structural and functional abnormality in COPD is briefly described here, but for more detail the reader is directed to the recently updated American Thoracic Society Statement on skeletal muscle dysfunction in COPD (Maltais et al., 2014).

Attention was drawn to the function of the skeletal muscles by observations that patients often cite muscle fatigue as the limiting symptom to exercise rather than breathlessness (Killian et al., 1992) and that weight loss and muscle wasting are a common manifestation of advancing COPD with adverse implications for symptoms and mortality (Vestbo et al. 2006; Marquis et al., 2002). Studies of the exercise response in COPD indicated an early and accelerated rise in lactate, suggesting an over-reliance on anaerobic (non-oxidative), and by implication a reduction in the use of mitochondrial (oxidative), energy sources (Maltais et al., 1998). This is supported by studies of muscle biopsy samples from COPD patients, which have consistently shown reduced concentrations of oxidative enzymes, reduced type I fibre cross-sectional area, and reduced capillary and mitochondrial density compared with similar-aged healthy controls (Gosker et al. 2007; Maltais 2000; Whittom et al. 1998). At peak exercise, dephosphorylation of phosphocreatine, depletion of adenine nucleotides, and accumulation of lactate is similar in patients with COPD to age-matched healthy controls, despite substantially lower absolute peak exercise intensities (Steiner et al., 2003). Excessive anaerobic energy production in COPD is not simply a function of reduced oxygen delivery, as it occurs in non-hypoxaemic patients, but is also dependent on mitochondrial substrate availability. For example, pharmacological activation of the pyruvate dehydrogenase complex (which promotes pyruvate entry to the tricarboxylic acid cycle) results in increased exercise capacity with reduced lactate accumulation in patients with COPD (Calvert et al., 2008). Taken together, these observations suggest that the muscles of patients with COPD exhibit an 'anaerobic' phenotype, which has implications for physical capacity. These characteristics are modifiable by aerobic exercise training (see section below), which also improves performance in patients with COPD, suggesting they have functional relevance.

Reduced quadriceps muscle mass and strength have been shown to be predictors of mortality in COPD independent from the severity of the underlying lung disease (Schols et al., 2005; Marquis et al., 2002). A reduced fibre cross-sectional area and a shift in composition to a greater proportion of type II fibres and fewer type I fibres has been observed in quadriceps biopsy samples in patients with COPD compared with similar-aged healthy controls. COPD patients with skeletal muscle dysfunction demonstrate reduced contractile endurance and a tendency to exhibit low-frequency quadriceps fatigue after an exercise task (Man et al., 2003; Swallow et al., 2007).

The cause of skeletal muscle dysfunction in COPD is probably multifactorial and may variably include systemic inflammation, oxidative stress, hypoxia, drug therapy (such as steroids) and nutritional abnormalities. However, the available evidence suggests that inactivity and deconditioning are the key drivers of muscle dysfunction in respiratory disease. For example, there is an anatomic predilection for skeletal muscle abnormalities to affect the locomotor muscles with relative sparing of the upper limb or respiratory muscles. In addition, structural changes observed in the muscles of patients with COPD mirror those seen in other immobilisation states.

Therapeutic approaches to improving exercise performance in CRD

The principle topic of this chapter is the role of exercise interventions in the treatment of CRDs, and this is covered in subsequent sections. However, treatment of the underlying pulmonary pathology may influence exercise performance, and may act synergistically with exercise therapies, so these are briefly considered here. In general terms, where there is a pathological constraint to ventilation during exercise, performance can be improved either by treatment that lifts this ventilatory constraint by improving lung function, or by a reduction in the ventilatory load such that more exercise can be performed within the pre-existing ventilatory limit (Casaburi and Petty, 1993). Exercise rehabilitation works through the latter mechanism, and, as we will describe in later sections, this is the most effective means to improve performance and reduce exercise-induced breathlessness in CRD.

For many diseases, reversing or substantially improving lung physiology has proved difficult, but some diseases (such as asthma) are highly responsive to anti-inflammatory therapy such as corticosteroids. In COPD, airflow obstruction is largely irreversible, but improvements in exercise performance can result from bronchodilator therapy through improvements in airway calibre and lung emptying during exercise. These improvements are generally of small magnitude compared with exercise rehabilitation, but may act synergistically with exercise training by increasing training intensities during rehabilitation (Casaburi et al., 2005). Recent studies have suggested that bronchodilators are more effective in those with a respiratory locus of symptom limitation in whom exercise fails to induce contractile fatigue in the locomotor muscles. In other words, those with a genuine respiratory limit to exercise will gain more from bronchodilation (Deschenes et al., 2008).

A proportion of patients with CRD will develop sustained or exercise-induced hypoxaemia, which requires supplementary oxygen therapy. In those with hypoxaemia at rest, this is given principally because it confers a survival benefit, but there is clear evidence that oxygen supplementation improves exercise performance in those who desaturate during physical activity. Portable oxygen systems are available in the UK and other health systems to assist patients with mobility (Hardinge et al., 2015). Although these are designed to be lightweight, in some cases the burden of carrying the equipment can outweigh the benefit of the supplementary oxygen, and an individual assessment of patient needs and preferences is advisable.

Some patients with advanced respiratory disease are candidates for surgical therapies. Transplantation may be a suitable therapy for some patients with severe disease; this results in a radical improvement in lung function with commensurate alleviation of breathlessness. However, chronic rejection of the donor organ (despite intensive immunosuppressive therapy) is a common longer-term problem, which causes progressive small airways obstruction (obliterative bronchiolitis), resulting in death by five years post procedure in 40–50 per cent of transplant recipients (ISHLT, n.d.). Moreover, other studies have indicated that, despite the restoration of lung function to near normal values, exercise performance does not recover to the same degree (Levy et al., 1993). This is probably in part because of the wider pre-transplant systemic effects of CRD on the skeletal musculature as described above. Lung volume reduction surgery (LVRS) is a technique that aims to reduce hyperinflation in emphysema by removing the most severely affected part of the lung. Evidence from a large multicentre trial of this procedure suggested that, in appropriately selected candidates, LVRS can improve exercise performance and quality of life (Fishman et al., 2003). Incorporation of pulmonary rehabilitation into the preparation for LVRS is crucial to ensure the patient is at optimal physical fitness before undergoing surgery, to ensure that the decision about undergoing the procedure is made at the point when maximal functional capacity for that individual has been achieved, and to allow the patient to make use of any increase in ventilatory capacity that results from surgery. More recently, potentially less invasive endobronchial techniques (e.g. valves and coils) have been tested and appear to be effective in selected individuals (Shah and Herth, 2014). The ideal place and long term effectiveness of these novel approaches is the subject of ongoing study (Shah and Hopkinson, 2012).

Exercise therapy in respiratory disease

Current disease management guidelines highlight the central role of exercise therapies in the context of pulmonary rehabilitation (PR) in the care of patients with respiratory disease (NICE, 2010; Vestbo et al., 2013). PR extends beyond a 'physical activity' or exercise intervention per se; rather, it delivers exercise training as part of a multicomponent package of support and education. This section will concentrate on the principles underlying physiological adaptation to exercise training. The largest body of evidence concerning exercise rehabilitation has been collected on COPD, and, therefore, the focus of this section will be on COPD. However many of the principles discussed will apply to other CRDs.

Adaptation to aerobic training

Long regarded as the cornerstone of PR programmes, aerobic training modalities such as walking and cycling exercise have proven benefits for patients. For most healthy sedentary individuals, adoption of an aerobic training programme involving regular bouts of moderate intensity continuous exercise (e.g. thirty minutes brisk walking, five times per week) will prompt physiological adaptation that can be quantified in terms of peak exercise performance. The benchmark assessment of aerobic capacity is a progressive exercise test to exhaustion performed on a treadmill or cycle ergometer with analysis of oxygen uptake throughout the test (a peak oxygen uptake [$\dot{V}O_{2peak}$] test). In contrast to apparently healthy participants, many patients with COPD are unable to increase $\dot{V}O_{2peak}$ after an aerobic training programme because of constraints to training intensity due to a pathological limit to ventilation. This is a factor which cannot readily be modified by training.

How, then, does aerobic training modify pathophysiology and deliver benefit to patients with COPD? It is possible to demonstrate adaptation in the musculature following aerobic training in COPD (see below), even in the absence of a change in peak exercise capacity and oxygen consumption. For the patient, this translates into improvement in sub-maximal exercise tests of endurance performance, which are more sensitive to a training intervention change than tests of maximal exercise performance (Spruit et al., 2013). In addition, perceived effort and task-related dyspnoea are reduced at an equivalent exercise workload after training, compared with the untrained state.

As discussed in the previous section, the capacity to perform prolonged exercise is impaired in COPD due to reduced muscle mitochondrial density and aerobic capacity, leading to metabolic acidosis at low absolute exercise intensities. Acidosis during exercise prompts premature fatigue and also places additional load on ventilation, therefore exacerbating dyspnoea. The mitochondria are the ultimate consumers of oxygen in muscle and are therefore key to sustainable aerobic energy delivery. The abundance of skeletal muscle mitochondria (quantified by citrate synthase activity), maximal rates of mitochondrial oxygen consumption, and the abundance of mitochondrial enzymes such as 3–hydroxyacyl–CoA dehydrogenase (HAD) are enhanced by aerobic training in COPD (Maltais et al., 1996). In the trained state, the greater efficiency of the mitochondrial energy systems and aerobic metabolism reduces the reliance on glycolytic metabolism and hydrogen ion accumulation at a given work rate. Compared to the untrained state, COPD patients experience less blood lactate accumulation and lower ventilatory demand (at the same absolute intensity) following a vigorous aerobic training regime (Casaburi et al., 1991).

Additional adaptations to aerobic training in COPD patients include an increase in the cross-sectional area of type I oxidative muscle fibres (see Maltais et al., 2014 for a summary). This increase in fibre area is matched by an increase in the capillary density of the muscle, thus ensuring that the capacity of the muscle to use oxygen is matched by the capacity to deliver oxygen to contracting fibres. Although the cross-sectional area of different fibre types may alter, it does not appear that the overall fibre type proportion is changed by aerobic training. As noted above, the pathological ventilatory constraint to maximum exercise performance restricts training intensities for many patients. However, for this reason also, patients with COPD are still able to train at high relative exercise workloads (as a proportion of VO_{2peak}); indeed, such high relative training intensities may be needed to provoke a physiological training response in the musculature. For example, patients with COPD are capable of training at 85 per cent of their baseline maximum walking speed, and this intensity is utilised as the standard in many UK PR programmes. It is important to recognise that, despite achieving such high relative intensities, absolute exercise workloads in this patient population may be low because of pre-existing exercise limitation.

Adaptation to resistance training

There is now substantial evidence that skeletal muscle mass and strength (particularly of the locomotor muscles) is lower in patients with COPD compared with age-matched healthy controls, and that this contributes to morbidity and mortality independently from the impairment of lung function. Thus, there is a strong theoretical rationale for providing resistance training during rehabilitation programmes, and indeed there is now clear evidence that resistance training is an effective means of improving muscle strength and mass in this population. The translation of these increases to gains in functional performance and health status is less clear cut but there is some evidence that this may occur (O'Shea et al., 2004). The mechanisms for the gains in muscle mass and strength following resistance training in COPD are the subject of ongoing research, but the available evidence suggests that training influences signalling pathways known to regulate muscle growth and atrophy leading to hypertrophy. Whole-body lean mass, trained-limb lean mass, muscle cross-sectional area, and muscle fibre size are all increased after exercise involving resistance training.

In some rehabilitation programmes, resistance training is prioritised for patients who are severely ventilatory limited or acutely unwell. By training smaller muscle volumes, resistance training places lower demand on the cardiorespiratory system, and therefore induces less dyspnoea than whole-body training.

Behavioural adaptation

Whilst there is clear evidence for physiological adaptation following training in COPD if trained at appropriate intensities, it is also recognised that there is a significant behavioural component underpinning the efficacy of exercise and rehabilitation therapies. Patients with chronic respiratory disease frequently avoid physical activity because it provokes dyspnoea and many have developed significant anxiety about undertaking exercise, fearing that it may worsen their condition or put them at risk of harm. One of the major benefits of exercise therapy is overcoming these fears and demonstrating that exercise is both safe and beneficial for symptoms and future health. Thus, patients may become 'desensitised' to the sensation of dyspnoea during exercise, feel more confident about undertaking exercise, and therefore increase performance through greater utilisation of pre-existing physiological capacity (Leidy, 1994). This benefit can accrue without physiological adaptation, but may be enhanced by it.

A key objective of rehabilitation programmes in lung disease is behaviour change leading to the adoption of a more active lifestyle, because the benefits of a short period of rehabilitation (such as those provided by most health services) will not be sustained unless this occurs. The impact of PR on daily physical activity behaviour varies considerably between individuals. Most patients will improve their exercise capacity but not all will use this additional capacity to increase the amount of physical activity undertaken in their daily lives. Others will continue their pre-rehabilitation activity level but benefit from reduced dyspnoea and fatigue during these activities.

Exercise prescription

As in health, in order to maximise the benefit of a training programme for patients with respiratory disease, it is important that exercise intensity and progression are prescribed appropriately. Below, we provide information about the prescription of both aerobic and resistance training in patients with respiratory disease, which should inform the planning of an exercise programme according to the FITT principles (Frequency, Intensity, Time, and Type of exercise). The frequency, time (duration), and type of exercise recommended for pulmonary rehabilitation are discussed in the next section of this chapter. Whilst it is important to consider the specific needs of the individual when prescribing exercise (for example which activities of daily living cause the most difficulty, and which type of exercise might best address these needs), many rehabilitation programmes provide a generic and broad range of exercise training. Some programmes tailor the mode of training to the physiological characteristics of the population (for example, the degree of muscle weakness or ventilatory limitation), but evidence at the population level that this approach improves outcomes is lacking. It is important, however, that the intensity and progression requires individual prescription based on a baseline measure of exercise capacity. A description of key exercise performance measures in PR can be found in the next section of this chapter. Throughout training, exercise intensity should be progressed as the patient adapts, for example by extending walking time or by increasing the resistance level. It is not imperative to formally reassess maximal exercise capacity in order to progress training. Patient-reported exertion and dyspnoea scores (Borg Scales – described below) provide a useful guide indicating when it is time to progress.

Aerobic training

Patients with COPD are advised to perform aerobic (or endurance) exercise three to five times per week. A minimum training intensity of 60 per cent of peak performance is recommended in the latest British Thoracic Society guidelines for the provision of pulmonary rehabilitation (Bolton et al., 2013). However, as discussed above, exercising at a higher intensity is likely to be of greater physiological benefit. In health, a common and effective way of monitoring exercise intensity is to measure heart rate. However, due to the influence of a ventilatory limit to exercise in many patients with respiratory disease and the influence of medication, heart rate is a poor means of monitoring exertion in this population. More reliable measures are task-related symptom scores such as the Borg Breathlessness Scale and Rating of Perceived Exertion (RPE) scale (Figure 3.2) (Borg, 1982; Kendrick et al., 2000). Breathlessness scores of 4 to 6 and RPE scores of 12 to 14 have been suggested as a suitable training intensity (Spruit et al., 2013).

The modified Borg scale breathlessness	
0	No breathlessness at all
0.5	Very, very slight (just noticeable)
1	Very slight
2	Slight breathlessness
3	Moderate
4	Somewhat severe
5	Severe breathlessness
6	
7	Very severe breathlessness
8	
9	Very, very severe (almost maximal)
10	Maximal

The Borg scale for ratings of received exertion	
6	
7	Very, very light
8	
9	Very light
10	
11	Fairly light
12	
13	Somewhat hard
14	
15	Hard
16	
17	Very hard
18	
19	Very, very hard
20	

Figure 3.2 Borg scales of breathlessness and perceived exertion. Reproduced from Borg (1982) and Kendrick et al. (2000) with permission from Elsevier.

Evidence suggests that sessions lasting between twenty minutes to an hour are of sufficient duration to elicit physiological changes. The primary mode of aerobic training is usually lower-limb walking or cycling. Walking is the most accessible form of exercise, as it requires no specific or expensive equipment, and has also been found to be the most meaningful activity to patients. The aim is to achieve thirty minutes of continuous exercise per session. For individuals who are not able to tolerate long duration of continuous aerobic training (for example, those with more severe disease and a ventilatory limit to exercise), interval training (short bouts of high intensity exercise interspersed with short periods of recovery), has been found to have similarly beneficial effects in terms of exercise capacity and health-related quality of life (HRQoL). The available evidence does not indicate superiority of either interval or continuous aerobic training in the broad population of patients with COPD referred for PR. Despite the relative preservation of upper-limb function, due to the involvement of the upper limbs in many activities of daily living, there may be benefits in incorporating upper-limb training as part of an exercise programme. This may be part of a resistance training programme, but aerobic training such as arm cycles can also be employed.

Resistance training

The American Thoracic Society (ATS)/European Respiratory Society (ERS) guidelines (Spruit et al. 2013) suggest that resistance training in a PR setting should follow the same principles as those defined for healthy individuals, taken from the American College of Sports Medicine (ACSM) model. To target improvements in muscle strength, the ACSM recommends one to three sets of eight to twelve repetitions, which should be undertaken on two to three days each week. Initial loads should be equivalent to 60–70 per cent of the one repetition maximum (1–RM). The 1–RM is the maximum load that can be moved with the proper technique for one repetition only over the full range of motion. Using RM training loads is appropriate for machine weights or free weights. However, other modes of resistance exercise are available, including elastic resistance bands and using body weight (callisthenics). The choice of equipment is dependent upon what is locally available and the risk assessment of the patient. RT is generally progressed by increasing the resistance/weight whilst keeping the number of sets and repetitions the same (i.e. low).

Alternatives and adjuncts to exercise training

Traditional aerobic and resistance exercises have proven benefits and should form the basis of most clinical exercise training programmes (see below). There is, however, recognition that not all patients are able to attend or complete a programme of training, and, therefore, alternative or additional training methodologies have been studied as therapeutic interventions in respiratory disease. This may be as an adjunct to conventional training, or possibly as an alternative for patients who due to a period of acute illness, comorbidities, or severe disease and deconditioning are unable to perform traditional exercise. An overview of some of the most commonly-reported alternatives and adjuncts to traditional exercise training can be found in Table 3.1.

Table 3.1 Alternatives and adjuncts to exercise training

Method	Basic principles	Possible effects and benefits	Strength of recommendation
Neuromuscular electrical stimulation (NMES)	A non-volitional method of activating the muscles where contraction is stimulated by a small electrical current delivered via electrodes placed on the skin.	May increase muscle mass, strength, and walking performance, particularly in patients with severe disability without inducing dyspnoea. Potentially applicable to settings where whole body exercise is impractical e.g. acute illness. Optimal stimulation intensity and duration yet to be established.	Promising evidence suggesting efficacy in improving muscle function in patients with low exercise tolerance.
Respiratory Muscle Training (RMT)	Techniques involve breathing through a device that applies variable resistance or threshold loading to inhalation or voluntary eucapnic hyperventilation.	Improves respiratory muscle strength and endurance and may reduce dyspnoea. Unclear whether the benefits of whole-body exercise training are augmented when IMT added.	Not currently recommended for inclusion in a general PR programmes. May have an application for selected individuals with respiratory muscle weakness.
Walking aids	A rollator or similar device to assist with ambulation stabilises the upper body and allows the adoption of a forward-leaning posture during walking, thus improving ventilatory mechanics.	Improves functional exercise performance and reduces exertional dyspnoea in selected patients. Most likely to benefit those with low exercise capacity and general frailty. For patients requiring ambulatory oxygen, provides a means of transporting the cylinder.	Appropriate for recommendation to patients with severely reduced functional exercise performance.
Vibration platform training	Patient stands/squats on a mechanical platform that vibrates at high frequency.	Preliminary evidence that whole-body vibration training improves 6-minute walk distance. Optimal prescription (frequency, amplitude, and direction of vibration) yet to be established.	Further evidence from additional larger-scale trials required before recommendations can be made regarding use in clinical practice.
Balance training	Specific exercise programme that aims to rectify the balance deficit and reduce falls risk in COPD patients.	Improves functional balance. May be of benefit in selected patients particularly those at risk of falls.	Not currently widely provided and evidence for routine use in clinical practice not yet available.

Nutrition

Attention to macro- and micro-nutrient intake during exercise training programmes has become routine in the fields of sports and athletics. In respiratory disease, body composition abnormalities are recognised as important clinical manifestations of the disease (both nutritional depletion and obesity). There has therefore been considerable study of nutritional interventions both to enhance exercise therapies and to improve nutritional status. A summary of the literature and recommendations for nutritional therapies can be found in the ERS statement on nutritional therapies in COPD (Schols et al., 2014). For patients with low fat-free mass, nutritional supplementation combined with exercise training can improve nutritional status in COPD. However, it is less clear that nutritional therapy is effective as an ergogenic aid to improve physical performance or the outcome of exercise training.

Practical provision of exercise rehabilitation in respiratory disease

Role of pulmonary rehabilitation

Pulmonary rehabilitation (PR) is the most frequent setting in which exercise therapy is provided to patients with respiratory disease. In COPD, PR is an established, evidence-based intervention, which is enshrined in UK and international disease management guidelines (NICE 2010; Vestbo et al., 2013). There is grade A evidence to support the benefits of PR in this population, and this group constitutes the most prevalent disease among those referred to PR (McCarthy et al., 2015). However, there is accumulating evidence in populations with other chronic respiratory diseases (for example interstitial lung disease, bronchiectasis, and chronic asthma). PR has been defined in the ATS and ERS statement as:

> An evidence-based, multidisciplinary, and comprehensive intervention for patients with chronic respiratory diseases who are symptomatic and often have decreased daily life activities. Integrated into the individualised treatment of the patient, pulmonary rehabilitation aims to reduce symptoms, optimise functional status, increase participation in society, and reduce health care costs through stabilising or reversing systemic manifestations of the disease.
>
> (Spruit et al., 2013)

PR is a multicomponent intervention in which an individual patient's needs are addressed, and whose objectives are largely achieved with a combination of supervised exercise sessions and an education programme delivered by a multi-professional team. The process of pulmonary rehabilitation is summarised in Figure 3.3. Recognition of the effectiveness of PR has resulted in the development and publication of UK and international statements providing guidance on the evidence-based provision of PR for healthcare organisations and practitioners to which the reader is directed for more information (Spruit et al., 2013; Bolton et al., 2013). In addition, the British Thoracic Society has published quality standards for the provision of pulmonary rehabilitation to assist commissioners, providers, and practitioners in delivering high quality

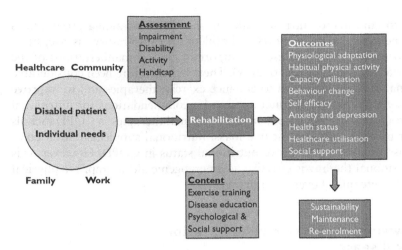

Figure 3.3 **The process of pulmonary rehabilitation.**

rehabilitation services and informing patients about the care they should expect to receive (British Thoracic Society, 2014).

PR is ideally provided as part of an integrated disease management pathway that addresses management of the disease in both the stable state and during acute crises. A schematic diagram of how PR is incorporated into the wider long-term management of COPD is provided in Figure 3.4. Support for self-management of the condition is a key component of the success of such integrated programmes. The intensity of support required will vary according to the complexity of the condition, the individual needs of the patient, and the security of the patient's social and family support.

In the remainder of this chapter we outline best practice in the provision and content of pulmonary rehabilitation. The clear effectiveness of PR in the management of COPD is enshrined in national and international guidelines and quality standards, which provide evidence-based recommendations for its provision. For more detailed information, the reader is directed to these resources.

Referral to pulmonary rehabilitation

Current guidelines recommend that PR is offered to stable patients with COPD who are functionally limited by breathlessness (Medical Research Council grades 3–5) (Fletcher et al., 1959). The requirement for PR should be reviewed regularly, ideally annually. In addition, it is recommended that patients who have been hospitalised with an exacerbation of COPD, are offered PR to assist with recovery and restoration of pre-admission fitness and activity. There is evidence that this is effective if PR is commenced within one month of discharge (Puhan et al., 2011). The safety and efficacy of exercise training during the hospitalisation episode itself remains uncertain (Greening et al., 2014). Early rehabilitation following hospitalisation is safe, delivers significant improvements in exercise capacity and quality of life, and may reduce the short-term risk of re-admission to hospital. However, it is also clear that, despite

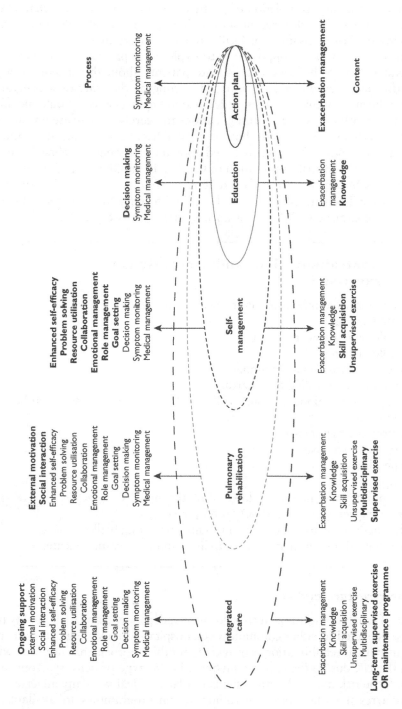

Figure 3.4 A tiered approach to the integrated management of patients with COPD. Reproduced from Wagg (2012) with permission from Sage Publications Ltd.

these benefits, uptake and completion of post-exacerbation pulmonary rehabilitation (PEPR) remains poor. The ideal setting and timing of exercise rehabilitation to assist recovery following hospitalisation for COPD remains uncertain.

The point of referral is the opportunity to explore the patient's understanding of PR, address concerns or barriers, and educate patients about the benefits of a programme. Informed decision making and goal setting at the start of a programme improves uptake and completion rates. A detailed initial assessment should include an evaluation of comorbidities and contraindications to exercise. There are few absolute contraindications to exercise therapy, but a suggested list of contraindications and precautions is shown in Box 3.2. These are based upon international guideline documents (Holland, et al., 2014; British Association of Cardiac Rehabilitation, 2006; American College of Sports Medicine, 2009). If exercise is contraindicated, the educational element of PR can still be offered. It may be beneficial to refer for treatment of comorbidities prior to commencing PR, for instance to manage anxiety and depression.

Box 3.2 Contraindications and precautions to exercise in PR

- Acute myocardial infarction (in the last five days)
- Unstable angina
- Unstable or acute heart failure
- Unstable diabetes
- New or uncontrolled arrhythmias
- Resting or uncontrolled tachycardia
- Resting systolic blood pressure (BP) >200mmHg or resting diastolic BP >120mmHg
- Symptomatic hypotension
- Severe aortic stenosis
- Febrile illness
- Syncope
- Acute pulmonary embolus or lower-limb thrombosis
- Resting oxygen saturation (SpO_2) ≤ 85 per cent
- Orthopaedic or neurological impairments preventing walking
- Psychological impairments leading to an inability to communicate.

Programme structure and venue

The benefits of rehabilitation appear to be location independent, and high-quality treatment can be delivered in either community- or hospital-based settings. In some parts of Europe, in-patient rehabilitation is provided, but this approach has not been widely adopted in the UK due to the expense involved in this type of delivery. Appropriate venues should be risk-assessed with systems in place to deal with any adverse events (e.g. cardiac arrests). Cohort-based or rolling-format programmes are available, and there is no evidence to support one approach above the other. The choice will depend on local needs, and there are pros and cons to both approaches. For instance, a cohort programme might be easier to manage for teams who are working in the community and need to provide PR groups in several localities. This approach, however, is not flexible in terms of allowing for people who have an exacerbation and need to 'catch up' on missed sessions.

Exercise training can be effective with limited equipment in improving exercise capacity and health-related quality of life in people with COPD. Basic equipment could include a chair for each patient, space for walking, a stopwatch, hand weights, and Borg scales. In addition, the provision of oxygen and pulse oximetry would be a requirement to control for exercise-induced de-saturation (defined as a fall in SpO_2 of 4 per cent to a value < 90 per cent), or to accommodate for those on long-term oxygen therapy (LTOT). Additional gym-based equipment may be utilised if available (e.g. leg/arm bike, treadmill, resistance machines).

In the UK, PR usually extends over six to eight weeks; a minimum of two supervised sessions per week is recommended in addition to home training. This is in line with advice for the general population, who should accumulate 150 minutes of moderate intensity activity per week (e.g. thirty minutes on five days of the week). A minimum of twelve supervised PR sessions is suggested. Although a supervised programme is recommended, a structured home-based programme may be considered for selected patients where access to a conventional programme cannot be achieved (e.g. due to transport difficulties). In this instance, remote support mechanisms (e.g. web-based solutions) and access to home equipment are factors to consider.

Components of pulmonary rehabilitation

There is a large body of evidence which demonstrates that aerobic (interval or continuous training) and resistance exercise result in clinically meaningful improvements in endurance and strength. As stated earlier in this chapter, exercise training should be individually tailored and progressed using the FITT principle. The educational component of PR is also key, with the aim being to support and promote lifestyle and behavioural change, which is required to sustain the benefits of PR and to assist the patient's wider understanding and self-management of the condition. Examples of topics frequently covered are: pulmonary anatomy and physiology, medication including oxygen, smoking cessation, managing breathlessness and chest-clearance techniques. The educational needs of the patient may be established prior to enrolment using various questionnaires (e.g. the Bristol COPD Knowledge Questionnaire, see White et al., 2006). This allows for the individual tailoring of the education and may also be used to assess the effectiveness of the education programme. The breadth of content and professional mix of educators remains uncertain and variable across PR programmes. As the diversity of the patient population referred to PR broadens, it is likely that education programmes will become more individualised and supported by written and online material.

Outcome assessments

Due to the multi-component nature of PR, numerous measures are used to capture its diverse benefits (Figure 3.3). Conventional outcome measures include those reflecting a change in exercise capacity, health related quality of life (HRQoL) (e.g. Chronic Respiratory Disease Questionnaire), symptoms (e.g. MRC dyspnoea grade, for which see Fletcher et al., 1959), and levels of anxiety and depression (e.g. Hospital Anxiety and Depression Scale) which can be measured at baseline and at the end of the programme. In recent years, physical activity measures (questionnaires or pedometers/accelerometers) have also gained considerable interest as reduced physical activity has been linked with reduced survival, poorer quality of life, and increased healthcare utilisation. Nutritional status (e.g. fat-free mass) and frailty measures (e.g. Short Physical Performance Battery) are also becoming increasingly popular in the COPD population due to their prognostic influence.

It is not the intention of this chapter to cover all of these outcomes in detail. As this textbook is focused on exercise, aerobic exercise, and strength-testing outcomes in PR are described in more detail below.

Aerobic exercise testing

Measuring exercise tolerance is important for assessing capacity, prescribing exercise, and evaluating responses to treatment. Laboratory-based tests are the gold standard measure of cardio-respiratory fitness. Cycle ergometry or treadmill tests are the most commonly employed. These tests are usually incremental in nature, meaning that a low work load is set at the start, and is gradually increased at regular intervals throughout the test. This is continued until the individual is no longer able to maintain the speed. These tests can also allow the individual to be monitored more closely for vital signs and observations of exercise limitation, such as ventilatory, cardiac, or leg fatigue. Laboratory exercise tests can be used to characterise the detailed physiological response to exercise, but (at least in the UK) they are rarely used in clinical rehabilitation programmes because of lack of access, expense, and technical support requirements. Field-based tests of exercise capacity that permit a measurement of capacity and facilitate exercise prescription have been developed as an alternative. These tests are largely based upon walking, which is a common and acceptable form of exercise for patients with CRD. Information about the choice and conduct of field exercise tests is provided in the ATS/ERS standard on field testing in chronic respiratory disease (Holland et al., 2014).

The most frequently employed field tests in patients with CRD are the self-paced six-minute walk test (6MWT), the externally-paced incremental shuttle walk test (ISWT), and the endurance shuttle walk test (ESWT). These field walking tests are able to test maximal performance, which is comparable to laboratory-based tests. However the pattern of response differs between self-paced and externally-paced tests. The 6MWT is a self-paced walking test over a 30m course. Patients are asked to walk as far as possible in six minutes, and the distance in metres is recorded. Patients are permitted to rest if required. Exercise intensity can be prescribed from the 6MWT, but is not particularly accurate because the speed of walking is variable during the 6MWT. Typically, 80 per cent of maximum is chosen as the training intensity. For instance, if a patient walked 300m, then: $300 \times 10 \div 1000 = 3.0$ km/hour (hr) and 80 per cent of 3.0 km/hr = 2.4 km/hr.

The ISWT is an externally-paced maximal test in which the speed of the test is controlled by a series of pre-recorded bleeps (Singh et al., 1992). Patients are required to walk around the 10m course; the speed increases every minute and continues until the patient can walk no further. The distance to the nearest 10m is recorded. The ESWT speed is calculated from the maximal ISWT and represents 85 per cent of peak performance (see Figure 3.5, and Revill et al., 1999). Time is recorded in seconds and patients are asked to walk for as long as possible up to a twenty-minute limit.

The minimum clinical important difference (MCID) is a statistically-derived measure that attempts to identify the smallest change in an outcome that a patient would identify as important or meaningful. The MCID for walking test outcomes following PR have been calculated using several methods. The MCID for the 6MWT lies between 25 and 33m, and the MCID for the ISWT is 48m (Singh et al., 2008). For the ESWT, an MCID has been derived for bronchodilator response (65 seconds) and estimated for change after rehabilitation (180 seconds) (Pepin et al., 2011). However, it is important to remember that the MCID is only applicable to the specific measure and relates to the population as a whole rather than an individual's threshold of change.

The 6MWT, ISWT, and ESWT are valid, reliable, and responsive to change (Holland et al., 2014). Due to a learning effect, it is important that two tests are conducted for the 6MWT and ISWT, and a rest period of at least thirty minutes is required between tests. A practice walk is not required for the ESWT. Heart rate, oxygen saturation, and Borg scales should be monitored during the test. If exercise-induced de-saturation (as defined earlier) is identified during exercise testing, this can be used to prompt an assessment for ambulatory home oxygen.

Muscle strength testing

The aims of measuring muscle function in patients with COPD are: to identify and quantify impairment, to prescribe an appropriate exercise programme, and to evaluate the response to treatment (such as resistance training). Strength can be measured using non-volitional or volitional techniques. Non-volitional testing using nerve stimulation is not effort-dependent but is intrusive for patients, and is therefore generally reserved for research use rather than clinical practice. Volitional techniques require maximum effort by the subject and can be affected by operator encouragement. Volitional strength

1   Predicted $VO_{2\,peak}$ (ml/min/kg) = 4.19
    + (0.025 × ISWT) distance
2   Endurance capacity at 85%
3   Identify speed to test endurance capacity

Example:

1   ISWT distance = 200m, predicted
    $VO_{2\,peak}$ = 9.2ml/min/kg
2   85% = 7.8ml/min/kg
3   Endurance walking speed = 3.3km/hr
4   ESWT level 7 (round up to 3.6km/hr)

Revill et al. (1999) *Thorax,* 54: 213–222

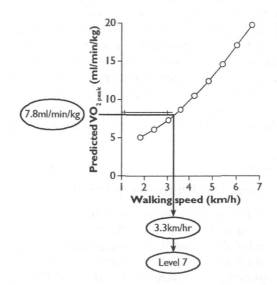

Figure 3.5 The calculation of ESWT speed derived from a maximal ISWT. Reproduced from Revill et al. (1999).

can be assessed using static (isometric) or dynamic (isotonic/isokinetic) contractions, and measured manually using resistance machines, with portable devices (e.g. handheld dynamometers [HHD]), cable tensiometers), and using computerised dynamometers.

The 1–RM measurement of strength can be used to measure isotonic strength, and is a safe and reliable measure of strength in patients with COPD. 1–RM testing is practical and may better reflect functional movements compared to other testing methods. To achieve the maximum, weight should be incrementally increased by 1–5kg at intervals of 1–5 minutes.

Maintenance of the benefits of pulmonary rehabilitation

As with most other interventions, not all eligible patients accept referral to PR or complete the programme. Post-exacerbation PR is particularly affected by poor uptake and high attrition because patients often feel vulnerable in terms of their health and ability to exercise at the time of referral, but also because exacerbations may be repeated and cyclical (Hurst et al., 2009). Lack of access to transport and lack of perceived benefit have been shown to most affect the uptake to PR. In addition, current smokers and patients who are depressed are at increased risk of non-completion.

The benefits of PR, for those who do complete, decline over time but remain higher than baseline at one year. The decline in aerobic exercise capacity and HRQoL may follow a different time-course. Patients may require further courses of rehabilitation, particularly after a disease exacerbation, and benefits following repeated programmes appear similar to those achieved after the first attendance. The British Thoracic Society guidelines and quality standards recommend that repeat programmes should be considered at one year if significant exercise limitation persists (Bolton et al. 2013; British Thoracic Society, 2014). The continuation of physical activity beyond the supervised component of PR is also recommended, as there is evidence to suggest that maintenance programmes offer advantages in preserving the benefits of PR. Community-based interventions following PR may be effective in maintaining the benefits of PR. These may include exercise on referral schemes, 'BLF Active', local clubs, etc. A written action plan for the continuation of exercise beyond PR, which is co-written by the patient and the health care professional, is recommended as best practice (British Thoracic Society, 2014). However, uncertainty remains about the best strategy to maintain the benefits of PR (repeated courses vs. ongoing supervised exercise). In many European centres, a significantly longer course of initial PR is offered (e.g. six months), but evidence that this confers greater benefit and preservation of performance is lacking.

Box 3.3 Pulmonary rehabilitation case study

David is a seventy five year-old outpatient who attends a secondary care clinic with symptoms of COPD and bronchiectasis. He was referred to pulmonary rehabilitation (PR) by his respiratory consultant as he was struggling with symptoms of breathlessness during daily life. His inhaled medication had been optimised prior to referral. He attended PR hoping that the benefits would prevent deterioration in the active lifestyle that he had.

David attended two supervised sessions per week, each with one hour of exercise and one hour of education. His exercise involved cycling and walking on a treadmill and overground, which was supervised by PR healthcare professionals who encouraged David to set targets to progress his exercises – a challenge that he found encouraging. In addition to the supervised sessions, David exercised at home and completed a home exercise diary.

The educational component of the course helped David to understand more about his condition: 'I've learnt about new breathing techniques, inhaler techniques and how to manage my exacerbations. I also keep myself active, putting into practice the skills I learnt during pulmonary rehabilitation'.

Following PR David's exercise capacity improved by 120 metres on the Incremental Shuttle Walking Test (ISWT) and his walking endurance increased by more than ten minutes on the Endurance Shuttle Walk Test (ESWT). David's health status also improved, particularly in the area of mastery (a person's feeling of control over their symptoms).

'When I first started I wasn't able to walk more than three minutes on the treadmill, but now I do up to forty five minutes.'

Throughout David's course of PR he was encouraged and helped to make formal plans for ongoing exercise and, at completion of the programme, he was also offered a referral to an Active Lifestyle Scheme.

After completing his course of PR, David returned as a volunteer and now mentors others on the course.

Summary

Physical activity limitation is one of the hallmarks of chronic respiratory disease, with significant consequences for patients, their families, and wider society. In diseases where the underlying pulmonary pathology is frequently irreversible, exercise therapies such as pulmonary rehabilitation offer major benefits to this patient population, both in terms of symptom reduction and preservation of longer-term health. The evidence base for the provision of pulmonary rehabilitation is incontestable, and whilst the intervention now has a central place in the management of these conditions, service provision in the UK remains suboptimal. This is despite robust evidence that pulmonary rehabilitation is one of the highest value therapies available for these diseases.

Future research

There is grade A evidence that exercise therapy in the context of pulmonary rehabilitation (PR) is effective for patients with respiratory disease. Therefore, future work should concentrate on refinement, enhancement, and delivery of the programme as outlined below.

- Refinement: The current format of PR is largely a 'one size fits all' approach and has therefore been successfully implemented in other chronic conditions (such as heart failure). However, it is uncertain whether personalising the intervention by tailoring training to individual physiological or functional deficits (e.g. training of smaller muscle groups, or involuntary training techniques for patients with a predominant ventiliatory limitation) would enhance efficacy. It may be that, in the future, we can identify different phenotypes who respond differently to the various components of PR, and we can stratify care accordingly. The optimal format of pulmonary rehabilitation could be explored further to identify the most important components of pulmonary rehabilitation, the ideal length of a programme, and the intensity of training required.

- Enhancement: Although a number of pharmacological and nutritional adjuncts to PR have been shown to have potential efficacy in improving the outcome of exercise training, most have not become part of routine practice. Larger-scale trials of effectiveness in large, well-characterised populations are needed to understand whether these improved, important health outcomes are needed, for instance neuromuscular electrical stimulation to preserve muscle function when patients are hospitalised with an exacerbation of COPD.

- Delivery: A key health service aim is to improve access to exercise therapies to ensure that all people who might benefit from a rehabilitation programme receive it. An understanding of the role of more diverse programme formats is required, for example, home-based treatment supported by written or online material self-management packages. The challenge is to ensure that sufficient choice is offered without sacrificing the efficacy of the intervention. This may require an understanding of individual patient capability to undertake progressive exercise without supervision. Further research to maximise sustainable behaviour change following a programme is required, with specific reference to the optimal frequency and mode of delivery for maintenance exercise models and repeated programmes.

Study tasks

1   Belinda is a sixty two-year-old woman who has recently been diagnosed with COPD after experiencing recurrent chest infections during the winter months. She experiences dyspnoea on exertion and finds that she now has to stop for breath when she is walking her dogs, particularly when climbing a slight hill. Belinda has never heard of pulmonary rehabilitation and is unsure about accepting a referral. Explain what benefits she might experience by participating in a rehabilitation programme.

2   Patrick attends his first assessment for pulmonary rehabilitation and performs an incremental shuttle walking test. At rest his blood oxygen saturation (SpO_2) is 96 per cent. After walking 240m his SpO_2 has dropped to 87 per cent and the assessor terminates the test. Suggest what impact this might have on Patrick's attendance at pulmonary rehabilitation, and what course of action you might recommend be taken before Patrick starts attending classes.

3   Using the literature from the 'Further reading' section of this chapter as a starting point, draft an outline exercise programme for

  a   An overweight patient with normal muscle mass and strength
  b   An underweight patient with reduced muscle mass and function (sarcopenia).

Both patients are attending pulmonary rehabilitation.

4 Thomas has been referred to your pulmonary rehabilitation programme following an exacerbation of his COPD which caused him to be hospitalised for four
days. He is seventy six years old, has severe airflow obstruction, low body mass
(BMI 19.0 kg/m²), and weak muscles (unable to rise from a chair without using
his arms for assistance). He is only able to walk 10m unaided, but is motivated to
improve his physical function so that he can be more independent. Consider what
exercises and adjuncts to rehabilitation might be appropriate for Thomas as he
starts a rehabilitation programme, and which tests of exercise capacity might be
appropriate when he attends his first assessment.

Further reading

British Thoracic Society (BTS) guidance and quality standards on Pulmonary Rehabilitation provision:

Bolton, C. E., Bevan-Smith, E. F., Blakey, J. D., Crowe, P., Elkin, S. L., Garrod, R., Greening, N. J.,
Heslop, K., Hull, J. H., Man, W. D., Morgan, M. D., Proud, D., Roberts, C. M., Sewell, L.,
Singh, S. J., Walker, P. P. and Walmsley, S. (2013). British Thoracic Society guideline on pulmonary rehabilitation in adults. *Thorax*, 68(suppl. 2), ii1–30: https://www.brit-thoracic.org.
uk/guidelines-and-quality-standards/pulmonary-rehabilitation-quality-standards/

Review of the complex interaction between ventilatory limitation and exercise intolerance in COPD:

O'Donnell, D. E. (2001). Ventilatory limitations in chronic obstructive pulmonary disease.
Medicine and Science in Sports and Exercise, 33, S647–55.

Detailed information about detection, assessment, and therapy for skeletal muscle dysfunction in COPD:

Maltais, F., Decramer, M., Casaburi, R., Barreiro, E., Burelle, Y., Debigaré, R., Dekhuijzen,
P. N., Franssen, F., Gayan-Ramirez, G., Gea, J., Gosker, H. R., Gosselink, R., Hayot, M.,
Hussain, S. N., Janssens, W., Polkey, M. I., Roca, J., Saey, D., Schols, A. M., Spruit, M. A.,
Steiner, M., Taivassalo, T., Troosters, T., Vogiatzis, I. and Wagner, P. D. (2014). An official
American Thoracic Society/European Respiratory Society statement: update on limb muscle
dysfunction in chronic obstructive pulmonary disease. *American Journal of Respiratory and
Critical Care Medicine*, 189, e15–62.

Comprehensive overview and technical standard for performing field walking tests:

Holland, A. E., Spruit, M. A., Troosters, T., Puhan, M. A., Pepin, V., Saey, D., McCormack,
M. C., Carlin, B. W., Sciurba, F. C., Pitta, F., Wanger, J., MacIntyre, N., Kaminsky, D. A.,
Culver, B. H., Revill, S. M., Hernandes, N. A., Andrianopoulos, V., Camillo, C. A., Mitchell,
K. E., Lee, A. L., Hill, C. J. and Singh, S. J. (2014). An official European Respiratory Society/
American Thoracic Society technical standard: field walking tests in chronic respiratory dis-
ease. *European Respiratory Journal*, 44, 1428–46.

Cochrane reviews on pulmonary rehabilitation, self-management, and nutritional support in COPD:

McCarthy, B., Casey, D., Devane, D., Murphy, K., Murphy, E. and Lacasse, Y. (2015).
Pulmonary rehabilitation for chronic obstructive pulmonary disease. *Cochrane Database of
Systematic Reviews*, 2, CD003793.

Puhan, M.A., Gimeno-Santos, E., Scharplatz, M., Troosters, T., Walters, E.H. and Steurer, J. (2011). Pulmonary rehabilitation following exacerbations of chronic obstructive pulmonary disease. *Cochrane Database of Systematic Reviews*, 10, CD005305.

Zwerink, M., van der Palen, J., van der Valk, P., Brusse-Keizer, M. and Effing, T. (2014). Self-management for patients with chronic obstructive pulmonary disease. *Cochrane Database of Systematic Reviews*, 3, CD002990.

Meta-analysis reviewing changes in physical activity following pulmonary rehabilitation:

Cindy Ng, L. W., Mackney, J., Jenkins, S. and Hill, K. (2012). Does exercise training change physical activity in people with COPD? A systematic review and meta-analysis. *Chronic Respiratory Disease*, 9, 17–26.

Practical advice on how to adapt a pulmonary rehabilitation for conditions other than COPD:

Holland, A. E., Wadell, K. and Spruit, M. A. (2013). How to adapt the pulmonary rehabilitation programme to patients with chronic respiratory disease other than COPD. *European Respiratory Review*, 22, 577.

References

American College of Sports Medicine (2009). *Guidelines for Exercise Testing and Prescription.* 8th ed. Baltimore, Maryland: Lippincott Williams and Wilkins.

Bolton, C. E., Bevan-Smith, E. F., Blakey, J. D., Crowe, P., Elkin, S. L., Garrod, R., Greening, N. J., Heslop, K., Hull, J. H., Man, W. D., Morgan, M. D., Proud, D., Roberts, C. M., Sewell, L., Singh, S. J., Walker, P. P. and Walmsley, S. (2013). British Thoracic Society guideline on pulmonary rehabilitation in adults. *Thorax*, 68(suppl. 2), ii1–30.

Borg, G. A. (1982). Psychophysical bases of perceived exertion. *Med. Sci. Sport. Exerc.*, 14, 377–81.

British Association of Cardiac Rehabilitation (2006). *Phase IV exercise instructor training manual.* Farnham, BACPR.

British Thoracic Society. Quality standards for pulmonary rehabilitation in adults. (2014): https://www.brit-thoracic.org.uk/document-library/clinical-information/pulmonary-rehabilitation/bts-quality-standards-for-pulmonary-rehabilitation-in-adults/

Casaburi, R., Kukafka, D., Cooper, C. B., Witek Jr., T. J. and Kesten, S. (2005). Improvement in exercise tolerance with the combination of tiotropium and pulmonary rehabilitation in patients with COPD. *Chest*, 127, 809–17.

Casaburi, R., Patessio, A., Ioli, F., Zanaboni, S., Donner, C.F. and Wasserman, K. (1991). Reductions in exercise lactic acidosis and ventilation as a result of exercise training in patients with obstructive lung disease. *Am. Rev. Respir. Dis.*, 143, 9–18.

Casaburi, R. and Petty, T. L. (1993). *Principles and practice of pulmonary rehabilitation.* Philadelphia: W. B. Saunders.

Calvert, L. D., Shelley, R., Singh, S. J., Greenhaff, P. L., Bankart, J., Morgan, M. D. and Steiner, M. C. (2008). Dichloroacetate enhances performance and reduces blood lactate during maximal cycle exercise in chronic obstructive pulmonary disease. *Am. J. Respir. Crit. Care Med.*, 177, 1090–94.

Cooper, C. B. (2009). Airflow obstruction and exercise. *Respir. Med.*, 103, 325–34.

Deschenes, D., Pepin, V., Saey, D., LeBlanc, P. and Maltais, F. (2008). Locus of symptom limitation and exercise response to bronchodilation in chronic obstructive pulmonary disease. *J. Cardiopulm. Rehabil. Prev.*, 28, 208–14.

Fishman, A., Martinez, F., Naunheim, K., Piantadosi, S., Wise, R., Ries, A., Weinmann, G. and Wood, D. E. (2003). A randomized trial comparing lung-volume-reduction surgery with medical therapy for severe emphysema. *N. Engl. J. Med.*, 348, 2059–73.

Fletcher, C. M., Elmes, P. C., Fairburn, M. B. and Wood, C. H. (1959). The significance of respiratory symptoms and the diagnosis of chronic bronchitis in a working population. *BMJ*, 5147, 257–66.

Gosker, H. R., Zeegers, M. P., Wouters, E. F. and Schols, A. M. (2007). Muscle fibre type shifting in the vastus lateralis of patients with COPD is associated with disease severity: a systematic review and meta-analysis. *Thorax*, 62, 944–49.

Greening, N. J., Williams, J. E., Hussain, S. F., Harvey-Dunstan, T. C., Bankart, M. J., Chaplin, E. J., Vincent, E. E., Chimera, R., Morgan, M. D., Singh, S. J. and Steiner, M. C. (2014). An early rehabilitation intervention to enhance recovery during hospital admission for an exacerbation of chronic respiratory disease: randomised controlled trial. *BMJ*, 349, g4315.

Hardinge, M., Annandale, J., Bourne, S., Cooper, B., Evans, A., Freeman, D., Green, A., Hippolyte, S., Knowles, V., MacNee, W., McDonnell, L., Pye, K., Suntharalingam, J., Vora, V. and Wilkinson, T. (2015). BTS guidelines for home oxygen use in adults. *Thorax*, 70(Suppl 1), i1–43.

Holland, A. E., Spruit, M. A., Troosters, T., Puhan, M. A., Pepin, V., Saey, D., McCormack, M. C., Carlin, B. W., Sciurba, F. C., Pitta, F., Wanger, J., MacIntyre, N., Kaminsky, D. A., Culver, B. H., Revill, S. M., Hernandes, N. A., Andrianopoulos, V., Camillo, C. A., Mitchell, K. E., Lee, A. L., Hill, C. J. and Singh, S. J. (2014). An official European Respiratory Society/ American Thoracic Society technical standard: field walking tests in chronic respiratory disease. *Eur. Respir. J.*, 44, 1428–46.

Hurst, J. R., Donaldson, G. C., Quint, J. K., Goldring, J. J., Baghai-Ravary, R. and Wedzicha, J. A. (2009). Temporal clustering of exacerbations in chronic obstructive pulmonary disease. *Am. J. Respir. Crit. Care Med.*, 179, 369–74.

The International Society for Heart and Lung Transplantation (ISHLT): www.ishlt.org/regis tries/heartLungRegistry.asp

Kendrick, K. R., Baxi, S. C. and Smith, R. M. (2000). Usefulness of the modified 0–10 Borg scale in assessing the degree of dyspnea in patients with COPD and asthma. *J. Emerg. Nurs.*, 26, 216–22.

Killian, K. J., Summers, E., Jones, N. L. and Campbell, E. J. (1992). Dyspnea and leg effort during incremental cycle ergometry. *Am. Rev. Respir. Dis.*, 145, 1339–45.

Leidy, N. K. (1994). Using functional status to assess treatment outcomes. *Chest*, 106, 1645–6.

Levy, R. D., Ernst, P., Levine, S. M., Shennib, H., Anzueto, A., Bryan, C. L., Calhoon, J. H., Trinkle, J. K., Jenkinson, S. G. and Gibbons, W. J. (1993). Exercise performance after lung transplantation. *J. Hear. Lung Transplant*, 12, 23–33.

Maltais, F. (2000). Oxidative enzyme activities of the vastus lateralis muscle and the functional status in patients with COPD. *Thorax*, 55, 848–53.

Maltais, F., Decramer, M., Casaburi, R., Barreiro, E., Burelle, Y., Debigaré, R., Dekhuijzen, P. N., Franssen, F., Gayan-Ramirez, G., Gea, J., Gosker, H. R., Gosselink, R., Hayot, M., Hussain, S. N., Janssens, W., Polkey, M. I., Roca, J., Saey, D., Schols, A. M., Spruit, M. A., Steiner, M., Taivassalo, T., Troosters, T., Vogiatzis, I. and Wagner, P. D. (2014). An official American Thoracic Society/European Respiratory Society statement: update on limb muscle dysfunction in chronic obstructive pulmonary disease. *Am. J. Respir. Crit. Care. Med.*, 189, e15–62.

Maltais, F., Jobin, J., Sullivan, M. J., Bernard, S., Whittom, F., Killian, K. J., Desmeules, M., Bélanger, M. and LeBlanc, P. (1998). Metabolic and hemodynamic responses of lower limb during exercise in patients with COPD. *J. Appl. Physiol.*, 84, 1573–80.

Maltais, F., LeBlanc, P., Simard, C., Jobin, J., Bérubé, C., Bruneau, J., Carrier, L. and Belleau, R. (1996). Skeletal muscle adaptation to endurance training in patients with chronic obstructive pulmonary disease. *Am. J. Respir. Crit. Care Med.*, 154, 442–7.

Man, W. D., Soliman, M. G., Gearing, J., Radford, S. G., Rafferty, G. F., Gray, B. J., Polkey, M. I., Moxham, J. (2003). Symptoms and quadriceps fatigability after walking and cycling in chronic obstructive pulmonary disease. *Am. J. Respir. Crit. Care Med.*, 168, 562–7.

Marquis, K., Debigaré, R., Lacasse, Y., LeBlanc, P., Jobin, J., Carrier, G. and Maltais, F. (2002). Midthigh muscle cross-sectional area is a better predictor of mortality than body mass index in patients with chronic obstructive pulmonary disease. *Am. J. Respir. Crit. Care Med.*, 166, 809–13.

McCarthy, B., Casey, D., Devane, D., Murphy, K., Murphy, E. and Lacasse, Y. (2015). Pulmonary rehabilitation for chronic obstructive pulmonary disease. *Cochrane Database Syst. Rev.*, 2, CD003793.

National Institute for Health and Care Excellence (NICE) (2010). Management of chronic obstructive pulmonary disease in adults in primary and secondary care (partial update): www.nice.org.uk/guidance/cg101/resources/guidance-chronic-obstructive-pulmonary-disease-pdf

O'Donnell, D. E. (2006). Hyperinflation, dyspnea, and exercise intolerance in chronic obstructive pulmonary disease. *Proc. Am. Thorac. Soc.*, 3, 180–4.

O'Shea, S. D., Taylor, N. F. and Paratz, J. (2004). Peripheral muscle strength training in COPD: a systematic review. *Chest*, 126, 903–14.

Pepin, V., Laviolette, L., Brouillard, C., Sewell, L., Singh, S. J., Revill, S. M., Lacasse, Y. and Maltais, F. (2011). Significance of changes in endurance shuttle walking performance. *Thorax*, 66, 115–20.

Puhan, M. A., Gimeno-Santos, E., Scharplatz, M., Troosters, T., Walters, E. H., Steurer, J. (2011). Pulmonary rehabilitation following exacerbations of chronic obstructive pulmonary disease. *Cochrane Database Syst. Rev.*, CD005305 doi:10.1002/14651858.CD005305.pub3.

Revill, S. M., Morgan, M. D. L., Singh, S. J., Williams, J. and Hardman, A. E. (1999). The endurance shuttle walk: a new field test for the assessment of endurance capacity in chronic obstructive pulmonary disease. *Thorax*, 54, 213–22.

Schols, A. M., Broekhuizen, R., Weling-Scheepers, C. A. and Wouters, E. F. (2005). Body composition and mortality in chronic obstructive pulmonary disease. *Am. J. Clin. Nutr.*, 82, 53–9.

Schols, A. M., Ferreira, I. M., Franssen, F. M., Gosker, H. R., Janssens, W., Muscaritoli, M., Pison, C., Rutten-van Mölken, M., Slinde, F., Steiner, M. C., Tkacova, R. and Singh, S. J. (2014). Nutritional assessment and therapy in COPD: a European Respiratory Society statement. *Eur. Respir J.*, 44(6), 1504–20.

Shah, P. L. and Herth, F. J. F. (2014). Current status of bronchoscopic lung volume reduction with endobronchial valves. *Thorax*, 69, 280–6.

Shah, P. L. and Hopkinson, N. S. (2012). Bronchoscopic lung volume reduction for emphysema: where next? *Eur. Respir. J.*, 39, 1287–9.

Singh, S. J., Jones, P. W., Evans, R. and Morgan, M. D. (2008). Minimum clinically important improvement for the incremental shuttle walking test. *Thorax*, 63, 775–7.

Singh, S. J., Morgan, M. D., Scott, S., Walters, D. and Hardman, A. E. (1992). Development of a shuttle walking test of disability in patients with chronic airways obstruction. *Thorax*, 47, 1019–24.

Spruit, M. A. Singh, S. J., Garvey, C., ZuWallack, R., Nici, L., Rochester, C., Hill, K., Holland, A. E., Lareau, S. C., Man, W. D., Pitta, F., Sewell, L., Raskin, J., Bourbeau, J., Crouch, R., Franssen, F. M., Casaburi, R., Vercoulen, J. H., Vogiatzis, I., Gosselink, R., Clini, E. M., Effing, T. W., Maltais, F., van der Palen, J., Troosters, T., Janssen, D. J., Collins, E., Garcia-Aymerich, J., Brooks, D., Fahy, B. F., Puhan, M. A., Hoogendoorn, M., Garrod, R., Schols, A. M., Carlin, B., Benzo, R., Meek, P., Morgan, M., Rutten-van Mölken, M. P., Ries, A. L., Make, B., Goldstein, R. S., Dowson, C. A., Brozek, J. L., Donner, C. F. and Wouters, E. F. (2013). An official American Thoracic Society/European Respiratory Society statement: key concepts and advances in pulmonary rehabilitation. *Am. J. Respir. Crit. Care Med.*, 188, e13–64.

Steiner, M. C., Patel, P., Singh, S. J., Greenhaff, P. L. and Morgan, M. D. (2003). Exercise induced metabolic stress in the skeletal muscles of COPD patients. *Eur. Respir. J.*, 22, 204s.

Swallow, E. B., Gosker, H. R., Ward, K. A., Moore, A. J., Dayer, M. J., Hopkinson, N. S., Schols, A. M., Moxham, J. and Polkey, M. I. (2007). A novel technique for nonvolitional assessment of quadriceps muscle endurance in humans. *J. Appl. Physiol.*, 103, 739–46.

Thomas, M., Decramer, M. and O'Donnell, D. E. (2013). No room to breathe: the importance of lung hyperinflation in COPD. *Pri. Care Respir J.*, 22, 101–11.

Vestbo, J., Hurd, S. S., Agustí, A. G., Jones, P. W., Vogelmeier, C., Anzueto, A., Barnes, P. J., Fabbri, L. M., Martinez, F. J., Nishimura, M., Stockley, R. A., Sin, D. D. and Rodriguez-Roisin, R. (2013). Global strategy for the diagnosis, management, and prevention of chronic obstructive pulmonary disease: GOLD executive summary. *Am. J Respir. Crit Care Med.*, 187, 347–65.

Vestbo, J., Prescott, E., Almdal, T., Dahl, M., Nordestgaard, B. G., Andersen, T., Sørensen, T. I. and Lange, P. (2006). Body mass, fat-free body mass, and prognosis in patients with chronic obstructive pulmonary disease from a random population sample: findings from the Copenhagen City Heart Study. *Am. J Respir. Crit Care Med.*, 173, 79–83.

Wagg, K. (2012). Unravelling self-management for COPD: what next? *Chron. Respir. Dis.*, 9, 5–7.

White, R., Walker, P., Roberts, S., Kalisky, S. and White, P. (2006). Bristol COPD Knowledge Questionnaire (BCKQ): testing what we teach patients about COPD. *Chron. Respir. Dis. 3*, 123–31.

Whittom, F., Jobin, J., Simard, P. M., Leblanc, P., Simard, C., Bernard, S., Belleau, R. and Maltais, F. (1998). Histochemical and morphological characteristics of the vastus lateralis muscle in patients with chronic obstructive pulmonary disease. *Med. Sci. Sport. Exerc*, 30, 1467–74.

World Health Organisation (WHO) (2014). The top 10 causes of death: www.who.int/ mediacentre/factsheets/fs310/cn/.

Chapter 4

Physical activity for type 2 diabetes

Thomas Yates and Andrew Scott

Introduction

Diabetes is a chronic disease whereby the body is not able to adequately regulate the amount of glucose in the blood, leading to hyperglycaemia. Diabetes leads to many serious co-morbidities, including a greatly elevated risk of cardiovascular disease, and can reduce life expectancy by up to nine years if developed at a young age (Roper et al. 2001). The prevalence and economic cost of diabetes is staggering; globally, there are 382 million people who have diabetes, which is expected to increase to 592 million by 2035. Around 11 per cent of total global health care expenditure is dedicated to the treatment of diabetes, and in the United Kingdom this is projected to increase to 17 per cent by 2030 (Hex et al. 2012). It is therefore essential that efficacious and cost-effective methods of preventing and managing diabetes are investigated and disseminated globally. Diabetes takes several forms, of which the most common are type 1 diabetes and type 2 diabetes mellitus (T2DM). Type 1 diabetes accounts for less than 10 per cent of all cases of diabetes, whilst type 2 diabetes accounts for around 90 per cent. These forms of diabetes have distinct pathophysiologies, which have important considerations for the use of physical activity. This chapter focuses on the role of physical activity as a therapy in T2DM.

T2DM is generally characterised by deteriorating insulin sensitivity, which initially forces the pancreas to produce more insulin to maintain homeostasis. However, in those who go on to develop T2DM, the pancreas cannot match the continuing demand and the beta cells begin to fail, thus producing an imbalance between insulin sensitivity and insulin secretion, leading to ever more poorly-controlled blood glucose levels. The deteriorating insulin sensitivity that is the hallmark of the early phases of progression to T2DM is largely attributable to lifestyle and environmental factors. Indeed, it has been estimated that 80–90 per cent of all cases of T2DM are linked to lifestyle and health behaviours such as inactivity, a poor diet, and, consequently, obesity (Mozaffarian et al. 2009). The strength of the link between lifestyle and T2DM is emphasised vividly by looking at the extent to which its prevalence has changed with industrialisation. In traditional hunter-gatherer and rudimentary agricultural societies, T2DM is virtually unknown, yet T2DM is estimated to have increased sixfold during the 20th Century (Booth et al. 2000). Given the strength of this link, the use of lifestyle therapy should be the cornerstone in the prevention and treatment of T2DM. Of all the factors related to a healthy lifestyle, none are more important or advantageous to global health than physical activity.

Physical activity

Physical activity is a powerful hormonal regulator; hence, metabolic regulation is highly sensitive and finely tuned to the amount of daily movement undertaken and the degree of cardiorespiratory fitness gained from daily activity levels. Indeed, some of the strongest evidence for the importance of physical activity to health comes directly from T2DM related research. We now have all the different levels of evidence needed, from epidemiological, through mechanistic to interventional research, to confirm a direct and powerful causal relationship between the amount of physical activity undertaken and our ability to adequately regulate blood glucose levels, both in the prevention and treatment of T2DM.

Epidemiological evidence

Epidemiological data has consistently reported that physical activity is inversely associated with the risk of developing T2DM. For example, compared to those who are inactive, those who meet the current physical activity recommendation of around 150 minutes of moderate-intensity physical activity per week have a 30–60 per cent reduction in the risk of developing T2DM (Bassuk and Manson 2005). For example, in a meta-analysis involving 301,221 participants and 9,367 incident cases of T2DM, participation in moderate-intensity physical activity was associated with a 31 per cent reduction in the relative risk of T2DM (Jeon et al. 2007). Data from the Finnish Diabetes Prevention Study suggested that these associations may be even stronger in those who already have a high risk of developing T2DM. For example, compared to those who walked for less than one hour per week for leisure, those who walked for more than 2.5 hours had around a 60 per cent relative risk of T2DM (Laaksonen et al. 2005).

Physical activity is also associated with a reduced risk of all-cause mortality and cardiovascular disease (CVD) morbidity and mortality in those diagnosed with T2DM. For instance, data from the Aerobics Center Longitudinal Study found that the risk of all-cause mortality was four times greater in those in the least fit quartile when compared to those in the most fit quartile after adjustment for known confounding factors, including BMI (Church, et al. 2004). Another study reported that individuals with T2DM who walked for at least two hours per week had a 39 per cent lower all-cause mortality rate and a 34 per cent lower CVD mortality rate compared to those who reported no walking (Hu et al. 2001). Increased participation in vigorous intensity physical activity (Williams and Franklin, 2007), and even walking (Williams, 2008), is associated with a decreased risk of the development of chronic diseases, including T2DM, as evidenced by reduced use of prescribed medications. In habitual runners, increasing weekly running distance above $64 \text{ km} \cdot \text{wk}^{-1}$ is associated with a reduced use of anti-diabetes medications by 69 per cent for males and 55 per cent for females compared to those completing distances equivalent to recommended physical activity guidelines ($16 \text{ km} \cdot \text{wk}^{-1}$) (Williams and Franklin, 2007). Most of the reductions in medication use were associated more with improved fitness than weekly running distance.

For individuals who are starting a new physical activity programme or who do not find running appealing, increased walking distance and/or intensity significantly reduces anti-diabetes medication use (Williams, 2008). Men and women whose self-reported walking speed was > 2.1 m·s^{-1} compared to those who self-reported walking at <1.2 m·s^{-1} decreased the odds for using anti-diabetes medications by 68 per cent and 59 per cent respectively, independently of BMI and total distance. Increased total cumulative distance walked per week (45 km·wk^{-1} vs. < 5 km·wk^{-1}) is associated with reduced odds of anti-diabetes medication by 64 per cent in women and 53 per cent in men, which is largely related to lower BMI in men who walk the most, but independent of BMI in females (Williams, 2008). Furthermore, the longest usual weekly walk is a stronger discriminator of medication status, where a single 4–6 km walk each week was associated with significantly lower odds for antidiabetic medication use in men and women, regardless of total weekly distance. However, the participants included in this study were recruited from a walking magazine's subscription list and may reflect a more active sample than the general population; therefore, similar health improvements, as evidenced by lower medication use, may be feasible through lower intensities and walking durations.

Intervention studies

Intervention studies have demonstrated a positive effect on glycaemic control, the primary goal in the prevention and management of T2DM. Physical activity interventions in those identified with a high risk of T2DM have shown that the risk of developing T2DM can be reduced by up to 60 per cent, and that efficacy is similar to multifactorial interventions that also target diet and weight loss (Gillies et al. 2007). Physical activity interventions have been shown to be equally powerful in the management of T2DM. For example, a recent meta-analysis of forty seven randomised controlled trials found that supervised aerobic exercise training studies reduced levels of glysated haemoglobin (HbA1c), a marker of long-term glycaemic control, by 0.79 per cent (Umpierre et al. 2011). A comparable clinical effect has also been seen over the longer term (two years) following a walking-based intervention in Italy (Di Loreto et al. 2003). This magnitude of effect on glycaemic control is similar to many pharmaceutical-based therapies and data from the United Kingdom Prospective Diabetes Study (UKPDS) has shown that this scale of improvements in HbA1c is associated with significant reductions in T2DM-related clinical end points and mortality (UKPDS, 1998). Furthermore, in terms of glucose control, it has been found that the scale of improvements following a physical activity intervention are dependent on the starting level of glucose control, with greater benefits observed with worse baseline glucose control (Jenkins and Hagberg 2011; Umpierre et al. 2011). This demonstrates that, as with some pharmaceutical agents, those with worse glucose control have the most to gain from undertaking physical activity.

Along with aerobic exercise, resistance training has also been extensively researched in the management of T2DM. Resistance training helps maintain, or increase, lean body mass, which has an important role in increasing insulin sensitive tissue, thereby reducing peripheral insulin resistance and increasing glucose storage capacity (as glycogen). Resistance training has been shown to be an effective mode of exercise for improving glycaemic control to similar levels to aerobic exercise (Umpierre et al. 2011). Some studies have found that the combination of both resistance training and aerobic physical activity provide optimal benefit (Church et al. 2010), although this is yet to be systematically confirmed (Umpierre et al. 2011).

Mechanisms

Multiple physiological mechanisms linking physical activity to improved glucose transport have been identified (Hawley 2004; Hawley and Gibala 2009; Telford 2007). Acute and long-term changes in insulin action and fuel utilisation occur through mitochondrial biogenesis, increased fatty acid oxidation, and increased expression and translocation of key signalling proteins involved in the insulin mediated glucose uptake pathway, particularly specific glucose transporter proteins (GLUT-4) (Hawley and Gibala 2009; Hawley 2004). For example, exercise increases the translocation of GLUT-4 to the membrane surface, which facilitates the diffusion of circulating glucose into muscle cells out of the circulation and into storage as glycogen. Interestingly, increased GLUT-4 translocation is initiated by both insulin-dependent and insulin-independent pathways, meaning the effects of physical activity are not solely reliant on the upstream actions of insulin. For example, muscular contractions lead to an up-regulation of adenosine monophosphate (AMP)-activated kinase (AMPK) activity (Hawley and Gibala 2009). However, insulin-independent pathways are likely to be transient and only affected by the last bout of physical activity, whereas both acute and chronic adaptations are observed in insulin mediated pathways.

Although blood glucose control is the primary pathology and the main focus of therapy, it is not the only health outcome associated with T2DM that can be addressed through increasing physical activity. Aerobic exercise was described over thirty years ago as

> an agent with lipid-lowering, antihypertensive, positive inotropic, negative chronotropic, vasodilating, diuretic, anorexi-genic, weight-reducing, cathartic, hypoglycemic, tranquilizing, hypnotic and antidepressive qualities.
>
> (Roberts, 1984)

Therefore, physical activity has polypharmaceutical properties that have a more widespread effect than anti-hyperglycaemic medication, which include thermogenic, myogenic, anti-hypertensive, lipid-lowering, fibrinolytic, anti-inflammatory, and mood-enhancing adaptations (Fiuza-Luces et al., 2013). The further advantages of physical activity over a polypill, besides the number of pills that would be required to equal the effects of physical activity, are that chronic adaptations are also promoted as well as maintaining the acute effects provided by the previous exercise bout. Many of these positive adaptations are associated with, or directly caused by, improved glucose control.

How much is enough?

General physical activity recommendations for adults have typically specified engaging in at least 150 minutes per week of moderate-intensity physical activity, or 75 minutes of vigorous-intensity physical activity in bouts of at least ten minutes in length. These recommendations have been nuanced by the American Diabetes Association for the management of T2DM, where recommendations state that aerobic exercise of at least moderate-intensity should be accumulated in bouts of at least ten minutes on at least three days per week (with no more than two consecutive days between bouts) accumulating a total of at least 150 minutes per week (Colberg et al. 2010). In addition, regular resistance training targeting the major muscle groups is also recommended. All current physical activity recommendations for those with T2DM or the general population are based on physical activity undertaken at a moderate to vigorous intensity. Physical activity intensity is commonly defined in terms of metabolic equivalent tasks (METs). METs denote intensity as a multiple of estimated resting metabolic rate. For example, sitting quietly is assigned a MET value of 1, whilst running can result in a MET value of 10 or higher depending on the pace (Ainsworth et al. 2011); thus, running requires at least ten times more energy than sitting per unit of time. A MET value 3 to 6 is defined as moderate intensity, whilst a value of greater than 6 is taken to count as vigorous intensity.

Along with the total amount of physical activity, the timing may also be particularly important in the management of T2DM. Physical activity undertaken shortly before or after a meal can substantially blunt postprandial glucose excursions (Høstmark et al. 2006). Blood glucose levels following a meal or glucose challenge can be two to three times higher in those with T2DM, and remain elevated for much longer than in individuals without diabetes. These postprandial excursions in glucose regulation are strongly linked to cardiovascular disease and other diabetes-related complications (Cavalot et al. 2006). Therefore, not only can physical activity be used to improve overall glycaemic control, but also to target and blunt postprandial glucose levels, which is likely to provide a substantial added value to the health of those with T2DM.

Another important consideration that is becoming increasingly clear is that there is no threshold effect in the link between physical activity and health. Many studies that have used objective methods of measuring fitness and activity have found a linear relationship; that is, the degree of benefit is directly proportional to the amount of activity undertaken. For example, the association between fitness and all-cause or cardiovascular mortality has been shown to be linear in the general population and those with T2DM. Every MET increase in fitness is associated with a 10–20 per cent reduction in mortality and morbidity outcomes (Kodama et al. 2009). In another study of over 9000 individuals with impaired glucose regulation and high cardiovascular disease risk, every 2000 step-per-day increase in walking activity over a twelve-month period was associated with an 8 per cent reduction in the risk of cardiovascular morbidity and mortality (Yates et al. 2014). These linear relationships have two important conclusions: first, failure to meet the minimum recommendations for health does not imply that the level of physical activity undertaken has no benefit; rather the benefit will simply be smaller. Second, the return in investment on health does not drop off when achieving above the minimum recommendation; doing twice as much will deliver twice the benefit. This was recently confirmed in a meta-analysis of exercise training studies in those with T2DM where interventions that increased physical activity by more than 150 minutes per week resulted in substantially greater improvements in glycaemic control (Umpierre et al. 2011). Therefore, doing something is better than doing nothing, but the more that is done, the better the metabolic health benefit.

Screening and risk stratification

Moderate-intensity physical activity is an extremely safe therapy in the management of T2DM and has few, if any, harmful side effects beyond the slightly elevated risk of musculoskeletal injury. However, the progressive nature of T2DM leads to specific challenges in the safe promotion of physical activity, which become more pronounced as diabetes control worsens. Diabetes-related complications such as retinopathy, peripheral neuropathy, autonomic neuropathy, and nephropathy all present specific challenges to the patient and their health care team in the promotion of physical activity. However, none of these conditions should require the cessation of physical activity by the patient or lead to contraindication if adequately managed and supported (Colberg et al. 2010). For example, with severe peripheral neuropathy, non-weight bearing exercise should be recommended, or with autonomic neuropathy it is recommend that patients should undergo cardiac investigation before initiating increased moderate or vigorous physical activity (Colberg et al. 2010). In addition to microvascular dysfunction, long-term impaired glucose control can precipitate macrovascular dysfunction, and when combined with neuropathy this can create a perfect storm for silent angina or myocardial infarction (MI). As previously stated, T2DM progression is directly proportional to the development of CVD, which predisposes to MI and sudden cardiac death. However, diabetic neuropathy can impair sensor neurone activity and inhibit pain feedback when suffering exertional angina or MI, hence the term 'silent'.

Risk stratification for individuals with T2DM who are beginning a new physical activity programme is based on the above complications, which indicate an increased risk of exercise-induced cardiac event or musculoskeletal injury, and also the level of expert supervision that is required during exercise. Generally, the main risk associated with exercise in T2DM is of cardiovascular origin rather than hypoglycaemia in this patient group; however, many patients with poorly-controlled T2DM are eventually prescribed insulin, and hypoglycaemia then becomes a risk with exercise. As a result of these varying complications, individuals with T2DM can be classified as low, moderate, or high risk, depending on the progression of their diabetes. Two such risk stratification tools available for this purpose are the Irwin and Morgan traffic light system (Irwin and Morgan, 2003) and the PARMed-X (Riddell and Burr, 2011). These tools ascribe risk based on symptoms and the level of treatment required. The Irwin and Morgan tool, suggested for use in UK exercise referral services by the BHF, stratifies exercise risk for individuals with T2DM as follows: low risk: diet controlled; medium risk: medication controlled; high risk: presenting autonomic neuropathy or advanced retinopathy. These are overt surrogate indicators of the progression of T2DM and are used to indicate the types of exercise and degree of exercise supervision that may be warranted. Furthermore, the ACSM risk stratification algorithm is also applied to indicate risk associated with family history, CVD risk factors, and lifestyle, such as smoking, physical activity, and obesity (Pescatello et al., 2013). This additional stratification level may result in individuals with T2DM increasing risk categories from low to moderate or even from moderate to high. Individuals in the low risk category may be treated as a client without limitations and provided with general exercise guidance and minimal supervision based on their limited CVD risk, with no medication considerations. Individuals in the moderate risk category may need advice on performing physical activities, and may benefit from supervision in an exercise referral service from individuals with expertise in exercise and diabetes. Individuals in the high risk category are likely to be required to be referred for specialist services, if these are not already provided. Support from a dietician should be sought to help to manage blood glucose to reduce further regression of micro- and macro-vascular function, and from the diabetology team to optimise medications. Ideally, individuals deemed high risk who wish to perform at least moderate-intensity physical activity, should perform an ECG exercise test carried out by an exercise physiologist (Angadi and Gaesser, 2009). Such tests can be used to identify abnormal cardiac rhythms in response to incremental exercise intensities, e.g. signs of silent ischaemia that would otherwise be undetected. If cardiovascular function is determined to be sufficiently impaired then referral to cardiac rehabilitation to treat the more significant cardiac condition would be the most appropriate course of action.

Although controversial, only high-risk patients with T2DM need to be referred for further evaluation or exercise testing, because otherwise pre-activity screening processes may delay the uptake of health-enhancing physical activities without adding much benefit (Whitfield et al., 2014).

Beyond weight loss

A crucial consideration in using physical activity as a therapeutic agent in the management of T2DM is whether benefits are dependent on weight loss; that is, do physical activity interventions have to induce weight loss in order to be effective? This is an important question, because interventions aimed at physical activity behaviour change are often judged by their success or failure at initiating weight loss, particularly in T2DM given the symbiotic association with obesity. However, despite this confusion, there is overwhelming evidence, supported by numerous adiposity-independent mechanisms, that increased physical activity promotes metabolic health and improves glycaemic control without the need for weight loss (Telford 2007). This has been consistently demonstrated in meta-analyses of the evidence where exercise training studies have been shown to improve glycaemic control without weight loss (Boulé et al. 2001, Umpierre et al. 2011). Epidemiological studies have also consistently demonstrated associations with morbidity and mortality outcomes independently to body weight (Church et al. 2004; Yates et al. 2014). Indeed, if weight loss was an important mechanism for mediating benefit, physical activity would make a poor therapy. It is well established that achieving levels of physical activity that are consistent with the minimum recommendations for health do not result in meaningful weight loss. Recent physical activity recommendations advise that around sixty minutes per day of moderate-intensity physical activity is needed to initiate and maintain weight loss (Department of Health, 2011). Although effects on body weight are weak, physical activity does appear to alter the distribution of body fat. For example, exercise training has been shown to reduce visceral and hepatic adipose tissue without impacting on overall weight (Johnson et al. 2009). Therefore, by changing their physical activity levels, those with T2DM may undergo positive alterations to their fat distribution, but experience no discernible change to their body weight.

Whilst the benefits of physical activity in the treatment of type 2 diabetes are well established, both in terms of improving glycaemic control and associations with a reduced risk of cardiovascular disease, the effect of weight loss in those with type 2 diabetes are much more controversial. Dietary interventions that have induced weight loss have been shown to result in modest improvements to glycaemic control (Terranova et al. 2015; Ajala et al. 2013). However, weight change in type 2 diabetes is not associated with a reduced risk of cardiovascular disease; indeed, higher levels of body weight have been shown to be protective whilst weight loss – not weight gain – has been linked to higher mortality risk (Doehner et al. 2012; Carnethon et al. 2012). The equivocal nature of body weight in the treatment of type 2 diabetes was further highlighted in the recent Look AHEAD trial (Wing et al. 2013). Look AHEAD is the largest and longest lifestyle intervention ever conducted in those with type 2 diabetes, with a strong focus on initiating and maintaining weight loss. Although the intervention reached its goal by achieving sustained weight loss, changes to fitness were small and not clinically meaningful. This study, therefore, provides a good model for the long-term effect of weight loss in the absence of clinically-meaningful changes to fitness. The primary outcome from the trial revealed that the intervention did not affect the risk of developing cardiovascular disease over the longer term (Wing et al. 2013).

In conclusion, physical activity should be promoted for its own sake and not solely for the end product of weight loss. Indeed, physical activity is likely to be a more clinically-effective focus for lifestyle intervention, especially in relation to cardiovascular disease.

Sedentary behaviour

Physical activity research and the recommendations based on this research have predominantly focused on moderate- to vigorous-intensity physical activity. However, there is emerging and compelling evidence that the focus on the upper end of the intensity spectrum has distracted attention from the impact of sedentary behaviour on metabolic health. Sedentary behaviour is defined as any sitting or lying behaviour conducted during waking hours, at an intensity of less than 1.5 METs. The distinction between sedentary and non-sedentary behaviour therefore exists at the interface between sitting/lying and standing, rather than purposeful exercise or movement. This is quantitatively different to 'inactivity', which has traditionally been conceptualised as the failure to meet the minimum moderate- or vigorous-intensity physical activity recommendations for health. Thus, it is possible to be 'active' but still engage in high levels of sedentary time, and also to not be sedentary but without overtly meeting physical activity recommendations. Recent evidence suggests that human physiology, particularly in the regulation of metabolic health, is highly sensitive to the amount of sedentary behaviour undertaken, and that these effects and associations are independent of MVPA. For example, compared to those who sit the least, those who sit the most have around a two-fold increased risk of developing T2DM, cardiovascular disease, or all-cause mortality (Wilmot et al. 2012). Associations were independent of obesity and MVPA and strongest and most consistent for T2DM. Others have shown that every two-hour increase in TV viewing time is associated with a 20 per cent increased risk of developing T2DM (Grøntved and Hu 2011). Studies with objective measurement (accelerometers) of sedentary time have even suggested that sedentary behaviour is a stronger determinant of, and thus explains more variance in, glucose and lipid regulation than MVPA in those at risk of, or diagnosed with, T2DM (Henson et al. 2013; Cooper et al. 2012). This epidemiological data is supported by emerging experimental research. Using laboratory studies, Australian researchers have reported that breaking sedentary behaviour with light-intensity ambulation throughout the day substantially improved glucose control in participants who were overweight or obese (Dunstan et al. 2012). The same group found providing office workers with standing desks and ensuring 50 per cent of working hours were spent standing also improved postprandial glucose regulation (Thorp et al. 2014).

The strong epidemiological data and emerging corroborating experimental evidence support the hypothesis that sedentary behaviour is a highly plausible behavioural target in the promotion of metabolic health, particularly glucose regulation. Whilst the importance of moderate- to vigorous-intensity physical activity remains, a paradigm shift is needed in targeting how the rest of our waking hours are spent, with greater emphasis on helping individuals spend more time on their feet in standing or in light ambulatory activities and less time sitting. Such approaches may substantially increase the efficacy of traditional physical activity interventions. Furthermore, standing and light-intensity activity can be undertaken by the vast majority of individuals.

Promoting increased physical activity

Although the benefits of physical activity to the general population, as well as those with T2DM, have been well established for decades, finding effective methods of promoting physical activity behaviour change has proved much more challenging. To date, the most effective methods of promoting metabolic health through physical activity in T2DM have involved interventions utilising supervised exercise training protocols in lab- or gym-based environments (Umpierre et al. 2011). This evidence for T2DM is reflected more widely by new National Institute for Health and Care Excellence (NICE) guidance for exercise on referral schemes, which continues to support their use in clinical, but not non-clinical, populations.

In contrast to supervised exercise training, behavioural counselling interventions supporting patients with T2DM to become more active in their own environments have been less effective at promoting behaviour change or improving metabolic health (Umpierre et al. 2011). This reflects the reality of trying to change individual behaviour in industrialised environments that actively discourage physical activity whilst making sedentary behaviour the most attractive default. However, despite this discouraging evidence base, there are behaviour-change techniques that have been shown to be effective in those with T2DM. For example, a recent meta-analysis included 1520 individuals with T2DM who had taken part in studies promoting physical activity behaviour change (Avery et al. 2012). Although a modest reduction in HbA1c of 0.32 per cent was reported overall following physical activity behaviour change interventions, the inclusion of the following behaviour change techniques were associated with a 0.3 per cent or greater reduction in HbA1c: prompting generalisation of a target behaviour; use of follow-up prompts; goal-setting (outcome such as HbA1c reduction); prompt rewards contingent on effort/progress toward behaviour; prompt review of behavioural goals; provide information on where and when to perform the behaviour, and plan social support/social change (Avery et al. 2012). The most effective behavioural intervention to date, incorporating these behaviour change techniques, demonstrated that behaviour counselling led to a 26 MET-hr/week increase in physical activity and a 0.6 per cent reduction in HbA1c over a two-year period, demonstrating that physical activity behaviour change can be maintained in those with T2DM through robust behaviour interventions (Di Loreto et al. 2003).

Goal-setting and self-monitoring have also consistently been demonstrated to be effective techniques for initiating physical activity behaviour change in the general population (Michie et al. 2009). An exemplar of the importance of these techniques is demonstrated by pedometers. Providing participants with step/day goals and pedometers for self-monitoring has consistently been shown to initiate behaviour change in a broad range of healthy and unhealthy adults and remains one of the most effective behavioural interventions for the promotion of physical activity (Bravata et al. 2007). In the first instance, sedentary individuals should be helped to determine their baseline levels of activity and then aim for an average increase in ambulatory activity of around 2000 steps per day. An increase of this magnitude represents around twenty minutes per day of increased moderate-intensity walking activity, and is therefore largely consistent with the current recommendations of 150 minutes of moderate-intensity activity per week (Tudor-Locke and Bassett Jr, 2004). Furthermore, an increase of 2000 steps per day has been associated with an 8 per cent reduction in cardiovascular morbidity and mortality (Yates et al. 2014). Goals should be broken down into small regular changes, such as an increase of 500 steps every fortnight up to 10,000 steps per day. Categories of ambulatory activity, highlighted and summarised in Table 4.1, have also been proposed to aid public health initiatives and interventions incorporating pedometers. Here, the first priority should be to help individuals move up to a higher activity category.

Of particular relevance to T2DM is combining structured education with pedometer use, which has been shown to substantially increase the effectiveness of promoting increased physical activity over twelve months, compared to structured education only (Yates et al. 2009). In this context, structured education refers to group-based educational programmes promoting behaviour change and self-management that include evidence-based curricula, standardised educator training, and quality assurance pathways. NICE recommends that all individuals with T2DM should receive some form of structured education at the time of diagnosis, and as such this type of intervention is now commonly delivered within primary care (National Institute for Health and Clinical Excellence. 2003). Combining such programmes with pedometer use provides a feasible and evidence-based strategy for ensuring that physical activity becomes an essential part of T2DM management pathways.

Table 4.1 Physical activity categories based on steps per day

Category	Steps per day
Sedentary	< 5000
Low (typical of habitual daily activity excluding any recreational, transport or occupational physical activity).	5000–7499
Moderate (likely to incorporate the equivalent of around thirty minutes per day of moderate-intensity physical activity).	7500–9999
High (likely to incorporate the equivalent of around forty five minutes per day of moderate-intensity physical activity).	10000–12499
Very High (likely to incorporate the equivalent of over forty five minutes per day of moderate-intensity physical activity.	>12500

(adapted from Tudor-Locke and Bassett 2004)

Box 4.1 Case study

Mr Malik, originally from Pakistan, visited his GP to request tablets to 'cure' him as he thinks his general health is 'not good' after feeling 'weak' and more thirsty recently. He was not sure what might be wrong but revealed that his older brother was diagnosed with diabetes last year. Both of his parents suffer from diabetes; his father had a myocardial infarction in his early sixties and is being treated for angina while his mother also has hypertension. Mr Malik does not drink alcohol, but smokes fifteen to twenty cigarettes per day; he is not physically active and works night shifts as a taxi driver. He eats rice, curry, and vegetables on most days, has sugar with his tea, and consumes 'full fat' cola and chocolate in his taxi.

The doctor administered a medical examination; his pulse was 75 b·min^{-1} and regular; his blood pressure was 135/80 mmHg, his body mass index (BMI) was 28.0 kg·m^2 (Ht 169 cm, BM 80 kg) and waist circumference 105 cm. A random blood glucose test was 16 mmol·L^{-1} (< 11.1 mmol·L^{-1} is normal). The next week, a fasting blood test revealed a blood glucose of 8.9 mmol·L^{-1}, indicating Mr Malik to be suffering T2DM. The GP emphasised that Mr Malik can do much himself to control the disease and prevent the development of cardiovascular disease, so he is not providing medication at this stage for at least three months and has advised lifestyle change.

The GP has referred Mr Malik to you as an exercise specialist to provide appropriate guidance to help to modify his health concerns prior to prescribing medication. What approaches would you take to encourage Mr Malik to be more physically active; what would be your priorities for improving his health outcomes, and who else might you want to involve to support him?

Future research

Much research in the area of exercise and medical conditions is based on the dogmatic research of yesteryear, which is also based on apparently-healthy participant samples. The varied pathology and presentation of T2DM means that whilst this is good information, and the health benefits of physical activity for health in general are relevant, physical activity prescriptions need to be specific to the individual. Therefore, the following research areas need to be explored:

- Whilst T2DM is largely associated with a sedentary lifestyle and being overweight, there are a number of individuals presenting the 'lean T2DM phenotype'. Any hope of addressing metabolic dysfunction through the generic 'must lose weight' mantra will not be effective in individuals who are normal weight for their height. However, if sarcopenic obesity is present, particularly in the presence of visceral obesity, there is an opportunity to increase muscle mass and decrease visceral fat through anabolic exercises such as resistance training to increase the volume of insulin-sensitive tissue. Research should be performed to study the effect of prolonged resistance training interventions on body composition and HbA1c in lean individuals with T2DM so that optimal training recommendations can be formulated.

- Recent research demonstrates that aerobic training and resistance training are both safe and independently associated with improvements in metabolic control in patients with T2DM, and that those who perform both modalities gain additive improvements. Research should aim to discover whether both modalities should be combined together in the same sessions or whether the same positive responses and adaptations can be accrued from separate sessions of aerobic training and resistance training during the week.
- With relatively recent evidence-based physical activity recommendations (O'Donovan et al. 2010; Garber et al. 2011) advocating the avoidance or breaking of periods of sedentary time in addition to performing more structured physical activity, metabolic health outcomes are one of the more common outcome measures in research (Wilmot et al. 2012). This is important for individuals with T2DM, since maintained daily metabolic control (HbA1c) is more important than the initial lowering of blood glucose in response to a single exercise session. Therefore, future research should investigate the individual responses to breaking from sitting or avoiding sitting, compared to participating in structured exercise sessions, and also long-term adaptations so that appropriate physical activity prescriptions can be developed for individuals daunted at the thought of intentional exercise.
- The previous research recommendations assume that individuals with T2DM are cognisant of the need to be physically active, have an intrinsic desire to be physically active, and will willingly take part in research studies. In many instances, this is not the case. Therefore, just like with apparently healthy individuals, methods for engaging and facilitating PA for the newly- and ongoing-diagnosed need to be developed and researched with greater fervour than physiological studies. The health benefits of physical activity are largely mapped; however, we live in an increasingly sedentary culture that needs to be addressed. Whether such interventions are through health trainers, exercise scientists, publicly funded exercise practitioners, information being provided by GPs/nurses/consultant diabetologists, leaflets, poster campaigns, increasing the physical activity component of structured education sessions such as DESMOND, or improved working relationships between medical and exercise professionals, interventions need to be developed and tested to facilitate greater levels of physical activity in this patient group. This may help to encourage NICE to include PA alongside medication and diet modification in the primary management of T2DM in their clinical guidance.

Summary

Physical activity is a safe and cost-effective therapy in the management of T2DM, with wide ranging clinical benefits, including improved glucose regulation to levels that are similar to pharmaceutical intervention. Health care and physical activity professionals should ensure that the promotion of physical activity is actively included within T2DM management pathways. Abstaining from physical activity should not be advocated by medical professionals to high-risk patients, but the risks of such activities must be acknowledged and mitigated by responsible exercise specialists and relayed to their clients. The benefits of physical activity are not solely reliant on reductions in body weight, and inability to change weight with an exercise programme should not be deemed as an unsuccessful venture by the client-exercise specialist team. Both aerobic and resistance training modalities appear beneficial for T2DM but still require further research, particularly methods for facilitating such physical activities.

The value of avoiding sedentary behaviours should also not be overlooked, particularly for clients who feel too deconditioned to partake in structured activities or have little interest in such activities, but who might be inclined to fit in energy-expending bursts throughout the day. Many individuals with T2DM do want to actively take control of their condition, and rely on health professionals to communicate together to provide information on physical activity and relevant opportunities to become physically active, which remains a key challenge.

Study tasks

1   In your role as an exercise specialist, an overweight client has been referred to you to help them to manage their T2DM. What objectives and goals would you set to facilitate this aim, and how would you agree and develop a safe and effective physical activity programme with the client?
2   A patient has been referred to you to help manage their T2DM, but a family member has read that 'diabetes causes hypoglycaemia, which can be fatal'. How would you counsel the patient so that they do not avoid being physically active?
3   A patient has been referred to you by their GP with peripheral neuropathy in their feet and autonomic neuropathy. How might these complications impact upon the way you prescribe and monitor their physical activities?

Further reading/resources

The DESMOND Collaborative is a nationwide quality-controlled network of education days delivered by diabetes nurse specialists for individuals with newly diagnosed T2DM:
http://www.desmond-project.org.uk/

Colberg, S. R., Sigal, R. J., Fernhall, B., Regensteiner, J. G., Blissmer, B. J., Rubin, R. R., Chasan-Taber, L., Albright, A. L. and Braun, B. (2010). Exercise and type 2 diabetes: the American College of Sports Medicine and the American Diabetes Association: joint position statement. *Diabetes Care*, 33(12), E147–67.
O'Hagan, C., De Vito, G. and Boreham, C. A. (2013). Exercise prescription in the treatment of type 2 diabetes mellitus: current practices, existing guidelines and future directions. *Sports Medicine*, 43(1), 39–49. doi: 10.1007/s40279-012-0004-y.
Yang, Z., Scott, C.A., Mao, C., Tang, J., and Farmer, A.J. (2014). Resistance exercise versus aerobic exercise for type 2 diabetes: a systematic review and meta-analysis. *Sports Medicine*, 44(4), 487–99. doi: 10.1007/s40279-013-0128-8.
Yates, T., Davies, M. J., Henson, J., Troughton, J., Edwardson, C., Gray, L. J. and Khunti, K. (2012). Walking away from type 2 diabetes: trial protocol of a cluster randomised controlled trial evaluating a structured education programme in those at high risk of developing type 2 diabetes. *BMC Family Practice*, 13, 46. doi: 10.1186/1471-2296-13-46.
Yates, T., Henson, J., Edwardson, C., Dunstan, D., Bodicoat, D. H., Khunti, K. and Davies, M. J. (2015). Objectively measured sedentary time and associations with insulin sensitivity: importance of reallocating sedentary time to physical activity. *Preventive Medicine*, 76, 79–83. doi: 10.1016/j.ypmed.2015.04.005.

References

Ainsworth, B. E., Haskell, W. L., Herrmann, S. D., Meckes, N., Bassett, D. R., Jr, Tudor-Locke, C., Greer, J. L., Vezina, J., Whitt-Glover, M. C. and Leon, A. S. (2011). 2011 compendium of physical activities: a second update of codes and met values. *Medicine* and *Science in Sports* and *Exercise*, 43(8), 1575–81.

Ajala, O., English, P. and Pinkney, J., 2013. Systematic review and meta-analysis of different dietary approaches to the management of type 2 diabetes. *American Journal of Clinical Nutrition*, 97(3), 505–16.

Angadi, S. S., Gaesser, G. A. (2009). Pre-exercise cardiology screening guidelines for asymptomatic patients with diabetes. *Clinics in Sports Medicine*, 28, 379–92.

Avery, L., Flynn, D., Van Wersch, A., Sniehotta, F. F. and Trenell, M. I. (2012). Changing physical activity behavior in type 2 diabetes: a systematic review and meta-analysis of behavioral interventions. *Diabetes Care*, 35(12), 2681–9.

Bassuk, S. S. and Manson, J. E. (2005). Epidemiological evidence for the role of physical activity in reducing risk of type 2 diabetes and cardiovascular disease. *Journal of Applied Physiology (Bethesda, Md.: 1985)*, 99(3), 1193–1204.

Booth, F. W., Gordon, S. E., Carlson, C. J. and Hamilton, M.T. (2000). Waging war on modern chronic diseases: primary prevention through exercise biology. *Journal of Applied Physiology (Bethesda, Md.: 1985)*, 88(2), 774–87.

Boulé, N. G., Haddad, E., Kenny, G. P., Wells, G. A., and Sigal, R. J. (2001). Effects of exercise on glycemic control and body mass in type 2 diabetes mellitus: a meta-analysis of controlled clinical trials. *JAMA*, 286(10), 1218–27.

Bravata, D. M., Smith-Spangler, C., Sundaram, V., Gienger, A. L., Lin, N., Lewis, R., Stave, C. D., Olkin, I. and Sirard, J. R. (2007). Using pedometers to increase physical activity and improve health: a systematic review. *JAMA*, 298(19), 2296–2304.

Carnethon, M. R., De Chavez, P. J. D., Biggs, M. L., Lewis, C. E., Pankow, J. S., Bertoni, A. G., Golden, S. H., Liu, K., Mukamal, K. J. and Campbell-Jenkins, B. (2012). Association of weight status with mortality in adults with incident diabetes. *JAMA*, 308(6), 581–90.

Cavalot, F., Petrelli, A., Traversa, M., Bonomo, K., Fiora, E., Conti, M., Anfossi, G., Costa, G. and Trovati, M. (2006). Postprandial blood glucose is a stronger predictor of cardiovascular events than fasting blood glucose in type 2 diabetes mellitus, particularly in women: lessons from the San Luigi Gonzaga Diabetes Study. *The Journal of Clinical Endocrinology and Metabolism*, 91(3), 813–19.

Church, T. S., Blair, S. N., Cocreham, S., Johannsen, N., Johnson, W., Kramer, K., Mikus, C. R., Myers, V., Nauta, M. and Rodarte, R. Q. (2010). Effects of aerobic and resistance training on hemoglobin A1c levels in patients with type 2 diabetes: a randomized controlled trial. *JAMA*, 304(20), 2253–62.

Church, T. S., Cheng, Y. J., Earnest, C. P., Barlow, C. E., Gibbons, L. W., Priest, E. L. and Blair, S. N. (2004). Exercise capacity and body composition as predictors of mortality among men with diabetes. *Diabetes Care*, 27(1), 83–8.

Colberg, S. R., Sigal, R. J., Fernhall, B., Regensteiner, J. G., Blissmer, B. J., Rubin, R. R., Chasan-Taber, L., Albright, A. L. and Braun, B. (2010). Exercise and type 2 diabetes: the American College Of Sports Medicine and the American Diabetes Association: joint position statement. *Diabetes Care*, 33(12), E147–67.

Cooper, A., Sebire, S., Montgomery, A., Peters, T., Sharp, D., Jackson, N., Fitzsimons, K., Dayan, C. and Andrews, R. (2012). Sedentary time, breaks in sedentary time and metabolic variables in people with newly diagnosed type 2 diabetes. *Diabetologia*, 55(3), 589–99.

Department of Health (2011). *Start active, stay active: a report on physical activity from the four home countries' chief medical officers*. London: Department of Health.

Di Loreto, C., Fanelli, C., Lucidi, P., Murdolo, G., De Cicco, A., Parlanti, N., Santeusanio, F., Brunetti, P. and De Feo, P. (2003). Validation of a counseling strategy to promote the adoption and the maintenance of physical activity by type 2 diabetic subjects. *Diabetes Care*, 26(2), 404–8.

Doehner, W., Erdmann, E., Cairns, R., Clark, A. L., Dormandy, J. A., Ferrannini, E. and Anker, S. D. (2012). Inverse relation of body weight and weight change with mortality and morbidity in patients with type 2 diabetes and cardiovascular co-morbidity: an analysis of the proactive study population. *International Journal of Cardiology*, 162(1), 20–6.

Dunstan, D. W., Kingwell, B. A., Larsen, R., Healy, G. N., Cerin, E., Hamilton, M. T., Shaw, J. E., Bertovic, D. A., Zimmet, P. Z., Salmon, J. and Owen, N. (2012). Breaking up prolonged sitting reduces postprandial glucose and insulin responses. *Diabetes Care*, 35(5), 976–83.

Fiuza-Luces, C., Garatachea, N., Berger, N. A. and Lucia, A. (2013). Exercise is the real polypill. *Physiology (Bethesda)*, 28(5), 330–58. doi: 10.1152/physiol.00019.2013.

Garber, C. E., Blissmer, B., Deschenes, M. R., Franklin, B. A., Lamonte, M. J., Lee, I. M., Nieman, D. C. and Swain, D.P. (2011). American College of Sports Medicine position stand. Quantity and quality of exercise for developing and maintaining cardiorespiratory, musculoskeletal, and neuromotor fitness in apparently healthy adults: guidance for prescribing exercise. *Medicine* and *Science in Sports* and *Exercise*, 43(7), 1334–59. doi: 10.1249/MSS.0b013e318213fefb.

Gillies, C. L., Abrams, K. R., Lambert, P. C., Cooper, N. J., Sutton, A. J., Hsu, R. T. and Khunti, K. (2007). Pharmacological and lifestyle interventions to prevent or delay type 2 diabetes in people with impaired glucose tolerance: systematic review and meta-analysis. *BMJ*, 334(7588), 299.

Grøntved, A. and Hu, F. B. (2011). Television viewing and risk of type 2 diabetes, cardiovascular disease, and all-cause mortality: a meta-analysis. *JAMA*, 305(23), 2448–55.

Hawley, J. A. (2004). Exercise as a therapeutic intervention for the prevention and treatment of insulin resistance. *Diabetes/Metabolism Research and Reviews*, 20(5), 383–93.

Hawley, J. A. and Gibala, M. (2009). Exercise intensity and insulin sensitivity: how low can you go? *Diabetologia*, 52(9), 1709–13.

Henson, J., Yates, T., Biddle, S., Edwardson, C. L., Khunti, K., Wilmot, E., Gray, L., Gorely, T., Nimmo, M. A., Davies, M. (2013). Associations of objectively measured sedentary behaviour and physical activity with markers of cardiometabolic health. *Diabetologia*, 56(5), 1012–20.

Hex, N., Bartlett, C., Wright, D., Taylor, M. and Varley, D. (2012). Estimating the current and future costs of type 1 and type 2 diabetes in the UK, including direct health costs and indirect societal and productivity costs. *Diabetic Medicine*, 29(7), 855–62.

Høstmark, A. T., Ekeland, G. S., Beckstrøm, A. C. and Meen, H. D. (2006). Postprandial light physical activity blunts the blood glucose increase. *Preventive Medicine*, 42(5), 369–71.

Hu, F. B., Stampfer, M. J., Solomon, C., Liu, S., Colditz, G. A., Speizer, F. E., Willett, W. C. and Manson, J. E. (2001). Physical activity and risk for cardiovascular events in diabetic women. *Annals of Internal Medicine*, 134(2), 96–105.

Irwin D. and Morgan, O. (2003). Developing a Risk Tool. *Sportex*, 16–18.

Jenkins, N. T. and Hagberg, J. M. (2011). Aerobic training effects on glucose tolerance in prediabetic and normoglycemic humans. *Medicine* and *Science in Sports* and *Exercise*, 43(12), 2231–40.

Jeon, C. Y., Lokken, R. P., Hu, F. B. and Van Dam, R. M. (2007). Physical activity of moderate intensity and risk of type 2 diabetes: a systematic review. *Diabetes Care*, 30(3), 744–52.

Johnson, N. A., Sachinwalla, T., Walton, D. W., Smith, K., Armstrong, A., Thompson, M. W. and George, J. (2009). Aerobic exercise training reduces hepatic and visceral lipids in obese individuals without weight loss. *Hepatology*, 50(4), 1105–12.

Kodama, S., Saito, K., Tanaka, S., Maki, M., Yachi, Y., Asumi, M., Sugawara, A., Totsuka, K., Shimano, H. and Ohashi, Y. (2009). Cardiorespiratory fitness as a quantitative predictor of all-cause mortality and cardiovascular events in healthy men and women: a meta-analysis. *JAMA*, 301(19), 2024–35.

Laaksonen, D. E., Lindstrom, J., Lakka, T. A., Eriksson, J. G., Niskanen, L., Wikstrom, K., Aunola, S., Keinanen-Kiukaanniemi, S., Laakso, M., Valle, T. T., Ilanne-Parikka, P., Louheranta, A., Hamalainen, H., Rastas, M., Salminen, V., Cepaitis, Z., Hakumaki, M., Kaikkonen, H., Harkonen, P., Sundvall, J., Tuomilehto, J. and Uusitupa, M. (2005). Physical activity in the prevention of type 2 diabetes: the Finnish Diabetes Prevention Study. *Diabetes*, 54(1), 158–65.

Michie, S., Abraham, C., Whittington, C., Mcateer, J. and Gupta, S. (2009). Effective techniques in healthy eating and physical activity interventions: a meta-regression. *Health Psychology*, 28(6), 690.

Mozaffarian, D., Kamineni, A., Carnethon, M., Djoussé, L., Mukamal, K. J. and Siscovick, D. (2009). Lifestyle risk factors and new-onset diabetes mellitus in older adults: the Cardiovascular Health Study. *Archives of Internal Medicine*, 169(8), 798–807.

National Institute for Health and Clinical Excellence (NICE) (2003). *Guidance on the use of patient-education models for diabetes.* Available at: https://www.nice.org.uk/guidance/ta60.

O'Donovan, G., Blazevich, A. J., Boreham, C., Cooper, A. R., Crank, H., Ekelund, U., Fox, K. R., Gately, P., Giles-Corti, B., Gill, J. M., Hamer, M., McDermott, I., Murphy, M., Mutrie, N., Reilly, J. J., Saxton, J. M. and Stamatakis, E. (2010). The ABC of Physical Activity for Health: a consensus statement from the British Association of Sport and Exercise Sciences. *Journal of Sports Science*, 28(6), 573–91. doi: 10.1080/02640411003671212.

Pescatello, L. S., Arena, R., Riebe, D. and Thompson, P. D. (Eds.) (2013). *ACSM's guidelines for exercise testing and prescription.* 9th ed. Philadelphia, PA: Wolters Kluwer/Lippincott Williams and Wilkins Health.

Riddell, M. C. and Burr, J. (2011). Evidence-based risk assessment and recommendations for physical activity clearance: diabetes mellitus and related comorbidities. *Applied Physiology, Nutrition and Metabolism*, 36(suppl. 1), S154–89. doi: 10.1139/h11-063.

Roberts, W. C. (1984). An agent with lipid-lowering, antihypertensive, positive inotropic, negative chronotropic, vasodilating, diuretic, anorexigenic, weight-reducing, cathartic, hypoglycemic, tranquilizing, hypnotic and antidepressive qualities. *American Journal of Cardiology*, 53, 261–2.

Roper, N. A., Bilous, R. W., Kelly, W. F., Unwin, N. C., and Connolly, V. M. (2001). Excess mortality in a population with diabetes and the impact of material deprivation: longitudinal, population based study. *BMJ (Clinical Research Ed.)*, 322(7299), 1389–93.

Telford, R.D. (2007). Low physical activity and obesity: causes of chronic disease or simply predictors? *Medicine and Science in Sports and Exercise*, 39(8), 1233–40.

Terranova, C. O., Brakenridge, C. L., Lawler, S., Eakin, E. and Reeves, M. (2015). Effectiveness of lifestyle-based weight loss interventions for adults with type 2 diabetes: a systematic review and meta-analysis. *Diabetes, Obesity and Metabolism*, 17(4), 371–8.

Thorp, A. A., Kingwell, B. A., Sethi, P., Hammond, L., Owen, N., and Dunstan, D. W. (2014). Alternating bouts of sitting and standing attenuate postprandial glucose responses. *Medicine and Science in Sports and Exercise*, 46(11), 2053–61.

Tudor-Locke, C. and Bassett Jr, D.R. (2004). How many steps/day are enough? *Sports Medicine*, 34(1), 1–8.

UK Prospective Diabetes Study (UKPDS) Group (1998). Effect of intensive blood-glucose control with metformin on complications in overweight patients with type 2 diabetes (UKPDS 34). *The Lancet*, 352(9131), 854–65.

Umpierre, D., Ribeiro, P. A., Kramer, C. K., Leitão, C. B., Zucatti, A. T., Azevedo, M. J., Gross, J. L., Ribeiro, J. P., and Schaan, B. D. (2011). Physical activity advice only or structured exercise training and association with HbA1c levels in type 2 diabetes: a systematic review and meta-analysis. *JAMA*, 305(17), 1790–9.

Whitfield, G. P., Gabriel, K. K. P., Rahbar, M. H. and Kohl, III, H. W. (2014). Application of the AHA/ACSM adult preparticipation screening checklist to a nationally representative sample of us adults aged 40 and older from NHANES 2001–2004. *Circulation*, 129(10), 1113–20.

Williams, P.T. (2008). Reduced diabetic, hypertensive, and cholesterol medication use with walking. *Medicine and Science in Sports and Exercise*, 40(3), 433–43.

Williams, P. T. and Franklin, B. (2007). Vigorous exercise and diabetic, hypertensive and hypercholesterolemia medication use. *Medicine and Science in Sports and Exercise*, 39(11), 1933–41.

Wilmot, E., Edwardson, C., Achana, F., Davies, M., Gorely, T., Gray, L., Khunti, K., Yates, T. and Biddle, S. (2012). Sedentary time in adults and the association with diabetes, cardiovascular disease and death: systematic review and meta-analysis. *Diabetologia*, 55, 2895–2905.

Wing, R. R., Bolin, P., Brancati, F. L., Bray, G. A., Clark, J. M., Coday, M., Crow, R. S., Curtis, J. M., Egan, C. M., Espeland, M. A., Evans, M., Foreyt, J. P., Ghazarian, S., Gregg, E. W., Harrison, B., Hazuda, H. P., Hill, J. O., Horton, E. S., Hubbard, V. S., Jakicic, J. M., Jeffery, R. W., Johnson, K. C., Kahn, S. E., Kitabchi, A. E., Knowler, W. C., Lewis, C. E., Maschak-Carey, B. J., Montez, M. G., Murillo, A., Nathan, D. M., Patricio, J., Peters, A., Pi-Sunyer, X., Pownall, H., Reboussin, D., Regensteiner, J. G., Rickman, A. D., Ryan, D. H., Safford, M., Wadden, T. A., Wagenknecht, L. E., West, D. S., Williamson, D. F. and Yanovski, S. Z. (2013). Cardiovascular effects of intensive lifestyle intervention in type 2 diabetes. *The New England Journal of Medicine*, 369(2), 145–54.

Yates, T., Davies, M., Gorely, T., Bull, F. and Khunti, K. (2009). Effectiveness of a pragmatic education program designed to promote walking activity in individuals with impaired glucose tolerance: a randomized controlled trial. *Diabetes Care*, 32(8), 1404–10.

Yates, T., Haffner, S. M., Schulte, P. J., Thomas, L., Huffman, K. M., Bales, C. W., Califf, R. M., Holman, R. R., Mcmurray, J. J. and Bethel, M. A. (2014). Association between change in daily ambulatory activity and cardiovascular events in people with impaired glucose tolerance (Navigator Trial): a cohort analysis. *The Lancet*, 383(9922), 1059–66.

Physical activity for mental health

Naomi Ellis and Leon Meek

Mental health

The term 'mental health' has been defined as the emotional and spiritual resilience enabling people to enjoy life and cope with adversity (Faulkner and Taylor 2005). While mental health is used positively to indicate a state of psychological wellbeing (Pilgrim 2005), the term 'mental health problem' refers to a negative aspect indicating a disruption to how people think and feel (Mentality 2004). The terms 'mental health problems' and 'mental illness' are often used interchangeably. Yet, references made to 'mental health problems', rather than specific diagnoses (e.g. schizophrenia) or 'mental illness', are thought to be less stigmatising and reduce negative connotations (Pilgrim 2005). In this chapter 'mental health problems' is used as an umbrella term, but 'mental illness' is sometimes used when discussing specific clinical diagnoses.

Together, mental, neurological, and substance-use disorders account for 13 per cent of the total global burden of disease, with depression as the single largest cause of disability worldwide (World Health Organisation 2013). In the UK, 22.8 per cent of the total burden of disease was attributable to mental health problems (WHO 2008), with one in four adults experiencing them during their lifetime (Singleton et al. 2001). However, some studies suggest that the lifetime prevalence is higher (e.g. Kessler et al. 2005). Furthermore, mental health affects, and is affected by, other non-communicable diseases, such as cancer and cardiovascular disease (Royal College of Psychiatrists 2010), which also have common risk factors (e.g. low socio-economic status, alcohol use, and stress).

The scale of this disease carries a considerable economic cost. In England, the annual cost of poor mental health in 2009–10 was estimated at £105 billion, including health and social care, lost economic output, and human suffering (Centre for Mental Health 2011). And the problem is increasing: the 2009–10 figures marked a 36 per cent increase from 2002–03 (Centre for Mental Health 2011), with projections of a further 14 per cent increase in the number of people in England experiencing mental health problems by 2026 (McCrone et al. 2008). The cost of this growing prevalence is reflected most in health and social care costs, which rose from £12.5 billion to £21.3 billion between 2002–03 and 2009–10 (a 70 per cent rise; Centre for Mental Health 2011). Mental health problems account for almost a quarter of all primary care consultations (Department of Health 2004) and one third of all GP time (Social Exclusion Unit, 2004). This is compounded by the greater risk of comorbidities in this population group. People with mental health problems have a higher risk of physical health issues (WHO 2013), chronic disease (Brown et al. 2000; Connolly and Kelly 2005) and premature mortality (Harris and Barraclough 1998), placing even greater pressure on health services (Ansseau et al. 2004; The MaGPIe Research Group 2003).

In the context of a disproportionate need for health care, there is evidence that provision for those with mental health problems is inconsistent. Issues have been reported around access to services, effectiveness of interventions, poor holistic care, and a lack of attention to physical health needs (Mental Health Foundation 2013a). Traditionally, mental health problems have been treated through prescribed medication (Sin and Gamble 2003). However, the potential side effects (Haslam et al. 2004), low rates of adherence (Chue and Kovacs 2003), and subsequent relapse, are all concerns (Cramer and Rosenbeck 1998). This, combined with the cost of pharmacological treatments, prompted interest in alternative or adjunct therapies to help reduce the mental health burden (Lam and Kennedy 2004). Cognitive behavioural therapy (Haddad 2005) and other forms of psychotherapy are now offered to patients, although access is variable (Social Exclusion Unit, 2004). Ultimately, the rising cost of pharmacological and psychological interventions means that health services may soon be unable to meet the demands (Martinsen, 2000). Physical activity has come to the attention of researchers and practitioners alike as an alternative or adjunct therapy for mental health problems, because of wide ranging benefits for mental and physical health without the potential side effects of medication (Daley 2002; Priest 2007).

Physical activity and mental health

Physical inactivity is one of the leading risk factors for global mortality (World Health Organization 2010), with sedentary behaviour now recognised as a major public health issue (Health and Social Care Information Centre 2012). The benefits of being physically active are well documented (Biddle and Mutrie 2008) and include the prevention and management of mental health conditions (World Health Organization 2010). Despite awareness of the benefits of active lifestyles, a large proportion of the UK population are inactive. Only 56 per cent of adults are thought to meet the Chief Medical Officer's guidelines (HM Government 2014; Health and Social Care Information Centre 2012), although this is a likely over-estimate, as it is based on self-reported physical activity measurements. True levels of participation are likely to be much lower, as indicated by objectively measured physical activity data, which suggest that only 6 per cent of men and 4 per cent of women meet Government guidelines (NHS Information Centre for Health and Social Care 2009).

The economic cost of this widespread physical inactivity is considerable (British Heart Foundation National Centre 2013). Direct costs in the UK are estimated to be over £1 billion (Allender et al. 2007; Scarborough et al. 2011), which increases significantly when loss of productivity (in England £5.5 billion) and premature death of working age people (in England £1 billion) are taken into account (Ossa and Hutton 2002). Given the consistent evidence linking active lifestyles to health, increasing population physical activity levels would help to improve physical and mental health, and reduce the associated cost of hypokinetic chronic diseases (Department of Health 2011).

Physical activity has been shown to have both preventative and therapeutic benefits for mental health (Chen and Millar 1999; Walsh, 2011). Physically active individuals tend to report lower depression and symptoms of anxiety when compared with inactive participants (Cassidy et al. 2004; Hassmen et al. 2000; Pasco 2011). People whose activity levels fall below levels recommended for health benefit increase their risk of mental health problems (Lampinen et al. 2000). The reverse has also been observed; previously sedentary individuals can reduce their risk of mental health problems by taking up physical activity (Brown et al. 2005; Camacho et al. 1991; Chen and Millar 1999).

Physical activity for people with mental health problems

The mental health benefits of physical activity in the general population provide a rationale for therapeutic application in those with established mental health problems. Cross-sectional evidence linking physical activity and the risk of mental health problems is consistent (Harvey et al. 2010). Although there is not as much evidence of the cause-effect relationship (Morgan et al. 2013), it is broadly supportive (Ten Have et al. 2011; Strawbridge et al. 2002).

When we look to trials and intervention studies of exercise in clinical mental health populations, the therapeutic potential is apparent (Cooney et al. 2013; Ellis et al. 2007; Holley et al. 2011; Wolff et al. 2011). Often, researchers have focused on physical activity for reducing symptoms of depression and anxiety (Craft and Landers 1998; Craft and Perna 2004; Crone and Guy 2008; Hutchinson 2005; Pelham and Campagna 1991; Pelham et al. 1993; Priest 2007), but increases in self-confidence (Mind 2007), mood (Ellis et al. 2013; McDevitt et al. 2005; Randall et al. 2014), enjoyment (Fogarty and Happell 2005), and motivation (O'Kane and McKenna 2002), as well as reductions in positive symptoms of psychosis (Faulkner and Sparkes 1999), and stress (Carless and Douglas 2004).

In relation to some of the most prevalent or severe mental health problems, again, the evidence is supportive. For example, depression is a common condition, affecting 121 million people globally, and physical activity has been shown to help prevent its onset (Mammen and Faulkner 2013). A short ten-day aerobic exercise intervention targeting in- and out-patients diagnosed with major depressive disorder was associated with a decrease in depression (Dimeo et al. 2001). Hutchinson (2005) evaluated a twenty-week (which was long-term in comparison to most interventions) gym-based exercise intervention consisting of three 45-minute sessions per week. Follow-up data from 40 weeks identified a significant improvement, not only in cardiovascular fitness, but also in depression and participants' quality of life. There is also review-level evidence that physical activity can improve depression. A small but significant beneficial effect has been reported in children and adolescents (Brown et al. 2013), and in adults (Mead et al. 2008), although the latter review reported methodological limitations in many cases.

Another example is the use of exercise for the prevention and treatment of cognitive impairment and dementias. There is growing evidence that physical activity is a key modifiable risk factor that could be used to reduce the prevalence of Alzheimer's disease, as well as related comorbidities such as diabetes (Mehlig et al. 2014; Norton et al. 2014). A meta-analysis identified that action on seven modifiable risk factors could prevent around one third of global cases of Alzheimer's diseases, and that physical inactivity was the most potent factor (Norton et al. 2014). Indeed, there is growing review-level evidence that interventions that combine exercise with cognitive training can improve cognitive function, thereby helping to delay the age-related decline in mental ability, and reduce the prevalence of mild cognitive impairment and dementias (Law et al. 2014). Similarly, a review of exercise training for older people with cognitive impairment and dementia reported significant benefits for strength, fitness, functional and cognitive performance, and behaviour (Heyn et al. 2004). A later Cochrane review of exercise as a treatment for dementia did report benefits for the ability to perform activities of daily living and, possibly, for improving cognition, but also highlighted variation between results of trials warranting a degree of caution (Forbes et al. 2013).

Psychosis is an important group of severe mental health disorders, which encompasses schizophrenia, schizophreniform disorder, schizoaffective disorder, bipolar disorder, and major depression with psychotic features (Ehmann and Hanson 2002). Positive symptoms of such conditions, such as hallucinations and delusions, are particularly debilitating (American Psychiatric Association 1994). A 2007 review of exercise as an adjunct therapy for psychosis was generally supportive of a positive effect, but stated the need for more consistency to allow the benefits to be quantified and to identify the most successful types of intervention (Ellis et al. 2007). Subsequently, a review of RCTs supported the use of physical activity as part of a multidisciplinary treatment of schizophrenia (Vancampfort et al., 2012), with more recent calls for modern multimodal intervention approaches that include physical activity to improve psychopathology and cognitive symptoms in psychosis (Malchow et al. 2013).

As noted above, some researchers express a need for caution when interpreting evidence in this area. Where discrepancies in the strength and consistency of relationships are observed, there are various considerations, such as the small number of RCTs, typically small samples, short follow-up periods, and the heterogeneity of study populations and exercise programmes. This might explain why, for example, Pearsall et al. (2014) reported mixed findings from a recent systematic review and meta-analysis on RCTs, examining exercise interventions in those with serious mental health problems. This notwithstanding, there is broadly supportive evidence that exercise has therapeutic value for a range of mental health problems.

Additional benefits of physical activity in clinical mental health populations

The rationale for increasing physical activity within this population group extends beyond the psychological benefits. First, there are the physical health benefits. We have already noted the role of active lifestyles in promoting physical health and how those experiencing mental health problems are more likely to have comorbidities, such as diabetes and cardiovascular disease (Brown et al. 1999; Sokal et al. 2004). This is often the result of lifestyle behaviours, such as smoking, poor diet, and lack of exercise (Lambert et al. 2003; Wirshing 2004), and possible medication side-effects (Goff et al. 2005), which, again, affect this population group disproportionately. Second, and related to this, there is evidence that participation in physical activity, such as group exercise sessions, can improve motivation in mental health service users. Participants of these groups have reported feeling stimulated to take on other activities, even having increased impetus in other areas of their therapy (Fogarty and Happell 2005). This is a considerable benefit, given the common barriers of tiredness (from symptoms of disease or medication) and poor motivation, which prevent many from leading more healthy and active lives (Corry et al. 2004). Third, mental health problems are often associated with social exclusion and isolation (Hacking and Bates 2008). Again, evidence from studies of patients using adult mental health services has shown that physical activity groups can help to address unmet needs for company, daytime activities, and intimate relationships (Cleary et al. 2006). Case studies and interviews with service users have reported that physical activity groups can engage individuals with mental health services, promote normalising activities, and offer safe environments for social interaction (Carter-Morris and Faulkner 2003; Crone and Guy 2008; Faulkner and Sparkes 1999; Mental Health Foundation 2000; Wallcraft 1998). This can help to mitigate the risk of social isolation and stigma that is associated with impaired mental health.

For all of these reasons, it is not surprising that physical activity appears popular among people experiencing mental health problems. Over 75 per cent of those surveyed by the Social Exclusion Unit (2004) expressed a wish for better access to leisure services, which has been advocated by others who highlight the rights of service users to engage in such widely enjoyed recreational and leisure activities (Richardson et al. 2005).

Physical activity recommendations in mental health populations

Given the impact of inactivity on health, and the associated cost, HM Government (2014) recognises the importance of getting people active. Adults in the general population are recommended to accumulate at least 150 minutes of moderate-to-vigorous intensity activity weekly, ideally in bouts of ten minutes or more on a daily basis (Department of Health, 2011). There is also recognition that some groups in society are more likely to be inactive and therefore require specific, targeted approaches; this includes those with mental health problems. However, mental health problems often present in different ways, with symptoms of varying severity, which can differentially affect people's ability to engage in physical activity. As becomes clear later in this chapter, and as is highlighted in Chapter 11, each case must be treated individually, with a tailored approach specific to the individual. That said, earlier, we described how people with mental health problems can reap the same type of physical and mental health benefits from being physically active as the general population and, in fact, have greater needs given the increased presence of comorbidities. So it is logical that the current physical activity recommendations should be applicable both to those with and those without mental health problems (Rethorst and Trivedi 2013); the approach might be very different, but the target behaviour in terms of activity volume and intensity should be the same.

There is much debate around the type, intensity, and duration of physical activity to confer benefit in people with mental health problems. Findings from research in this area are by no means conclusive, limiting the evidence base to inform prescription guidelines (Morgan et al. 2013). To date, research has tended to focus on aerobic exercise, with few studies comparing, for example, aerobic, resistance, or mindful activity. Those that have report little difference (Rehor et al. 2001; Stathopoulou et al. 2006). Those undertaking an activity that is new to them (regardless of activity type) might benefit less because they need to learn a new skill (Rehor et al. 2001). A combination of aerobic- and resistance-based exercise has been proposed as preferable (Rethorst and Trivedi 2013) and feasible within a multidisciplinary team (Marzolini et al. 2009). However, it is noted that the type of exercise, and whether it is group or individual, might be less important than ensuring it is structured around their personal preferences (Morgan et al. 2013).

Research has focused on regular exercise, which is the ultimate behavioural target. However, within this population group, engagement in regular activity is not always feasible as opportunities for exercise may be limited, particularly for in-patients (Cormac et al. 2004). To better understand the effect of exercise (and the duration of benefits) some researchers have considered the impact of a single bout of activity. For some, where routine might be difficult, understanding the impact of just one session could prove useful in determining the frequency of sessions required to sustain benefit. Benefits have been shown immediately post exercise across a range of mental health diagnoses (Bartholomew et al. 2005; Ellis et al. 2013; Randall et al. 2014; Weinstein et al. 2010), with evidence that this might last for up to forty eight hours post-exercise (Randall, 2015). However, this was not supported elsewhere (Weinstein et al. 2010). Further research is required in this area to better support the structuring of exercise intervention.

Most evidence examines the impact of moderate-intensity exercise. This is a likely consequence of practicalities surrounding getting those experiencing mental health problems active, and the relatively low baseline activity levels from which many are starting. A minimum recommendation of thirty minutes of moderate-to-vigorous exercise three times per week has been suggested (Morgan et al. 2013). Although the authors advocate greater activity levels if possible, increasing to this level from a largely sedentary lifestyle will confer health benefits regardless of exercise intensity (Asztalos et al. 2010; Sparling et al. 2015; Wen et al. 2011). When considering exercise intensity, current fitness levels, and any comorbidity need to be taken into account, as exercise tolerance might be also lower in some mental health groups (Shah et al. 2007).

Physical activity in mental health services

The range of psychological, physical, and social benefits of physical activity make it an appealing and potentially low-cost mental health therapy (Daley 2002) that is often favourable to, or can provide a way to reduce, medication (Lautenschlager et al. 2004). The need for physical activity to be integrated into mental health services is recognised (Richardson et al. 2005; Walsh 2011). Health care professionals should be involved in the design and implementation of relevant activity programmes, and should include service users in the process (Cormac et al. 2004; Happell et al. 2012; NICE 2011, 2012). The Mental Health Foundation have recommended that all health professionals should understand the physical and psychological benefits that physical activity can offer, and should support people with mental health problems to become more active (Mental Health Foundation 2013b). Indeed, mental health nurses are often involved with intervention delivery, and are well placed to support patients with behaviour change interventions (Happell et al. 2012). These points are ech-oed by WHO (2013), who also recommend support from families and carers where appropriate.

Other important considerations for physical activity programmes within mental health services include, first, the need for regular communication between the exercise specialists and the care team (Cormac et al. 2004). Second, staff enthusiasm is key for successful engagement with, and encouragement of, service users (Cormac et al. 2004). Third, support networks are thought to play a fundamental role in any lifestyle behaviour change, particularly in this population group (NICE 2011). Where possible, these should be tailored to the individual, for example, the use of mobile devices and social media in young people (Killackey et al. 2011). Finally, basic practical considera-tions such as ensuring that people have appropriate clothes to exercise in is essential as they may have been an inpatient and sedentary for some time. A pre-exercise group is also suggested as it can provide patients with some of the skills and, therefore, increase confidence to exercise (Cormac et al. 2004).

Good practice for physical activity intervention in NHS mental health services

This section presents an example of good practice in an NHS mental health service. A number of stages are involved, from establishing an individual's suitability for physi-cal activity intervention, to gathering of initial information, identifying appropriate physical activity, and case formation. This is designed to be a practical guide and offers some key points for practitioners to consider at each stage. Figure 5.1 shows an exam-ple care plan pathway to be followed by the exercise specialist, who should be trained as a level 4 specialist exercise instructor, specifically in Mental Health, on the Register of Exercise Professionals (REPs).

All individuals accessing NHS mental health services should receive a physical health screen prior to any formal physical activity engagement, to identify comorbidi-ties and assess the initial disease risk classification of service users. This screening now follows the recommendations of the 2014 physical health CQUIN, (Commissioning for quality and innovation; NHS England/Commissioning Policy and Primary Care/Commissioning Policy and Resources, 2014; Shiers et al. 2014). Central to these rec-ommendations is the need to develop, in partnership with the service user, a personal-ised evidence-based recovery plan that is well supported by a multi-disciplinary team (NHS England et al. 2014).

Triage information gathering

The exercise specialist determines if the referral is appropriate for physical activity therapy or whether a different discipline (physiotherapy, occupational therapy) is more appropriate, although a multi-disciplinary approach is likely. The exercise spe-cialist should classify the priority of need (or risk level) for the identified problem and arrange to see the patient within a specific time period (Figure 5.1). The exercise specialist should make every effort to gather all pre-assessment information from the patient's GP, medical notes, family and friends, and significant others. Those closest to the individual will often have a valuable understanding of the patient and information

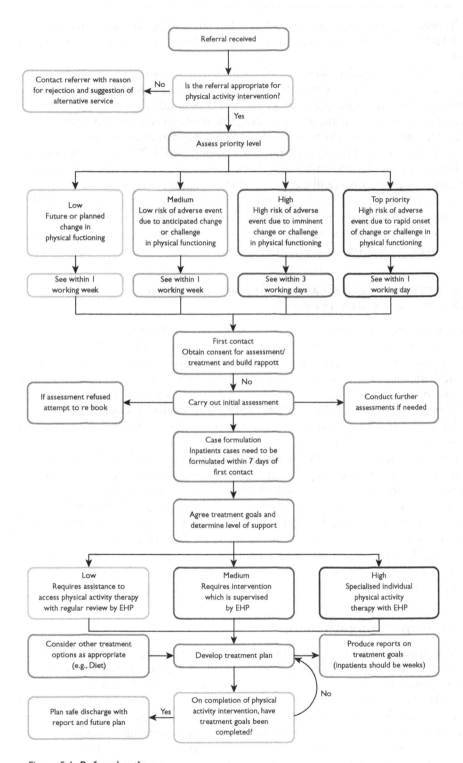

Figure 5.1 **Referral pathway.**

not otherwise disclosed to health care professionals. It is anticipated that the exercise specialist will have a thorough understanding of the concerns and needs of the patient prior to progressing to the next stage, 'first contact'.

First contact

At first contact, the exercise specialist should build a rapport with the patient, aiming to understand their interests and desire to engage in the process. It may also include further discussions with carers, relatives, and relevant professions to follow-up on any concerns arising at triage. At this point, patient consent is sought for subsequent assessment and treatment. The patient may not wish to engage, but this should not preclude further involvement. It is recognised that people with mental health problems are likely to have reduced levels of motivation and the exercise specialist should periodically re-engage with them as appropriate.

Assessment

Within one-week of first contact, there should be an initial assessment, completed in collaboration with the patient. This might take place over a number of meetings, dependent on the patient and the extent of their needs. The aim is to generate sufficient information for case formulation, so it requires consideration of both psychiatric and physical health concerns. The Lester Screening Tool offers a useful way to identify the physical health concerns of people with psychiatric illnesses, and presents guidance for appropriate interventions (Shiers et al. 2014). There is the potential to prioritise physical health needs at this stage. But, because the patient's mental illness will determine their ability to tackle such problems, practitioners should give sufficient credence to the mental health facets. This requires that practitioners understand patients' clinical diagnoses and identify constraints to participation in any physical activity intervention.

Case formulation

The exercise specialist should consider the level of support needed to address both the physical and mental health concerns, which are determined by the patient's classified risk (from triage and subsequent information gathering). At this stage, the exercise specialist should consider the design of an exercise and health care plan to guide the intervention. Exercise-specialist care plans are an integral component to the safe delivery of physical activity intervention and should reflect the specific needs of the individual. Principles of re-motivation and motivational interviewing, widely-used practices in the mental health arena (described in Chapter 13), might prove useful at this stage.

Depending on risk level and patient motivation, the intervention might take a number of forms. It could involve a supervised exercise specialist-led intervention, which involves a one-to-one specific structured intervention, including a thorough assessment of physiological and psychological changes, whereby the exercise specialist continually tailors the activity to the individual's needs (Figure 5.1; Box 5.1). However, such specialised supervised intervention might not be appropriate or necessary in an in-patient psychiatric hospital setting and, for many, physical activity interventions can be conducted within their own local community.

Box 5.1 Case study

The following case study describes an individual who has received an exercise and health intervention within an NHS mental health service in the UK.

The individual. Bobby is a twenty three year-old male who has been detained under Section 2 of the Mental Health Act (1983). This was his first admission to hospital and he was previously unknown to the local mental health service. Bobby was experiencing thoughts of paranoia, and was suspicious and guarded of those around him. He was continually seeking to leave the hospital. He has been referred to the exercise specialist for an assessment of his physical health needs as standard procedure following admission and he has indicated an interest in physical activity.

Triage gathering. His brother reported that Bobby had no known physical health concerns, but had not been screened or seen his GP for over three years. He stated that Bobby was a keen athlete until recently and regularly attended a local athletics club. Recently, Bobby's odd behaviour caused friends to distance themselves, leaving him isolated within the family home. The GP confirmed that there were no known physical health or heredity concerns.

First contact. First contact was made in the hospital ward. Bobby was obviously disturbed in his thought processes as he was observed to be responding to some internal stimuli. He was, however, able to respond to verbal direction from the exercise specialist and, whilst suspicious at first, appeared reassured and interested when given an explanation of exercise specialist role. Bobby confirmed the information provided by his brother, giving details of his athletics and physical activity participation. Bobby reported that he was predominantly interested in his physique and appearance, and regularly attended his local gym for resistance training. Bobby expressed motivation to participate in any physical activity intervention but wanted this to occur within his local community rather than the hospital.

Exercise health practitioner assessment. Bobby was happy to cooperate with all aspects of the assessment; however, given the disturbance in his thought processes, it was not practical to complete in one session. Consideration was given to Bobby's level of understanding at this time. Several visits also provided the opportunity to build rapport between practitioner and patient, ensuring Bobby's needs were fully considered.

Metabolic considerations
Smoking: < 10cigarettes a day
Lifestyle: happy with his own diet (predominantly protein-orientated)
Body Mass Index: 25–30 kg·m^2
Blood pressure: < 130/90 mmHg
Glucose regulation: < 5 mmol·L^{-1}
Blood lipids: total cholesterol < 5 mmol·L^{-1}

Mental health consideration. Whilst there was no formal diagnosis, Bobby's symptoms were similar to those of a psychotic-type illness (e.g., hallucinations, delusions, confused and disturbed thoughts, lack of insight and self-awareness). Further mental health consideration was Bobby's continual ambition to leave hospital, yet legally detained under Section 2 of the Mental Health Act. This means he was detained for up to twenty eight days for a mental health assessment and any treatment required.

Case formulation. Bobby's care plan was completed. All information was kept on record, reviewed, and updated to ensure the care plan remained relevant to his needs.

Development. Bobby engaged in the physical activity intervention on a 1:1 basis for two weeks with a focus on weight training. He remained conscious of his appearance and how others perceived him. Whilst it was assumed this was attributable to his mental illness, it became evident that Bobby had always held these thoughts. During the course of intervention, Bobby expressed additional interests, specifically in swimming. Although still detained under Section 2, Bobby had been prescribed Section 17 leave under the Mental Health Act, which allowed periods of supervised leave outside the hospital. Whilst not visibly at ease within a group environment, it was deemed fitting to offer Bobby the opportunity to participate in the swimming group in the local community, as he had not absconded from any previous leave and had formed good relations with the exercise specialist. Furthermore, he was now accepting his psychotropic medication. Consequently, Bobby used several periods of escorted leave to attend the local swimming facility. Over time, he was observed to be more trusting of others and able to interact socially within a group setting. Thereafter, Bobby was able to attend both individual and group intervention without the need for direct exercise specialist supervision or mental health escort. Bobby was subsequently discharged from hospital and referred to his local community mental health team.

Progression. Following discharge, Bobby did not seek the support services of his community mental health team, specifically his community psychiatric nurse. However, he remained keen to engage with available physical activity interventions and was referred to the exercise specialist attached to the local community mental health team. At this time, Bobby was avoiding any association with his mental health concerns. It was, therefore, important to extend the exercise specialist relationship to safeguard against deterioration in his mental health problem. Although exercise specialist intervention continued, Bobby was disengaged from other services and in denial of his psychiatric disorder. Consequently, his mental health began to deteriorate and he was subsequently admitted to hospital under Section 3 of the Mental Health Act. Someone detained under section 3 is done so if they are known to mental health services and require treatment in hospital for their own health or for the protection of other people.

Review. Bobby had become well known to his mental health services and occasionally needed admission to hospital. Whilst his mental health disorder impeded his thought processes, his previous relationships with exercise specialists ensured that he accepted the services provided. The exercise specialist continued to play a significant role in Bobby's acceptance of his mental health disorder.

For those not considered high risk, but who require supervised physical activity within the institutional setting, there are some important considerations. Some psychiatric hospitals fail to address the need for physical activity provision. Authors have suggested that management style, ethos, and culture in such places can contribute to socially-disengaged and inactive in-patients (Radcliffe and Smith 2007). Where barriers exist, one solution is that the activities are prescribed by the exercise specialist, but delivery is facilitated by other practitioners. This can afford greater frequency and flexibility of programmes, but requires that exercise specialists involve other professions in the design and creation of physical activity interventions.

Finally, those with lower risk levels and sufficient motivation might be able to implement their own activity plan, with regular reviews from the exercise specialist. In these instances, activity is most likely to occur within the community. While there are benefits, potential barriers to community-based physical activity to consider include social exclusion, access to facilities, and stigma (Social Exclusion Unit 2004). Support mechanisms to address such issues might involve buddying, a practice commonly used by mental health providers, which offers both emotional and practical peer support to help with engagement (e.g. introducing individuals to new groups or facilities, offering encouragement to attend sessions).

In all cases, ongoing assessment and review are important to ensure activities are appropriate and tailored to individual need, ultimately with a view to safe discharge with a plan for continued activity.

Future research

Several areas warrant further research:

- Greater understanding of the duration of psychological benefits of exercise would provide practitioners with the evidence base to inform the frequency of sessions;
- Use of objective physical activity measurement (e.g. accelerometry) would provide researchers with a more valid measure of physical activity frequency, intensity, and duration to allow exploration of dose-response in different conditions. However, it is acknowledged that using activity monitors is likely to present challenges beyond those experienced in studies of non-clinical populations, given the nature of certain mental health conditions (e.g. patients experiencing symptoms of paranoia);
- The challenges of working with populations who have clinical mental health diagnoses often result in studies and evaluations with relatively small sample sizes and short follow-up periods. Efforts to address this common limitation might require closer collaboration between mental health service providers and academic institutions to allow more routine and longer-term data collection.

Chapter summary

This chapter has introduced the scale of the challenge that mental health problems pose, globally and in the UK, in terms of health, health care provision, and the economic burden. The multiple benefits of physical activity for mental, physical, and social health, and the absence of side-effects, make it an appealing adjunct or alternative to pharmacological treatments. Although there are some limitations and inconsistencies in the evidence base, there is sufficient support to implement exercise interventions in those with mental health problems. We have tried to emphasise that the range and complexities of mental illnesses demand each individual be assessed and treated in a way that is appropriate to their need. As discussed in other chapters of this book, effecting behaviour change in the general population is a considerable challenge. With the additional complications and challenges that mental health problems present, effective intervention in this population group warrants careful consideration. The good practice example and case study outline some practical steps for practitioners and those involved in the design and delivery of mental health services, to help with the basic processes and factors for including physical activity as part of the care pathway in mental health service users.

Further reading

Cormac, I., Martin, D. and Ferriter, M. (2004). Improving the physical health of long-stay psychiatric in-patients. *Advances in Psychiatric treatment*, 10, 107–115.
Mental Health Foundation (2013) *Starting today: the future of mental health services*. London, Mental Health Foundation.
Pearsall, R., Smith, D. J., Pelosi, A. and Geddes, J. (2014). Exercise therapy in adults with serious mental illness: a systematic review and meta-analysis. *BMC Psychiatry*, 14, 117, doi:10.1186/1471-244X-14-117.
World Health Organisation (2013). *Mental health action plan 2013–2020*. Geneva, World Health Organisation.

Study tasks

1   Read the most recent mental health guidance documents (e.g. by organisations such as NICE, Mind, WHO, Mental Health Foundation) and summarise their advice relating to physical activity and exercise.
2   Choose a type of mental health problem (e.g. depression, schizophrenia) and review the evidence, commenting on both the strength of support for exercise interventions and a key area for future research.
3   Within your local area, identify what physical activity opportunities are available for mental health service users, and consider what challenges should be considered if trying to encourage attendance.

References

Allender, S., Foster, C., Scarborough, P. and Rayner, M. (2007). The burden of physical activity-related ill health in the UK. *Journal of Epidemiology and Community Health*, 61, 344–8.
American Psychiatric Association. (1994). *Diagnostic and statistical manual of mental disorders*. Washington, DC: American Psychiatric Association.
Ansseau, M., Dierick, M., Buntinkx, F., Cnockaert, P., De Smedt, J., Van Den Haute, M. and Vander Mijnsbrugge, D. (2004). High prevalence of mental disorders in primary care. *Journal of Affective Disorders*, 78(1), 49–55.
Asztalos, M., De Bourdeaudhuij, I. and Cardon, G. (2010). The relationship between physical activity and mental health varies across activity intensity levels and dimensions of mental health among women and men. *Public Health Nutrition*, 13(8), 1207–14.
Bartholomew, J. B., Morrison, D. and Ciccolo, J. T. (2005). Effects of acute exercise on mood and well-being in patients with major depressive disorder. *Medicine and Science in Sports and Exercise*, 37(12), 2032–7.

Biddle, S. J. H. and Mutrie, N. (2008). *Psychology of physical activity: determinants, well-being and interventions*. Abingdon: Routledge.

British Heart Foundation National Centre (2013). *Economic costs of physical inactivity*. Loughborough: British Heart Foundation National Centre.

Brown, H. E., Pearson, N., Braithwaite, R. E., Brown, W. J. and Biddle, S. J. H. (2013). Physical Activity Interventions and Depression in Children and Adolescents. *Sports Medicine*, 43(3), 195–206.

Brown, S., Barraclough, B. and Inskip, H. (2000). Causes of the excess mortality of schizophrenia. *British Journal of Psychiatry*, 177, 212–17.

Brown, S., Birtwistle, J., Roe, J. and Thompson, C. (1999). The unhealthy lifestyle of people with schizophrenia. *Psychological Medicine*, 29, 697–701.

Brown, W. J., Ford, J. H., Burton, N. W., Marshall, A. L. and Dobson, A. J. (2005). Prospective study of physical activity and depressive symptoms in middle-aged women. *American Journal of Preventive Medicine*, 29(4), 265–72.

Camacho, T. C., Roberts, R. E., Lazarus, N. B., Kaplan, G. A. and Cohen, R. D. (1991). Physical activity and depression: evidence from the Alameda County Study. *American Journal of Epidemiology*, 134(2), 220–31.

Carless, D. and Douglas, K. (2004). A golf programme for people with severe and enduring mental health problems. *Journal of Health Promotion*, 3(4), 26–39.

Carter-Morris, P. and Faulkner, G. (2003). A football project for services users: the role of football in reducing social exclusion. *Journal of Mental Health Promotion*, 2(2), 24–30.

Cassidy, K., Kotynia-English, R., Acres, J., Flicker, L., Lautenschlager, N. T. and Almeide, O. P. (2004). Association between lifestyle factors and mental health measures among community dwelling older women. *Australian and New Zealand Journal of Psychiatry*, 38, 940–47.

Centre for Mental Health (2011). *The economic and social costs of mental health problems in 2009/10*. Accessed via: www.centreformentalhealth.org.uk/pdfs/economic_and_social_costs_2010.pdf.

Chen, J. and Millar, W. J. (1999). Health effects of physical activity. *Health Reports*, 11(1), 21–30.

Chue, P. and Kovacs, C. S. (2003). Safety and tolerability of atypical antipsychotics in patients with bipolar disorder: prevalence, monitoring and management. *Bipolar Disorders*, 5 (suppl. 2), 62–79.

Cleary, M., Freeman, A., Hunt, G. E. and Walter, G. (2006). Patient and carer perceptions of need and associations with care-giving burden in an integrated adult mental health service. *Social Psychiatry and Psychiatric Epidemiology*, 41(3), 208–14.

Connolly, M. and Kelly, C. (2005). Lifestyle and physical health in schizophrenia. *Advances in Psychiatric Treatment*, 11, 125–32.

Cooney, G. M., Dwan, K., Greig, C. A., Lawlor, D. A., Rimer, J., Waugh, F. R., McMurdo, M. and Mead, G. E. (2013). Exercise for depression. *Cochrane Database Systematic Review*, 9:CD004366.

Cormac, I., Martin, D. and Ferriter, M. (2004) Improving the physical health of long-stay psychiatric in-patients. *Advances in Psychiatric treatment*, 10, 107–15.

Corry, P., Dru Drury, C. and Pinfold, V. (2004). *Lost and found. Voices from the forgotten generation*. London: Rethink.

Craft, L. L. and Landers, D. M. (1998). The effect of exercise on clinical depression and depression resulting from mental illness: a meta-analysis. *Journal of Sport and Exercise Psychology*, 20, 339–57.

Craft, L. L. and Perna, F. M. (2004). The benefits of exercise for the clinically depressed. *Primary Care Companion Journal of Clinical Psychiatry*, 6(3), 104–13.

Cramer, J. A. and Rosenbeck, R. (1998). Compliance with medication regimes for mental and physical disorders. *Psychiatric Services*, 49(2), 196–201.

Crone, D. and Guy, H. (2008). 'I know it's only exercise, but to me it is something that keeps me going': a qualitative approach to understanding mental health service users experiences of sports therapy. *International Journal of Mental Health Nursing*, 17(3), 197–207.

Daley, A. (2002) Exercise therapy and mental health in clinical populations: is exercise therapy a worthwhile intervention? *Advances in Psychiatric Treatment*, 8(4), 262–70.

Davies, S. C. (2014). *Annual report of the Chief Medical Officer, surveillance volume 2012: on the state of the public's health*. London: Department of Health.

Department of Health. (2001). *Making it happen: a guide to delivering mental health promotion*. London: HMSO.

Department of Health (2004). *At least five a week*. London: HM Government.

Department of Health (2011). *Start active, stay active: a report on physical activity for health from the four home countries' Chief Medical Officers*. London: HM Government.

Dimeo, F., Bauer, M., Varahram, I., Proest, G. and Halter, U. (2001). Benefits from aerobic exercise in patients with major depression: a pilot study. *British Journal of Sports Medicine*, 35, 114–17.

Ehmann, T. and Hanson, L. (2002). *Early psychosis: a care guide summary*. Vancouver: The University of British Columbia.

Ellis, N. J., Crone, D., Davey, R. and Grogan, S. (2007). Exercise interventions as an adjunct therapy for psychosis: A critical review. *British Journal of Clinical Psychology*, 46(1), 95–111.

Ellis, N. J., Randall, J. A. and Punnett, G. (2013). The effects of a single bout of exercise on mood and self-esteem in clinically diagnosed mental health patients. *Open Journal of Medical Psychology*, 2(3), 81–5.

Faulkner, G. and Sparkes, A. (1999). Exercise as a therapy for schizophrenia: an ethnographic study. *Journal of Sport and Exercise Psychology*, 21, 52–69.

Faulkner, G. and Taylor, A. H. (2005). Exercise and mental health promotion. In G. E. J. Faulkner and A. H. Taylor, eds., *Exercise, health and mental health: emerging relationships*. London: Routledge. Ch. 1.

Fogarty, M. and Happell, B. (2005). Exploring the benefits of an exercise program for people with schizophrenia: a qualitative study. *Issues in Mental Health Nursing*, 26, 341–51.

Forbes, D., Thiessen, E. J., Blake, C. M., Forbes, S. C. and Forbes, S. (2013). Exercise programs for people with dementia. *The Cochrane Library*, 12:CD006489.

Goff, D. C., Cather, C., Evins, E., Henderson, D. C., Freudenreich, O., Copeland, P. M., Bierer, M., Duckworth, K. and Sacks, F. M. (2005). Medical morbidity and mortality in schizophrenia: guidelines for psychiatrists. *Journal of Clinical Psychiatry*, 66(2), 183–94.

Hacking, S. and Bates, P. (2008). The inclusion web as a tool for person-centred planning and service evaluation. *Mental Health Review Journal: Research, Policy and Practice*, 13, 4–15.

Haddad, P. (2005). Weight change with atypical antipsychotics in the treatment of schizophrenia. *Journal of Psychopharmacology*, 19(6), 16–27.

Happell, B., Davies, C. and Scott, D. (2012). Health behaviour interventions to improve physical health in individuals diagnosed with a mental illness: a systematic review. *International Journal of Mental Health Nursing*, 21, 236–47.

Harris, E., C. and Barraclough, B. (1998). Excess mortality of mental disorder. *The British Journal of Psychiatry*, 173, 11–53.

Harvey, S. B., Hotopf, M., Øverland, S. and Mykletun, A. (2010). Physical activity and common mental disorders. *The British Journal of Psychiatry*, 197, 357–64.

Haslam, C., Brown, S., Atkinson, S. and Haslam, R. (2004). Patients' experiences of medication for anxiety and depression: effects on working life. *Family Practice*, 21(2), 204–12.

Hassmen, P., Koivula, N. and Uutela, A. (2000). Physical exercise and psychological well-being: a population study in Finland. *Preventive Medicine*, 30, 17–25.

Health and Social Care Information Centre (2012). *Health Survey for England 2012: health, social care and lifestyles*. London: HSCIC.

Heyn, P., Abreu, B. C. and Ottenbacher, K. J. (2004). The effects of exercise training on elderly persons with cognitive impairment and dementia: a meta-analysis. *Archives of Physical Medicine and Rehabilitation*, 85(10), 1694–1704.

HM Government (2014). *Moving more, living more: the physical activity Olympic and Paralympic legacy for the nation*. London: HM Government.

Holley, J., Crone, D., Tyson, P. and Lovell, G. (2011). The effects of physical activity on psychological well-being for those with schizophrenia: a systematic review. *British Journal of clinical Psychology*, 50(1), 84–105.

Hutchinson, D. S. (2005). Structured exercise for persons with serious psychiatric disabilities. *Psychiatric Services*, 56(3), 353–54.

Kessler, R. C., Berglund, P., Demler, O., Jin, R., Merikangas, K. R. and Walters, E. E. (2005). Lifetime prevalence and age-of-onset distributions of DSM-IV disorders in the National Comorbidity Survey Replication. *Archives of General Psychiatry*. 62(6), 593–602.

Killackey, E., Anda, A. L., Gibbs, M., Alvarez-Jimenez, M., Thompson, A., Sun, P. and Baksheev, G.N. (2011). Using internet enabled mobile devices and social networking technologies to promote exercise as an intervention for young first episode psychosis patients. *BMC Psychiatry*, 11, 80 doi:10.1186/1471-244X-11-80

Lam, R. and Kennedy, S. H. (2004). Evidence-based strategies for achieving and sustaining full remission in depression: focus on metaanalyses. *Canadian Journal of Psychiatry*, 49(suppl.1), 17–26S.

Lambert, T. J. R., Velakoulis, D. and Pantelis, C. (2003). Medical comorbidity in schizophrenia. *Medical Journal of Australia*, 178(suppl.), S67–70.

Lampinen, P., Heikkinen, R. L. and Ruoppila, I. (2000). Changes in intensity of physical exercise as predictors of depressive symptoms among older adults: an eight-year follow-up. *Preventive Medicine*, 30, 371–80.

Lautenschlager, N. T., Almeido, O. P., Klicker, L. and Janca, A. (2004). Can physical activity improve the mental health of older adults? *Annals of General Hospital Psychiatry*, 3(12), doi: 10.1186/1475-2832-3-12.

Law, L. L. F., Barnett, F., Yau, M. K. and Gray, M. A. (2014). Effects of combined cognitive and exercise interventions on cognition in older adults with and without cognitive impairment: a systematic review. *Ageing Research Reviews*, 15, 61–75.

Malchow, B., Reich-Erkelenz, D., Oertel-Knöchel, V., Keller, K., Hasan, A., Schmitt, A., Scheewe, T. W., Cahn, W., Kahn, R. S. and Falkai, P. (2013). The effects of physical exercise in schizophrenia and affective disorders. *European Archives of Psychiatry* and *Clinical Neuroscience*, 263(6), 451–67.

Mammen, G. and Faulkner, G. (2013). Physical activity and the prevention of depression: a systematic review of prospective studies. *American Journal of Preventive Medicine*, 45(5), 649–57.

Martinsen, E. W. (2000) Physical activity for mental health. *Tidaakr nor Laegeforen*, 120(25), 3054–6.

Marzolini, S., Jensen, B. and Melville, P. (2009). Feasibility and effects of a group-based resistance and aerobic exercise program for individuals with severe schizophrenia: a multidisciplinary approach. *Mental Health and Physical Activity*, 2(1), 29–36.

McCrone, P., Dhanasiri, S., Patel, A., Knapp, M. and Lawton-Smith, S. (2008). *Paying the price. The cost of mental health care in England to 2026*. London: The King's Fund.

McDevitt, J., Wilbur, J., Kogan, J. and Briller, J. (2005). A walking program for outpatients in psychiatric rehabilitation: a pilot study. *Biological Research for Nursing*, 7(2), 87–97.

Mead, G. E., Morley, W., Campbell, P., Greig, C. A., McMurdo, M. and Lawlor, D. A. (2008) Exercise for depression. *Cochrane Database of Systematic Reviews*, 4, CD004366.

Mehlig, K., Skoog, I., Waern, M., Miao Jonasson, J., Lapidus, L., Björkelund, C., Ostling, S. and Lissner, L. (2014). Physical activity, weight status, diabetes and dementia: a 34-year follow-up of the Population Study of Women in Gothenburg. *Neuroepidemiology*, 42(4), 252–9.

Mental Health Foundation. (2000). *Strategies for living: a report of user-led research into people's strategies for living with mental distress.* London: Mental Health Foundation.

Mental Health Foundation (2013a). *Starting today: the future of mental health services.* London, Mental Health Foundation.

Mental Health Foundation (2013b). *Let's get physical: the impact of physical activity on wellbeing.* London, Mental Health Foundation.

Mentality (2004). *Mental health promotion – implementing standard one of the National Service Framework for Mental Health.* London: SCMH.

Mind. (2007). *Ecotherapy: the green agenda for mental health.* London: Mind.

Morgan, A. J., Parker, A. G., Alvarez-Jimenez, M. and Jorm, A. F. (2013). Exercise and mental health: an Exercise and Sports Science Australia commissioned review. *Journal of Exercise Physiology online*, 16(4), 64–73.

National Institute for Clinical Excellence (NICE) (2011). *Service user experience in adult mental health: improving the experience of care for people using adult NHS mental health services.* NICE guidelines [CG136].

National Institute for Clinical Excellence (NICE) (2012). *Quality standard for patient experience in adult NHS services.* NICE guidelines [QS15].

NHS England/Commissioning Policy and Primary Care/Commissioning Policy and Resources (2014), *Commissioning for Quality and Innovation (CQUIN): 2014/15 guidance.* Leeds: Commissioning Policy and Primary Care.

NHS Information Centre for Health and Social Care. (2009). *Health survey for England 2008: physical activity and fitness.* London: NHS Information Centre for Health and Social Care.

Norton, S., Matthews, F. E., Barnes, D. E., Yaffe, K. and Brayne, C. (2014). Potential for primary prevention of Alzheimer's disease: an analysis of population-based data. *The Lancet Neurology*, 13(8), 788–94.

O'Kane, P. and McKenna, B. (2002). Five-a-side makes the difference. *Mental Health Nursing*, 22(5), 6–9.

Ossa, D. and Hutton, J. (2002). *The economic burden of physical inactivity in England.* London: MEDTAP International.

Pasco, J. A., Williams, L. J., Jacka, F. N., Henry, M. J., Coulson, C. E., Brennan, S. L., Leslie, E., Nicholson, G. C., Kotowicz, M. A. and Berk, M. (2011). Habitual physical activity and the risk for depressive and anxiety disorders among older men and women. *International Psychogeriatrics*, 23(2), 292–8.

Pearsall, R., Smith, D. J., Pelosi, A. and Geddes, J. (2014). Exercise therapy in adults with serious mental illness: a systematic review and meta-analysis. *BMC Psychiatry* 14, 117, doi: 10.1186/1471-244X-14-117.

Pelham, T. W. and Campagna, P. D. (1991). Benefits of exercise in psychiatric rehabilitation of persons with schizophrenia. *Canadian Journal of Rehabilitation*, 4(3), 159–68.

Pelham, T. W., Campagna, P. D., Ritvo, P. G. and Birnie, W. A. (1993). The effects of exercise therapy on clients in a psychotic rehabilitation program. *Psychosocial Rehabilitation Journal*, 16, 75–84.

Pilgrim, D. (2005). *Key concepts in mental health.* London: SAGE.

Priest, P. (2007). The healing balm effect; using a walking group to feel better. *Journal of Health Psychology*, 12(1), 36–52.

Radcliffe, J. and Smith, R. (2007). Acute in-patient psychiatry: how patients spend their time on acute psychiatric wards. *Psychiatric Bulletin*, 31, 167–70.

Randall, J. (2015). *The effect of a single bout of exercise on mood and self-esteem in individuals with a clinical mental health diagnosis*, Doctoral research, Staffordshire University.

Randall, J., Ellis, N., Gidlow, C. and Jones, M. (2014). Comparing mental health diagnoses: changes in mood and self-esteem following a single bout of exercise. *The Journal of Psychological Therapies in Primary Care*, 3(1), 34–6.

Rehor, P. R., Dunnagan, T., Stewart, G. and Cooley, D. (2001). Alteration of mood state after a single bout of non-competitive and competitive exercise programs. *Perceptual and Motor Skills*, 93, 249–56.

Rethorst, C. D. and Trivedi, M. H. (2013). Evidence-based recommendations for the prescription of exercise for major depressive disorder. *Journal of Psychiatric Practice*, 19(3), 204–12.

Richardson, C. R., Faulkner, G., McDevitt, J., Skrinar, G. S., Hutchinson, D. S. and Piette, J. D. (2005). Integrating physical activity into mental health services for persons with serious mental illness. *Psychiatric Services*, 56(3), 324–31.

Royal College of Psychiatrists (2010). *No health without mental health: the supporting evidence*. Royal College of Psychiatrists, London.

Scarborough, P., Bhatnagar, P., Wickramsinghe, K. K., Allender, S., Foster, C. and Rayer, M. (2011). The economic burden of ill health due to diet, physical inactivity, smoking, alcohol and obesity in the UK: an update to the 2006–2007 NHS costs. *Journal of Public Health*, 33(4) 527–35.

Shah, A., Alshaher, M., Dawn, B., Siddiqui, T., Longaker, R., Stoddard, M. F. and El-Mallakh, R. (2007). Exercise tolerance is reduced in bipolar illness. *Journal of Affective Disorders*, 104, 191–5.

Shiers, D. E., Rafi, I., Cooper, S. J., Holt, R. I. G. (2014). *Positive cardiometabolic health resource: an intervention framework for patients with psychosis and schizophrenia. 2014 update*. London: Royal College of Psychiatrists.

Sin, J. and Gamble, C. (2003). Managing side-effects to the optimum: valuing a client's experience. *Journal of Psychiatric and Mental Health Nursing*, 10(2), 147–53.

Singleton, N., Bumpstead, R., O'Brien, M., Lee A. and Meltzer, H. (2001). *Psychiatric morbidity among adults living in private households, 2000*. London: The Stationary Office.

Social Exclusion Unit (2004). *Mental health and social exclusion*. London: Office of the Deputy Prime Minister.

Sokal, J., Messias, E., Dickerson, F. B., Kreyenbuhl, J., Brown, C. H., Goldberg, R. W. and Dixon, L. B. (2004). Co-morbidity of medical illnesses among adults with serious mental illness who are receiving community psychiatric services. *Journal of Nervous Mental Diseases*, 192(6), 421–7.

Sparling, P. B., Howard, B. J., Dunstan, D. W. and Owen, N. (2015). Recommendations for physical activity in older adults. *British Medical Journal*, 350, h100.

Stathopoulou G., Powers, M. B., Berry A. C., Smits, J. A. J. and Otto, M. W. (2006). Exercise interventions for mental health: a quantitative and qualitative review. *Clinical Psychology (New York)*, 13, 179–93.

Strawbridge, W. J., Deleger, S., Roberts, R. E. and Kaplan, G. A. (2002). Physical activity reduces the risk of subsequent depression for older adults. *American Journal of Epidemiology*, 156(4), 328–34.

Ten Have, M., de Graaf, R. and Monshouwer, K. (2011) Physical exercise in adults and mental health status: findings from the Netherlands Mental Health Survey and Incidence Study (NEMESIS). *Journal of Psychosomatic Research*, 71, 342–8.

The MaGPIe Research Group (2003). The nature and prevalence of psychological problems in New Zealand primary care: a report on Mental Health and General Practice Investigation (MaGPIe). *The New Zealand Medical Journal*, 116, 1171.

Vancampfort, D., Probst, M., Helvik Skjaerven, L., Catalán-Matamoros, D., Lundvik-Gyllensten, A., Gómez-Conesa, A., Ijntema, R. and De Hert, M. (2012). Systematic review of the benefits of physical therapy within a multidisciplinary care approach for people with schizophrenia. *Physical Therapy*, 92, 11–23.

Wallcraft, J. (1998). *Healing minds: a report on current research, policy and practice concerning the use of complementary and alternative therapies for a wide range of mental health problems*. London: Mental Health Foundation.

Walsh, R. (2011). Lifestyle and mental health. *American Psychologist*, 66(7), 579–92.

Weinstein, A. A., Deuster, P. A., Francis, P. L., Beadling, C. and Kop, W. J. (2010). The role of depression in short-term mood and fatigue responses to acute exercise. *International Journal of Behavioral Medicine*, 17(1), 51–7.

Wen, C. P., Wai J. P. M., Tsai, M. K., Yi Yang, C., Cheng, T. Y. D., Lee, M.-C., Chan, H. T., Tsao, C. K., Tsai, S. P. and Wu, X. (2011). Minimum amount of physical activity for reduced mortality and extended life expectancy: a prospective cohort study. *The Lancet*, 378(9798), 1244–53.

Wirshing, D. A. (2004). Schizophrenia and obesity: impact of antipsychotic medications. *Journal of Clinical Psychiatry*, 65(18), 13–26.

Wolff E., Gaudlitz K., von Lindenberger B. L., Plag J., Heinz A., and Ströhle, A. (2011). Exercise and physical activity in mental disorders. *European Archives of Psychiatry and Clinical Neuroscience*, 261(suppl. 2), S186–91.

World Health Organisation (WHO) (2008). *Global burden of disease, 2004 update*. Geneva, World Health Organisation.

World Health Organisation (2010). *Global recommendations for physical activity for health*. Geneva, World Health Organisation.

World Health Organisation (2013). *Mental health action plan 2013–2020*. Geneva, World Health Organisation.

Chapter 6

Physical activity for cancer

Clare Stevinson, Anna Campbell, and Helen Crank

Introduction

Cancer is a group of diseases defined by disruption of the usual process of cellular turnover due to changes in the genetic information of cells. Instead of reproducing in an orderly, regulated manner, cancerous cells multiply uncontrollably, accumulating in a mass (known as a tumour or neoplasm). A cancerous (i.e. malignant) tumour will also invade the normal tissue surrounding it, and malignant cells can spread to others sites in the body through the bloodstream or lymphatic system, a process known as metastasis. Major organs such as the lung, brain, and liver, are common sites for metastasised cells. Cancer can develop in almost any part of the body, with more than 200 different types of cancer cell identified. However, the vast majority are classed as carcinomas, meaning that they originate from epithelial cells that cover the body's outer and inner surfaces. Other types of cancer cell include leukaemias (arising from blood cells), lymphomas (lymphatic system), and sarcomas (connective tissues such as muscle, bone, and cartilage).

Causes of cancer include endogenous (i.e. within the body) and exogenous (i.e. outside the body) factors. A small proportion (approximately 5–10 per cent) of cancer is attributed to inherited genes that increase the risk of developing the disease. Other endogenous causes are related to excessive exposure to oxidative stress, chronic inflammation, or hormones. Among exogenous factors, tobacco use is a known risk factor for multiple cancers, and is particularly associated with lung cancer. Others include infectious agents (e.g. viruses, bacteria, parasites), industrial chemicals (e.g. asbestos, arsenic, some pesticides), radiation, and food contaminants. Additional lifestyle factors such as poor diet (e.g. consumption of processed meat, insufficient vegetable and fruit), alcohol use, weight gain, and lack of physical activity are also implicated in contributing to some cancer cases (Parkin et al., 2011).

Cancer statistics

Each year, approximately 14.1 million new cases of cancer are diagnosed worldwide (Stewart and Wild, 2014). In the United Kingdom (UK), more than one in three people will develop cancer at some time during their lifetime, and the latest UK statistics show that more than 331,000 people were diagnosed with cancer in 2011 (Cancer Research UK, 2014). The most common sites of cancer diagnosis in the UK population are displayed in Figure 6.1. Breast cancer accounts for 15 per cent of all new cases, and lung, prostate, and bowel cancer each account for 13 per cent of cases.

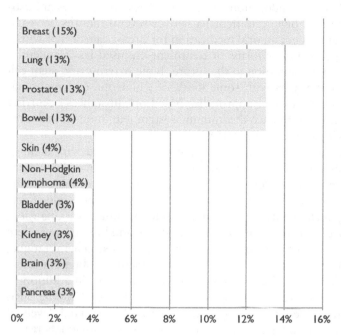

Figure 6.1 The ten most common sites of cancer diagnosis in the UK (percentage of cases).

Source: data from Cancer Research UK (2014). Cancer Statistics Report: Cancer Incidence and Mortality in the UK. Available at: http://publications.cancerresearchuk.org/ [accessed 22.07.14]

Cancer is more common in later life, with 53 per cent of cases diagnosed in people aged fifty to seventy four years, and 36 per cent after age seventy five years. Thanks to improved detection systems and more effective treatment options, cancer deaths have been reduced by 10 per cent in the last decade, with over half of patients living for at least ten years (Cancer Research UK, 2014). Estimated prevalence (the number of people alive following a cancer diagnosis) is currently approximately 3 per cent (representing about two million people) (Maddams et al., 2009). However, since the UK population is aging, cancer prevalence is projected to increase by 55 per cent in males and 35 per cent in females in the next two decades, resulting in more than four million people living with or beyond cancer by 2030 (Mistry et al., 2011).

Cancer treatment

The most common treatments for cancer are surgery, chemotherapy, radiation, and hormonal therapy. Many patients will receive more than one treatment approach. Surgery involves the excision of a localised tumour along with some of the surrounding healthy tissue, and sometimes associated lymph nodes. Chemotherapy is a systemic treatment approach using drugs to destroy cancer cells. It is commonly administered intravenously, or orally by taking tablets, over a number of cycles. Radiotherapy involves the use of high-energy X-rays or electron beams to deliver repeated small doses (known as fractions) of radiation to the site of cancer. Some patients can receive radiotherapy internally through radioactive liquids or implants. Hormone treatments are medications used to treat cancers that are hormone-sensitive (e.g. breast, ovarian, prostate), by altering the effects of endogenous hormones. These treatments are usually taken orally on a continuous or intermittent basis over several months or years. A well-known example is Tamoxifen, an oral medication for breast cancer that works by blocking oestrogen receptors. Other forms of treatment are used less frequently, although some may become more common in the future. Bone marrow and stem cell transplants are performed on patients with some kinds of leukaemia or lymphoma. Biological therapies refer to a number of approaches based on substances occurring naturally in the body that aim to influence the immune system (e.g. monoclonal antibodies, interferon, interleukin, and cancer vaccines).

Although effective in treating cancer, most therapies are associated with a range of side-effects, some of which are self-limiting and others longer-lasting. For example, following surgery, patients can suffer from infections or complications with the wound, post-operative pain, or lymphoedema. Some of the more common side-effects possible with chemotherapy include fatigue, nausea, appetite loss (anorexia), hair loss (alopecia), nerve damage (neuropathy), sore mouth (mucositis), and low red and white blood cell counts (anaemia and neutropenia). Radiotherapy can cause general fatigue, along with pain and other problems specific to the site of treatment (e.g. breathlessness or coughing after chest radiation, or diarrhoea after pelvic radiation). In addition to the direct side-effects of therapies, receiving a cancer diagnosis and undergoing difficult treatments can have a negative impact on psychological wellbeing. High levels of emotional distress are reported among cancer patients, with many individuals reaching clinical levels of anxiety and depression (Linden et al., 2012).

Evidence for exercise

Studies investigating the role of exercise for cancer patients have been accumulating since the 1980s, when several trials suggested that women who exercised during chemotherapy for breast cancer had superior physical functioning and mood than patients receiving usual care (Winningham and MacVicar, 1988; MacVicar et al., 1989; MacVicar and Winningham, 1986). In outlining their model of physical activity and cancer control, Courneya and Friedenreich (2007) identified key areas where exercise may have potential benefit. These included preparing for treatment, coping with the side-effects of cancer therapy, rehabilitating after treatment completion, and receiving palliative care. A summary of the current evidence base in these areas is provided.

Exercise pre-treatment

The potential value of performing exercise before the commencement of cancer therapy has been highlighted, since fitter individuals may be better able to tolerate difficult treatments (Silver and Baima, 2013). For other conditions, prehabilitation exercise ahead of surgery has been shown to reduce inpatient stays and post-treatment complications (Valkenet et al., 2011; see Chapter 10 for further information on prehabilitation). For cancer, a systematic review of eighteen intervention trials included ten randomised controlled trials (RCTs) of pre-surgery exercise prescriptions (Singh et al., 2013). The majority of trials involved lung cancer patients engaging in walking or supervised aerobic exercise. Although findings were mixed, there were some encouraging results for pulmonary and cardiovascular parameters, and shorter hospi-talisations. Results from four other trials suggested that pelvic floor exercises helped to reverse incontinence following prostatectomy.

Exercise during treatment

In one early RCT, seventy inpatients with solid tumours receiving high-dose chemo-therapy followed by stem cell transplantation were allocated to daily exercise on a supine cycle ergometer or to usual care (Dimeo et al., 1997). At discharge, exercisers recorded a significantly smaller decline in physical performance (14 per cent) than controls (19 per cent), and had been hospitalised for one and a half fewer days. Several treatment-related complications were lower among the exercise group, including pain, diarrhoea, thrombopenia, and neutropenia. A systematic review of eight RCTs of exer-cise interventions for cancer patients undergoing haematopoietic stem cell transplants reported some encouraging results (Wiskemann and Huber, 2008). Exercising during inpatient stays helped to prevent aerobic and muscular deconditioning, enhance qual-ity of life, and improve immune function. Exercise after discharge led to improvements in aerobic and muscular functioning, quality of life, and body composition.

A comprehensive systematic review published in 2010 summarised all randomised and non-randomised controlled trials involving exercise interventions for cancer pop-ulations (Speck et al., 2010). Based on thirty three trials involving exercise performed during treatment (usually chemotherapy or radiotherapy), significant small to moder-ate beneficial effects were evident for aerobic fitness, muscular strength, body fat per-centage, and anxiety. Subsequently, another systematic review focused solely on quality of life outcomes from trials of exercise performed during cancer treatment (Mishra et al., 2012a). Collectively, the results from fifty six RCT or quasi-randomised trials indicated an overall small improvement in global quality of life (standardised mean difference of 0.33) after exercise interventions, compared with control conditions.

Childhood cancer

Unsurprisingly, given that cancer is most common in later life, the majority of exer-cise research has focused on adults. Nonetheless a limited number of small-scale studies have addressed childhood cancers, and several systematic reviews have sum-marised the evidence to date. Observational studies suggest that physical activity levels are reduced during treatment periods, and may remain lower in the long-term, compared with healthy controls (Winter et al., 2010). Meanwhile, the results of intervention trials provide encouraging evidence that exercise can be feasible and safe for patients during treatment, and may lead to benefits in physical function, fatigue, and quality of life outcomes (Huang and Ness, 2011; Baumann et al., 2013; Braam et al., 2013).

Exercise post-treatment

A systematic review published in the *British Medical Journal* in 2012 (Fong et al., 2012) included thirty four RCTs of exercise performed after cancer treatment com-pletion. Meta-analysis of data suggested that when compared with non-exercising control groups, small improvements from exercise interventions existed for a range of clinical outcomes. These included cardiorespiratory fitness (increase in peak oxygen consumption of 2.2 ml·kg⁻¹·min⁻¹, and in 6-minute walk test of 29m), body composition (weight loss of 1.1kg), upper-body strength (6kg increase in one repetition maximum bench press), and lower-body strength (19kg increase in one repetition maximum leg press). Quality of life outcomes were also significantly improved.

Other systematic reviews have focused on specific outcomes. For cancer-related fatigue a review of fifty six RCTs indicated an overall significant reduction in fatigue following exercise interventions compared with no-exercise control conditions (Cramp and Byron-Daniel, 2012). Meta-analysis elicited larger effects for exercise performed post-treatment than during treatment (standardised mean difference of 0.44 versus 0.23). Another review of seventy RCTs concluded that exercise during treatment had a palliative effect, while after treatment the effect was recuperative (Puetz and Herring, 2012). Fatigue is a common side-effect of many cancer treatments, and is exacerbated by the deconditioning associated with excessive rest. The evidence suggests that appropriate levels of exercise during and post-treatment can help prevent the development of a vicious cycle of declining functional fitness and increasing fatigue (Figure 6.2).

Quality of life changes were examined in a review of forty RCTs or quasi-randomised trials of post-treatment exercise interventions (Mishra et al, 2012b). Pooling data suggested a moderate increase in global quality of life at the end of interventions that was maintained at later follow-up points. Depression symptoms were also significantly influenced by exercise to a modest degree, based on a meta-analysis of fifteen RCTs involving exercise interventions performed either during or after cancer therapy (Craft et al., 2012). Cardiorespiratory fitness outcomes were meta-analysed from six RCTs of supervised exercise training versus no-exercise controls (Jones et al., 2011). Significant increases in peak oxygen consumption were more pronounced for exercise performed

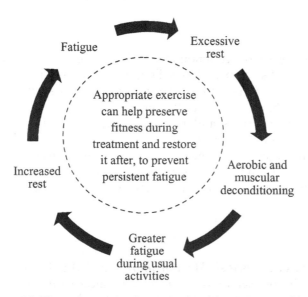

Figure 6.2 The vicious cycle of cancer-related fatigue, rest, and loss of functional fitness.

post-treatment ($3.4 \text{ ml} \cdot \text{kg}^{-1} \cdot \text{min}^{-1}$) than during treatment ($1.2 \text{ ml} \cdot \text{kg}^{-1} \cdot \text{min}^{-1}$). A review of eight trials of bone health outcomes (e.g. bone mineral density) concluded that studies were too few in number, and too inconsistent in methods and results, to determine the impact of exercise (Winters-Stone et al., 2010).

Exercise in palliative care

The benefits achievable through exercise are not limited to patients with good prognoses. Several systematic reviews of a small, but growing, body of evidence have concluded that exercise interventions may help maintain, or slow the decline in, quality of life and fatigue among patients with advanced cancer (Lowe et al., 2009; Beaton et al., 2009; Albrecht and Taylor, 2012). The strongest evidence has come from a large RCT involving 231 patients with incurable disease and short life expectancy (Oldervoll et al., 2011), comparing the effects of an eight-week supervised group exercise intervention with usual care. Unsurprisingly, given the population, the number of patients not completing the trial was high (36 per cent and 23 per cent in the exercise and control arms respectively). Nonetheless, encouraging results were reported, with significant increases in physical function outcomes (grip strength and walking performance) observed for the exercise group. These improvements can be very important for enabling the performance of activities of daily living.

Exercise for survival and disease progression

Although there is a substantial body of research relating to physical activity and the primary prevention of cancer (Clague and Bernstein, 2012), there is limited evidence on whether exercise influences prognosis. The first epidemiological study on this subject, published in 2005, reported outcomes for 2987 women diagnosed with breast cancer and followed up for an average of eight years (Holmes et al., 2005). The results indicated significant reductions in risk of all-cause mortality (relative risk [RR] of 0.65), breast cancer mortality (RR: 0.60), and breast cancer recurrence (RR: 0.74) for the most active women (≥ 24 metabolic equivalents × hours [MET-h] per week) compared with the least active (< 3 MET-h per week). Subsequent studies have generally supported these findings. A systematic review of studies of physical activity and disease outcomes included seventeen studies on breast cancer with follow-up periods ranging from three to thirteen years (Ballard-Barbash et al., 2012). Among nine studies assessing physical activity performed pre-diagnosis, most indicated a slightly lower risk of death from breast cancer and from any cause, although only one reached statistical significance. However, from eight studies assessing post-diagnosis physical activity, the results were stronger. Most studies found lower rates of all-cause mortality and breast cancer deaths for the most active women, with over half being significant results. The magnitude of the risk reduction was in the region of 40–50 per cent in some studies (Chen et al., 2011; Irwin et al., 2011; Holick et al., 2008), having adjusted for relevant risk factors such as age, cancer stage, menopausal status, body composition, and diet.

A more recent analysis was based on the follow-up data of 242 breast cancer patients who took part in a randomised trial of aerobic and resistance exercise interventions during their chemotherapy treatment (Courneya et al., 2007). Eight years later, disease-free survival was slightly higher for those who had exercised during the trial than those who had received usual care (83 per cent versus 76 per cent) (Courneya et al., 2014). Although not a statistically significant difference, the results are supportive of the earlier observational studies on survival after breast cancer survival. With several large intervention trials ongoing, future long-term follow-up data will be available to help clarify the effects of exercise on disease progression outcomes.

For other cancers, evidence is scarcer. Three studies that focused on the post-diagnosis physical activity of colorectal cancer patients indicated reductions in risk of all-cause mortality and cancer-specific mortality in the region of 50 per cent. Interestingly, the weekly volume of activity needed to achieve a significant reduction was ≥18 MET-h in a study of women (Mcyerhardt et al., 2006), but ≥ 27 MET-h in two other studies involving men (Meyerhardt et al, 2006; Meyerhardt et al., 2009). Effects of pre-diagnosis physical activity on survival were not evident (Meyerhardt et al., 2006; Haydon et al., 2006). Two studies of pre-diagnosis physical activity did not show an association with ovarian cancer mortality rates (Yang et al., 2008; Moorman et al., 2011).

One study of 2705 men with prostate cancer reported that the risk of death from prostate cancer was halved in men achieving ≥ 48 MET-h per week of activity compared with those achieving < 3 MET-h per week (Kenfield et al., 2011). For all-cause mortality, a significantly lower risk (30 per cent) was evident at 9 MET-h, but a greater one (60 per cent) was demonstrated at ≥ 48 MET-h per week. In a separate study involving 1455 prostate cancer patients (Richman et al., 2011), walking at a fast pace (≥ 3 miles per hour) led to a reduced risk of disease progression compared with walking slowly (< 3 miles per hour), regardless of the distance walked.

Two further studies focused on populations with poor prognosis. One included 243 patients with recurrent malignant brain tumours (Ruden et al., 2011), and observed a significantly longer survival (twenty two months) among those reporting higher physical activity (9 MET-h per week), than those who were less active (thirteen months). The other study, including 118 patients with inoperable lung cancer (Jones et al., 2012), had very similar results, with neither study reaching statistical significance. Nonetheless, in conjunction with evidence of higher fitness levels predicting lower mortality in this population after adjusting for other prognostic factors (Jones et al., 2010; Jones et al., 2012; Sui et al., 2010), there are promising signs that physical activity may influence survival.

There is some preliminary evidence that effects of exercise on recurrence and mortality outcomes may be partly mediated by tumour phenotype. The risk of mortality was reduced by 50 per cent among women with oestrogen receptor (ER) positive breast cancer tumours compared with a 9 per cent risk reduction for those with ER negative tumours (Holmes et al., 2005). The presence of other tumour markers such as p27, β-catenin, and prostaglandin-endoperoxide synthase 2 (PTGS2) may also be predictive of the influence of exercise on prognosis (Morikawa et al., 2011; Yamauchi et al., 2013).

Potential mechanisms of exercise

Postulated mechanisms by which physical activity might influence cancer progression include: modulation of the insulin pathway (e.g. effects on circulating levels of glucose, insulin, insulin-like growth factor 1 [IGF-1] and IGF binding proteins); improvements in cellular immune surveillance (e.g. numbers and lytic ability of natural killer cells); reduced systemic inflammation (through modulation of cytokines such as IL-6, TNF-α); modulation of sex steroid hormone levels (e.g. oestrogen); and reductions in oxidative damage (by counteracting production of reactive oxygen species). Although research into these postulated host pathways is in its infancy, there is emerging clinical and pre-clinical evidence of associations between exercise biomarkers and physical activity. One review (Betof et al., 2013) evaluated twenty four observational studies and RCTs of the effects of exercise training on blood-based biomarkers in cancer survivors. The most widely studied pathway was the insulin pathway, with the majority of the studies suggesting that exercise is associated with changes in levels of IGF1, its associated binding protein (IGFBP-3), and the IGF-1:IGFBP-3 ratio. Two RCTs, which specifically recruited sedentary obese breast cancer survivors, showed that the exercise group also experienced a borderline significant decrease in fasting insulin (Ligibel et al., 2008; Irwin et al., 2009). Nine studies investigating the effects of exercise on the inflammatory and immune systems have produced more variable results *in vitro* and *in vivo*. C-reactive protein (CRP), an acute phase protein linked with systemic inflammation, was most consistently shown to decrease with exercise in four trials with breast and prostate cancer survivors (Fairey et al., 2005; Galvão et al., 2010; George et al., 2010, Pierce et al., 2009). Two studies examined exercise in relation to oxidative damage to DNA, with one indicating reduced excretion of a marker of oxidative damage and tumour progression (8-oxo-dG) in colorectal cancer patients after treatment (Allgayer et al., 2008). In the other study, exercise increased levels of F2-isopostanes, eicosanoid markers of oxidative stress, in lung cancer patients (Jones et al., 2011). To date, no exercise studies in breast cancer survivors have measured changes in sex steroid hormones [SSH] as a primary outcome, despite a large number of RCTs in post-menopausal women showing significant effects of exercise on the SSH estradiol and free estradiol. An overview of the potential mechanisms is depicted in Figure 6.3. In order to examine whether exercise has a direct effect on tumour growth and metastasis through blood perfusion, angiogenesis, or other host related factors, research using animal models is now underway.

Exercise dimensions

The optimal volume or dimensions of exercise for achieving specific outcomes is difficult to establish and may vary for each individual. Below is a summary of existing evidence on the key dimensions of mode, intensity, duration, and frequency.

Mode of exercise

Although the majority of trials have involved aerobic forms of exercise, there is a growing number involving resistance training. Four systematic reviews have focused exclusively on trials involving resistance exercise interventions. The most recent review included fifteen RCTs of resistance training performed either during or post-treatment (Focht et al., 2013). Meta-analysis of data indicated significant overall effects on several outcomes in comparison with control conditions. Effects were large for increased

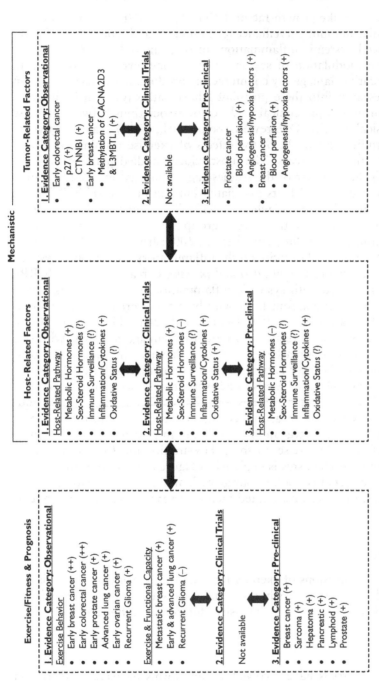

Figure 6.3 Overview of possible mechanisms of exercise on cancer progression. Reprinted with permission from Betof, A. S., Dewhirst, M. W., Jones, L. W. [2013]. Effects and potential mechanisms of exercise training on cancer progression: a translational perspective. *Brain Behaviour and Immunity* 30, S75–87. Copyright 2013, Elsevier.

Evidence-based representation of the known effects and mechanisms of exercise on tumor progression adopting a bi-directional translational research or scientific discovery (T0) paradigm. Exercise/fitness and prognosis, evidence supporting association between self-reported exercise behavior, objective measures of exercise capacity or functional capacity, and cancer prognosis; Host-Related Factors, postulated systemic (host-related) pathways mediating the association between exercise behavior and exercise/functional capacity and cancer prognosis; Tumor-Related Factors, intratumoral factors shown to mediate the association between exercise and prognosis or factors shown to be modulated in response to exercise. $+ +$, strong evidence; $+ +$, moderate evidence; $+$, weak evidence; $-$, null; ?, unknown at present.

muscular fitness, moderate for increased cardiorespiratory fitness, and small for improved body composition and quality of life. These finding supported those of the other reviews (De Backer et al., 2009; Cramp et al., 2010; Strasser et al., 2013).

One RCT was designed to directly compare the benefits of aerobic and resistance exercise training (Courneya et al., 2007). This study involved 242 women undergoing chemotherapy for breast cancer who were randomised to twelve weeks of supervised bicycle ergometry or progressive resistance training, or usual care. As expected, aerobic exercise led to greater improvements in cardiorespiratory fitness, with increases in peak oxygen consumption of 2.0 ml·kg^{-1}·min^{-1} over usual care, and 1.4 ml·kg^{-1}·min^{-1} over resistance exercise. Similarly, resistance training led to superior gains in upper and lower body muscle strength. Improvements in one-repetition maximum tests for bench and leg press were greater by 7.7 and 6.8kg respectively compared with usual care, and by 5.2 and 6.8kg compared with aerobic training. No differences were evident on weight and body composition parameters although resistance training led to a greater gain in lean tissue (1kg more than usual care), than aerobic training (0.3kg more than usual care). Similar increases in self-esteem were observed with the two modes of exercise. Another RCT compared aerobic and resistance training interventions with usual care over six months in 121 men receiving radiotherapy for prostate cancer (Segal et al., 2009). Both modes of training reduced fatigue, and resistance exercise also led to improvements in quality of life, cardiorespiratory fitness, and upper and lower body strength.

Several trials have reported positive results using a combined aerobic and resistance intervention (Milne et al., 2008; Galvão et al., 2010; Adamsen et al., 2009). One trial directly examined the effects of a combined approach against two volumes of aerobic training (25–30 minutes or 50–60 minutes). A sample of 301 women receiving chemotherapy for breast cancer were randomised to one of the three supervised exercise interventions for training three times weekly (Courneya et al., 2013). Upper and lower body muscular strength and endurance outcomes were all superior after combined training, while the higher volume of aerobic exercise limited some of the decline observed in cardiovascular fitness during chemotherapy. Fatigue increased in all three groups, and no changes in body composition were demonstrated.

Other modes of exercise investigated include yoga and tai-chi. A systematic review of eighteen RCTs of yoga interventions for women with breast cancer reported small benefits from the majority of studies for symptoms of depression, anxiety, or stress, and quality of life outcomes (Harder et al., 2012). Evidence was inconsistent for fatigue. Quality of life was also significantly improved by tai chi or qigong in a systematic review and meta-analysis of thirteen RCTs across various cancers (Zeng et al., 2014). Effects on depression, anxiety, body composition, and cortisol changes were not clearly demonstrated.

Intensity of exercise

The majority of exercise programmes have been described as moderate intensity (typically 50–70 per cent of maximum performance). However, one RCT examined the effects of a high-intensity multimodal exercise programme over six weeks compared with usual care in 269 cancer patients receiving chemotherapy (Adamsen et al, 2009). The intervention comprised a combination of aerobic exercise on stationary bicycles

(85–95 per cent of maximum heart rate), and resistance exercises (70–100 per cent of one repetition maximum), on three days a week, along with relaxation, body awareness, and massage on additional days. The intervention was safely completed by participants, and led to improvements on measures of aerobic capacity, muscular function, fatigue, and psychological wellbeing.

Few trials have directly compared interventions of different intensities. One RCT compared moderate-intensity aerobic exercise (40–60 per cent heart rate reserve) with low-intensity (25–40 per cent), and a no-exercise control arm in eighteen patients with breast or colon cancer over ten weeks (Burnham and Wilcox, 2002). Although no significant differences between the exercise groups existed on physical function outcomes, the small sample raises the likelihood of the trial being insufficiently statistically powered to detect differences. Another RCT involving seventy three women with breast cancer-related lymphedema, compared twelve weeks of high- and low-intensity resistance exercise (each including a moderate-intensity aerobic exercise component), with a usual care control group (Gibbs et al., 2011). Both interventions produced superior results than usual care for measures of physical function, fatigue, and body image, but there was little difference between the two intensities.

Duration and frequency of exercise

The majority of exercise interventions have lasted approximately three months, with a few having longer durations of six or twelve months. One non-randomised trial compared two combined aerobic and resistance exercise interventions (lasting three months versus six months) with usual care in 114 women with breast cancer (Sprod et al., 2010). Results were mixed, with some outcomes improving in all three groups and few differences evident between the two exercise durations. Studies comparing the effects of different frequencies are also lacking. Most trials have employed an exercise frequency of three to five days, compatible with public health guidelines for health-enhancing physical activity.

With few trials available, evidence is currently insufficient to determine whether specific volumes, modes, or intensities of exercise are optimal for influencing particular outcomes. However, a number of trials designed to examine some of these questions are ongoing (Buffart et al., 2014), from which the findings may lead to greater precision in future exercise prescription.

Evidence for nutrition

Some common side-effects of cancer treatments include nausea, vomiting, anorexia, altered taste and smell, and bowel disturbance that may lead to reduced nutrient intake. Specialist oncology dieticians can provide individualised guidance to patients in developing appropriate diet plans. The general aims are to prevent or correct nutritional deficiencies, achieve or maintain a healthy body weight, preserve lean mass, and prevent fat gain. Treatments for some cancers that affect the upper or lower gastrointestinal system (e.g. oesophageal, liver, pancreatic, stomach, colorectal cancers) may result in specific long-term alterations to dietary intake. For all patients after treatment completion, dietary advice is aimed at avoiding excess weight gain, and minimising foods associated with increased risk of recurrence. An evidence-based report from the World Cancer Research Fund provided a series of dietary recommendations with regard to preventing cancer that were also directed to people with a cancer diagnosis (World Cancer Research Fund, 2007). These included limiting consumption of energy-dense foods, avoiding sugary drinks, eating mostly foods of plant origin (e.g. vegetables, fruit, unprocessed grains), limiting red meat, avoiding processed meat, limiting alcoholic drinks, limiting salt, and avoiding dietary supplements (unless specifically prescribed). The American Cancer Society also provides a useful overview of evidence on nutrition for cancer survivors (Rock et al., 2012).

Exercise prescription

In 2010, the American College of Sports Medicine (ACSM) convened a multidisciplinary expert panel to provide guidelines on exercise for cancer survivors (Schmitz et al., 2010). The panel concluded that exercise is safe and effective during and after cancer treatment. This review concentrated on breast, colon, prostate, gynaecological, and haematological cancers and provided cancer-specific screening/contraindications criteria for starting and stopping an exercise programme. For example, they recommended that a colon cancer patient with an ostomy should receive permission from a health professional before participating in contact sports. Similarly, if a woman with breast cancer reported swelling in the arm or hand during exercise (indicating risk of lymphoedema), it was recommended that upper body exercise should be minimised until appropriate medical evaluation and action took place. Currently, there is no position statement on exercise testing and training in people with cancer. Nonetheless, a set of guidelines relating to safety considerations for cancer survivors have been published in the ACSM's Guidelines for Exercise Testing and Prescription (Pescatello et al., 2014). The recommendations concerning screening and participation eligibility are deliberately conservative and applicable to a clinical setting rather than most community-based settings. They also do not necessarily apply to every person with cancer, because of the diversity of this patient population. The general recommendations in the UK (Campbell et al., 2012) are that, as far as they are able, cancer patients and survivors should adhere to the current physical activity guidelines for adults of at least 150 minutes per week of moderate-intensity aerobic activity and twice weekly strength-building exercise. Clinicians should advise cancer patients and survivors to avoid inactivity, even for patients with existing diseases, or who are undergoing difficult treatments. It is also important that exercise recommendations are tailored to the individual, to account for exercise tolerance and cancer-specific side-effects. For example, prostate cancer patients on hormone treatment with osteoporosis may be advised to include weight training in order to avoid bone thinning and fractures, whereas those with bone metastases would be discouraged from undertaking specific high-intensity resistance training.

Unlike cardiac rehabilitation, there is currently no formal or structured referral pathway or phased rehabilitation programme for those living with cancer. A number of pilot schemes exist, such as brief behaviour change interventions in the hospital setting, self-referrals to community-based exercise programmes, and GP referrals to generic gym-based programmes. One example, Move More Scotland, is described in Box 6.1.

Box 6.1 Case study: Move More Scotland

Move More Scotland is an initiative through Macmillan Cancer Support designed to help those affected by cancer in Scotland to remain active, throughout their treatment and afterwards. There are currently three programmes to choose from, all designed specifically for people with cancer. All activities are free of charge.

The first option is adapted classes in chi gung, an ancient Chinese practice of aligning breath and physical activity with mental and spiritual awareness. It can be practiced seated, so is open to people of all ages and abilities. The second programme involves walking groups, which are led by a trained volunteer. The walks are low-intensity, short, and sociable. The only requirement is a comfortable pair of shoes. Finally, there are circuit-based exercise classes. These are delivered by fitness instructors with specialist training in cancer and exercise. Gardening is soon to be added to the menu of options to widen the range of opportunities and offer appropriate activities for all individuals. All programmes are led or supported by volunteers.

Working in partnership with local authorities has allowed Move More to be delivered within local venues such as libraries, municipal gyms, and community halls. Classes and groups are accessible and welcoming to all – some can even be attended by carers, family, or friends of the person affected by cancer.

If a cancer survivor requires supervision or needs guidance on safe procedures, referral to a physiotherapist or cancer exercise specialist can help. In the UK, a National Occupational Standards awarding body, SkillsActive, ensures that all training providers teaching fitness instructors to design, adapt, or review programmes for cancer patients are registered with them. Most qualified cancer specialist exercise instructors are also members of the Register of Exercise Professionals (REPS). CanRehab provides training for cancer exercise fitness instructors and oncology health professionals to help create workable referral pathways from the clinic to safe and effective community-based programmes (Campbell, 2014).

More hospital and cancer centres are linking with local municipal/community leisure services where staff in the gym setting may have experience of working with cancer survivors as part of their clinical exercise programmes. Box 6.2 outlines an example of a collaborative programme in South-West England.

Box 6.2 Case study: Bournemouth Cancer Survivorship Programme

This twelve-week programme is run through a partnership between Royal Bournemouth and Christchurch Hospitals NHS Foundation Trust and Bournemouth Borough Council Littledown Centre. Patients are identified by clinicians and clinical nurse specialists, as part of the assessment and care-planning process. On referral, patients attend two one-to-one appointments with an exercise consultant at the leisure centre.

The first session includes an introduction to the programme and information pack, along with a review of personal health, goals, motivation, and exercise barriers. Measurements are also taken of blood pressure, resting pulse, weight, and height, and any treatment complications that will influence exercise recommendations (e.g. shoulder function, lymphoedema, wound tenderness) are noted.

In the second session, individuals undergo an exercise tolerance test, and their goals are reviewed and formalised. Advice is provided on appropriate activity recommendations, guided by the FITT principles, along with information on educational talks, workshops, and community opportunities available.

During the programme, individuals receive a three week supportive telephone call and a six week (mid-term) review. At the end of the twelve weeks, all measurements are repeated and changes noted. Future activity plans are discussed, along with the opportunity to continue exercising at the leisure centre and join a 'Living Well Active' community that continues to provide news and information, and offers to support physical activity. A final supportive telephone call is received after six months.

When referring individuals to any exercise specialist or community-based facility, doctors and patients should enquire about the exercise practitioner's qualifications and experience of working with the cancer population. The translation of guidelines into clinical practice is challenging because the guidelines do not cover the many logistical issues that may arise in clinical practice or in a community settings (e.g. triage of patients with complex needs). This highlights the developing nature of the field with there still being substantial knowledge gaps relating to optimal prescription and programme implementation.

Future research

A key focus of future research is the potential role of physical activity in influencing direct disease-related outcomes (e.g. recurrence, metastasis, and survival), and associated biological endpoints (e.g. immunological and hormonal function). In particular, the volume or intensity of exercise associated with meaningful changes for different cancer types would need to be determined. Similarly, there is scope for better understanding of whether exercise impacts the effectiveness of cancer therapies, and the side-effects of treatment, both in the short term and for longer-term outcomes (e.g. bone, metabolic, and cardiopulmonary health). The potential value of pre-treatment exercise (e.g. to improve fitness ahead of surgery or chemotherapy) is also an area deserving research. Given that the majority of studies have involved women with early-stage breast cancer, there is need for more inclusion of participants with less-common cancer diagnoses and more advanced disease. In addition, other demographic groups (e.g. young people, older adults, ethnic minorities), should be investigated. For example, the importance of exercise for the long-term health of childhood cancer survivors is under-studied. As well as determining the benefits achievable through exercise, there also needs to be a greater focus on behaviour-change research in this context, to know how to best help people become regularly active. A final important consideration for future research is cost-effectiveness. If exercise is to be included within routine cancer care in the future, economic analyses must be included alongside studies of the clinical benefits of exercise following cancer diagnosis.

Chapter summary

Cancer is characterised by the uncontrollable reproduction of abnormal cells in any part of the body. Left untreated, cancerous cells may invade surrounding tissue and spread to major organs. The most common treatments for cancer are surgery, chemotherapy, radiation, and hormonal therapy. In the UK, the current prevalence of cancer is approximately 3 per cent (representing about two million people), with the most prevalent cancer sites being breast and prostate. Since cancer is most common in later life, and the population is growing older, cancer prevalence is projected to increase by 55 per cent in males and 35 per cent in females by 2030. Evidence for various benefits of exercise following cancer diagnosis is accumulating. Exercise performed during treatment helps to preserve some physical function and quality of life, and control fatigue. Exercising post-treatment leads to improvements in muscular and cardiorespiratory fitness, fatigue, and psychological wellbeing. Some of these benefits are also achieved by patients with advanced cancer receiving palliative care. Emerging evidence suggests that exercise after diagnosis is associated with lower risk of mortality for breast and colorectal cancer patients. There is insufficient information on the precise type and volume of physical activity that is optimal for improving cancer-related outcomes. Most recommendations are compatible with public health guidelines for physical activity, with various precautions built in for the limitations of individual patients.

Study tasks

1   Doctors and nurses are often asked by patients about ways of reducing the risk of cancer returning. Based on the evidence to date on physical activity and cancer recurrence or survival, write a summary for health professionals to inform them of the cancers that have some promising results in this area.

2   Henry is an overweight, inactive seventy-year-old man recently treated for prostate cancer. His GP wants him to start exercising, but Henry is unsure about the benefits and lacks confidence in his ability. Drawing on existing evidence, write a list of the potential benefits achievable through exercise post-treatment, and suggest ways that would help him initiate regular exercise.

3   Rachel is fifty five years old and terminally ill with metastatic ovarian cancer. Her doctor estimates her life expectancy to be no more than six months. She has always lived an active life and would like to be doing some exercise to help maximise her quality of life. However, her family are concerned about this, because she is constantly very tired and in some pain. They believe that she should be resting more. Decide what advice you would give to the family about the potential benefits of exercise for Rachel, and suitable ways of exercising without exacerbating her symptoms.

Further reading

A concise overview of the role of exercise in cancer survivorship written for the British Association of Sport and Exercise Sciences:

Campbell, A., Stevinson, C., Crank, H. (2012). The BASES expert statement on exercise and cancer survivorship. *Journal of Sports Sciences*, 30, 949–52.

A thorough review of the evidence and mechanisms for exercise on cancer progression and mortality:

Betof, A. S., Dewhirst, M. W., Jones, L. W. (2013). Effects and potential mechanisms of exercise training on cancer progression: a translational perspective. *Brain Behaviour and Immunity*, 30, S75–87.

A comprehensive discussion of issues relating to physical activity and nutrition following cancer diagnosis provided by the American Cancer Society:

Rock, C. L., Doyle, C., Demark-Wahnefried, W., Meyerhardt, J., Courneya, K. S., Schwartz, A. L., Bandera, E. V., Hamilton, K. K., Grant, B., McCullough, M., Byers, T, Gansler, T. (2012). Nutrition and physical activity guidelines for cancer survivors. *CA: A Cancer Journal for Clinicians*, 62, 243–74.

References

Adamsen, L., Quist, M., Andersen, C., Møller, T., Herrstedt, J., Kronborg, D., Baadsgaard, M. T., Vistisen, K., Midtgaard, J., Christiansen, B., Stage, M., Kronborg, M. T. and Rørth, M. (2009). Effect of a multimodal high intensity exercise intervention in cancer patients undergoing chemotherapy: randomised controlled trial. *British Medical Journal*, 339, b3410.

Albrecht, T. A. and Taylor, A. G. (2012). Physical activity in patients with advanced-stage cancer: a systematic review of the literature. *Clinical Journal of Oncology Nursing*, 16, 293–300.

Allgayer, H., Owen, R. W., Nair, J., Spiegelhander, B., Streit J., Reichel, C. and Bartsch, H. (2008). Short-term moderate exercise programs reduce oxidative DNA damage as determined by high-performance liquid chromatography-electrospray ionization-mass spectrometry in patients with colorectal carcinoma following primary treatment. *Scandinavian Gastroenterology*, 43, 971–8.

Ballard-Barbash, R., Friedenreich, C. M., Courneya, K. S., Siddiqi, S. M., McTiernan, A. and Alfano, C. M. (2012). Physical activity, biomarkers, and disease outcomes in cancer survivors: a systematic review. *Journal of the National Cancer Institute*, 104, 815–40.

Baumann, F. T., Bloch, W. and Beulertz, J. (2013). Clinical exercise interventions in pediatric oncology: a systematic review. *Pediatric Research*, 74, 366–74.

Beaton, R., Pagdin-Friesen, W., Robertson, C., Vigar, C., Watson, H. and Harris, S. R. (2009). Effects of exercise intervention on persons with metastatic cancer: a systematic review. *Physiotherapy Canada*, 61, 141–53.

Betof, A. S., Dewhirst, M. W. and Jones, L. W. (2013). Effects and potential mechanisms of exercise training on cancer progression: a translational perspective. *Brain Behaviour and Immunity*, 30, S75–87.

Braam, K. I., van der Torre, P., Takken, T., Veening, M. A., van Dulmen-den Broeder, E. and Kaspers, G. J. (2013). Physical exercise training interventions for children and young adults during and after treatment for childhood cancer. *Cochrane Database of Systematic Review*, 30(4), CD008796.

Buffart, L. M., Galvão, D. A., Brug, J., Chinapaw, M. J. and Newton, R. U. (2014). Evidence-based physical activity guidelines for cancer survivors: current guidelines, knowledge gaps and future research directions. *Cancer Treatment Reviews*, 40, 327–40.

Burnham, T. R. and Wilcox, A. (2002). Effects of exercise on physiological and psychological variables in cancer survivors. *Medicine and Science in Sports and Exercise*, 34, 1863–7.

Campbell, A., Stevinson, C. and Crank, H. (2012). The BASES expert statement on exercise and cancer survivorship. *Journal of Sports Sciences*, 30, 949–52.

Campbell, A. (2014). *Cancer rehabilitation* [online]. Available at: http://canrehab.co.uk/ [accessed 22.07.14].

Cancer Research UK. (2014). *Cancer statistics report: cancer incidence and mortality in the UK.* Available at: http://publications.cancerresearchuk.org/ [accessed 22.07.14].

Chen, X., Lu, W., Zheng, W., Gu, K., Matthews, C. E., Chen, Z., Zheng, Y. and Shu, X. O. (2011). Exercise after diagnosis of breast cancer in association with survival. *Cancer Prevention Research*, 4, 1409–18.

Clague, J. and Bernstein, L. (2012). Physical activity and cancer. *Current Oncology Reports*, 14, 550–8.

Courneya, K. S. and Friedenreich, C. M. (2007). Physical activity and cancer control. *Seminars in Oncology Nursing*, 23, 242–52.

Courneya, K. S., McKenzie, D. C., Mackey, J. R., Gelmon, K., Friedenreich, C. M., Yasui, Y., Reid, R. D., Cook, D., Jespersen, D., Proulx, C., Dolan, L. B., Forbes, C. C., Wooding, E., Trinh, L. and Segal, R. J. (2013). Effects of exercise dose and type during breast cancer chemotherapy: multicenter randomized trial. *Journal of the National Cancer Institute*, 105, 1821–32.

Courneya, K. S., Segal, R. J., Mackey, J. R., Gelmon, K., Reid, R. D., Friedenreich, C. M., Ladha, A. B., Proulx, C., Vallance, J. K. H., Lane, K., Yasui, Y. and McKenzie, D. C. (2007). Effects of aerobic and resistance exercise in breast cancer patients receiving adjuvant chemotherapy: a multicenter randomized controlled trial. *Journal of Clinical Oncology*, 25, 4396–4404.

Courneya, K. S., Segal, R. J., McKenzie, D. C., Dong, H., Gelmon, K., Friedenreich, C. M., Yasui, Y., Reid, R. D., Crawford, J. J. and Mackey, J. R. (2014). Effects of exercise during adjuvant chemotherapy on breast cancer outcomes. *Medicine and Science in Sports and Exercise*, 46(9), 1744–51.

Craft, L. L., Vaniterson, E. H., Helenowski, I. B., Rademaker, A. W. and Courneya, K. S. (2012). Exercise effects on depressive symptoms in cancer survivors: a systematic review and meta-analysis. *Cancer Epidemiology Biomarkers and Prevention*, 21, 3–19.

Cramp, F. and Byron-Daniel, J. (2012). Exercise for the management of cancer-related fatigue in adults. *Cochrane Database of Systematic Reviews*, 11, CD006145.

Cramp, F., James, A. and Lambert, J. (2010). The effects of resistance training on quality of life in cancer: a systematic literature review and meta-analysis. *Supportive Care in Cancer*, 18, 1367–76.

De Backer, I. C., Schep, G., Backx, F. J., Vreugdenhil, G. and Kuipers, H. (2009). Resistance training in cancer survivors: a systematic review. *International Journal of Sports Medicine*, 30, 703–12.

Dimeo, F. C., Fetscher, S., Lange, W., Mertelsmann, R. and Keul, J. (1997). Effects of aerobic exercise on the physical performance and incidence of treatment-related complications after high-dose chemotherapy. *Blood*, 90, 3390–4.

Fairey, A. S., Courneya, K. S., Field, C. J., Bell, G. J., Jones, L. W., Martin, B. and Mackey, J. R. (2005). Effect of exercise training on c-reactive protein in postmenopausal breast cancer survivors: a randomized controlled trial. *Brain, Behavior and Immunity*, 19, 381–8.

Focht, B. C., Clinton, S. K., Devor, S. T., Garver, M. J., Lucas, A. R., Thomas-Ahner, J. M. and Grainger, E. (2013). Resistance exercise interventions during and following cancer treatment: a systematic review. *Journal of Supportive Oncology*, 11, 45–60.

Fong, D. Y., Ho, J. W., Hui, B. P., Lee, A. M., Macfarlane, D. J., Leung, S. S., Cerin, E., Chan, W. Y., Leung, I. P., Lam, S. H., Taylor, A. J. and Cheng, K. K. (2012). Physical activity for cancer survivors: meta-analysis of randomised controlled trials. *British Medical Journal*, 344:e70, doi: 10.1136/bmj.e70.

Galvão, D. A., Taaffe, D. R., Spry, N., Joseph, D. and Newton, R. U. (2010). Combined resistance and aerobic exercise program reverses muscle loss in men undergoing androgen suppression therapy for prostate cancer without bone metastases: a randomized controlled trial. *Journal of Clinical Oncology*, 28, 340–7.

George, S. M., Neuhouser, M. L., Mayne, S. T., Irwin, M. L., Albanes, D., Gail, M. H., Alfano, C. M., Bernstein, L., McTiernan, A., Reedy, J., Smith, A. W., Ulrich, C. M. and Ballard-Barbash, R. (2010). Postdiagnosis diet quality is inversely related to a biomarker of inflammation among breast cancer survivors. *Cancer Epidemiology Biomarkers and Prevention*, 19, 2220–8.

Gibbs, Z. G., Galvao, D. A. and Newton, R. U. (2011). High versus low intensity resistance exercise in late stage breast cancer patients with lymphedema: a randomised controlled trial. *Asia-Pacific Journal of Clinical Oncology*, 7(suppl. 4), 118.

Harder, H., Parlour, L. and Jenkins, V. (2012). Randomised controlled trials of yoga interventions for women with breast cancer: a systematic literature review. *Supportive Care in Cancer*, 20, 3055–64.

Haydon, A. M., Macinnis, R. J., English, D. R. and Giles, G. G. (2006). Effect of physical activity and body size on survival after diagnosis with colorectal cancer. *Gut*, 55, 62–7.

Holick, C. N., Newcomb, P. A., Trentham-Dietz, A., Titus-Ernstoff, L., Bersch, A. J., Stampfer, M. J., Baron, J. A., Egan, K. M. and Willett, W. C. (2008). Physical activity and survival after diagnosis of invasive breast cancer. *Cancer Epidemiology Biomarkers and Prevention*, 17, 379–86.

Holmes, M., Chen, W. Y., Feskanich, D., Kroenke, C. H. and Colditz, G. A. (2005). Physical activity and survival after breast cancer diagnosis. *Journal of the American Medical Association*, 293, 2479–86.

Huang, T. T. and Ness, K. K. (2011). Exercise interventions in children with cancer: a review. *International Journal of Pediatrics*, 2011, 461–512.

Irwin, M. L., McTiernan, A., Manson, J. E., Thomson, C. A., Sternfeld, B., Stefanick, M. L., Wactawski-Wende, J., Craft, L., Lane, D., Martin, L. W. and Chlebowski, R. (2011). Physical activity and survival in postmenopausal women with breast cancer: results from the Women's Health Initiative. *Cancer Prevention Research*, 4, 522–9.

Irwin, M. L., Varma, K., Alvarez-Reeves, M., Cadmus, L., Wiley, A., Chung, G. G., Dipietro, L., Mayne, S. T. and Yu, H. (2009). Randomized controlled trial of aerobic exercise on insulin and insulin like growth factors in breast cancer survivors: the Yale exercise and survivorship study. *Cancer Epidemiology Biomarkers and Prevention*, 18, 306–13.

Jones, L. W., Eves, N. D., Spasojevic, I., Wang, F. and Il'yasova, D. (2011). Effects of aerobic training on oxidative status in postsurgical non-small cell lung cancer patients: a pilot study. *Lung Cancer*, 72, 45–51.

Jones, L. W., Hornsby, W. E., Goetzinger, A., Forbes, L. M., Sherrard, E. L., Quist, M., Lane, A. T., West, M., Eves, N. D., Gradison, M., Coan, A., Herndon, J. E. and Abernethy, A. P. (2012). Prognostic significance of functional capacity and exercise behavior in patients with metastatic non-small cell lung cancer. *Lung Cancer*, 76, 248–52.

Jones, L. W., Liang, Y., Pituskin, E. N., Battaglini, C. L., Scott, J. M., Hornsby, W. E. and Haykowsky, M. (2011). Effect of exercise training on peak oxygen consumption in patients with cancer: a meta-analysis. *Oncologist*, 16, 112–20.

Jones, L. W., Watson, D., Herndon, J. E. 2nd, Eves, N. D., Haithcock, B. E., Loewen, G. and Kohman, L. (2010). Peak oxygen consumption and long-term all-cause mortality in nonsmall cell lung cancer. *Cancer*, 116, 4825–32.

Kenfield, S. A., Stampfer, M. J., Giovannucci, E. and Chan, J. M. (2011.) Physical activity and survival after prostate cancer diagnosis in the health professionals follow-up study. *Journal of Clinical Oncology*, 29, 726–32.

Ligibel, J. A., Campbell, N., Partridge, A., Chen, W. Y., Salinardi, T., Chen, H., Adloff, K., Keshaviah, A. and Winer, E. P. (2008). Impact of a mixed strength and endurance exercise intervention on insulin levels in breast cancer survivors. *Journal of Clinical Oncology*, 26, 907–12.

Linden, W., Vodermaier, A., Mackenzie, R. and Greig, D. (2012). Anxiety and depression after cancer diagnosis: prevalence rates by cancer type, gender, and age. *Journal of Affective Disorders*, 141, 343–51.

Lowe, S. S., Watanabe, S. M. and Courneya, K. S. (2009). Physical activity as a supportive care intervention in palliative cancer patients: a systematic review. *Journal of Supportive Oncology*, 7, 27–34.

MacVicar, M. G. and Winningham, M. L. (1986). Promoting the functional capacity of cancer patients. *Cancer Bulletin*, 38, 235–9.

MacVicar, M. G, Winningham, M. L. and Nickel, J. L. (1989). Effects of aerobic interval training on cancer patients' functional capacity. *Nursing Research*, 38, 348–51.

Maddams, J., Brewster, D., Gavin, A., Steward, J., Elliott, J., Utley, M. and Møller, H. (2009). Cancer prevalence in the United Kingdom: estimates for 2008. *British Journal of Cancer*, 101, 541–7.

Meyerhardt, J. A., Giovannucci, E. L., Holmes, M. D., Chan, A. T., Chan, J. A., Colditz, G. A. and Fuchs, C. S. (2006). Physical activity and survival after colorectal cancer diagnosis. *Journal of Clinical Oncology*, 24, 3527–34.

Meyerhardt, J. A., Giovannucci, E. L., Ogino, S., Kirkner, G. J., Chan, A. T., Willett, W. and Fuchs, C. S. (2009). Physical activity and male colorectal cancer survival. *Archives of Internal Medicine*, 169, 2102–8.

Meyerhardt, J. A., Heseltine, D., Niedzwiecki, D., Hollis, D., Saltz, L. B., Mayer, R. J., Thomas, J., Nelson, H., Whittom, R., Hantel, A., Schilsky, R. L. and Fuchs, C. S. (2006). Impact of physical activity on cancer recurrence and survival in patients with stage III colon cancer: findings from CALGB 89803. *Journal of Clinical Oncology*, 24, 3535–41.

Milne, H. M., Wallman, K. E., Gordon, S. and Courneya, K. S. (2008). Effects of a combined aerobic and resistance exercise program in breast cancer survivors: a randomized controlled trial. *Breast Cancer Research and Treatment*, 108, 279–88.

Mishra, S. I., Scherer, R. W., Geigle, P. M., Berlanstein, D. R., Topaloglu, O., Gotay, C. C. and Snyder, C. (2012b). Exercise interventions on health-related quality of life for cancer survivors. *Cochrane Database Systematic Reviews*, 8, CD007566.

Mishra, S. I., Scherer, R. W., Snyder, C., Geigle, P. M., Berlanstein, D. R. and Topaloglu, O. (2012a). Exercise interventions on health-related quality of life for people with cancer during active treatment. *Cochrane Database Systematic Reviews*, 8, CD008465.

Mistry, M., Parkin, D. M., Ahmad, A. S. and Sasieni, P. (2011). Cancer incidence in the United Kingdom: projections to the year 2030. *British Journal of Cancer*, 105, 1795–1803.

Moorman, P. G., Jones, L. W., Akushevich, L. and Schildkraut, J. M. (2011). Recreational physical activity and ovarian cancer risk and survival. *Annals of Epidemiology*, 21, 178–87.

Morikawa, T., Kuchiba, A., Yamauchi, M., Meyerhardt, J. A., Shima, K., Nosho, K., Chan, A. T., Giovannucci, E., Fuchs, C. S. and Ogino S. (2011). Association of CTNNB1 (β-catenin) alterations, body mass index, and physical activity with survival in patients with colorectal cancer. *Journal of the American Medical Association*, 305, 1685–94.

Oldervoll, L. M., Loge, J. H., Lydersen, S., Paltiel, H., Asp, M. B., Nygaard, U. V., Oredalen, E., Frantzen, T. L., Lesteberg, I., Amundsen, L., Hjermstad, M. J., Haugen, D. F., Paulsen, Ø. and Kaasa, S. (2011) Physical exercise for cancer patients with advanced disease: a randomized controlled trial. *Oncologist*, 16, 1649–57.

Parkin, D. M., Boyd, L. and Walker, L. C. (2011). The fraction of cancer attributable to lifestyle and environmental factors in the UK in 2010. *British Journal of Cancer*, 105, S77–81.

Pescatello, L., Arena, R., Riebe, D. and Thompson, P. (eds) (2014). ACSM's *guidelines for exercise testing and prescription*, Philadelphia: Wolters Kluwer/Lippincott Williams and Wilkins Health.

Pierce, B. L., Neuhouser, M. L., Wener, M. H., Bernstein, L., Baumgartner, R. N., Ballard-Barbash, R., Gilliland, F. D., Baumgartner, K. B., Sorensen, B., McTiernan, A. and Ulrich, C. M. (2009). Correlates of circulating c-reactive protein and serum amyloid a concentrations in breast cancer survivors. *Breast Cancer Research Treatment*, 114, 155–67.

Puetz, T. W. and Herring, M. P. (2012). Differential effects of exercise on cancer-related fatigue during and following treatment: a meta-analysis. *American Journal of Preventive Medicine*, 43, e1–24.

Richman, E. L., Kenfield, S. A., Stampfer, M. J., Paciorek, A., Carroll, P. R. and Chan, J. M. (2011). Physical activity after diagnosis and risk of prostate cancer progression: data from the cancer of the prostate strategic urologic research endeavor. *Cancer Research*, 71, 3889–95.

Rock, C. L., Doyle, C., Demark-Wahnefried, W., Meyerhardt, J., Courneya, K. S., Schwartz, A. L., Bandera, E. V., Hamilton, K. K., Grant, B., McCullough, M., Byers, T. and Gansler, T. (2012). Nutrition and physical activity guidelines for cancer survivors. *CA Cancer Journal for Clinicians*, 62, 243–74.

Ruden, E., Reardon, D. A., Coan, A. D., Herndon, J. E. 2nd, Hornsby, W. E., West, M., Fels, D. R., Desjardins A., Vredenburgh, J. J., Waner, E., Friedman, A. H., Friedman, H. S., Peters, K. B. and Jones, L. W. (2011). Exercise behavior, functional capacity, and survival in adults with malignant recurrent glioma. *Journal of Clinical Oncology*, 29, 2918–23.

Schmitz, K. H., Courneya, K. S., Matthews, C., Demark-Wahnefried, W., Galvão, D. A., Pinto, B. M., Irwin, M. L., Wolin, K. Y., Segal, R. J., Lucia, A., Schneider, C. M., von Gruenigen, V. E. and Schwartz, A. L. (2010). American College of Sports Medicine roundtable on exercise guidelines for cancer survivors. *Medicine and Science in Sports and Exercise*, 42,1409–26.

Segal, R. J., Reid, R. D., Courneya, K. S., Sigal, R. J., Kenny, G. P., Prud'Homme, D. G., Malone, S. C., Wells, G. A., Scott, C. G. and D'Angelo, M. E. S. (2009). Randomized controlled trial of resistance or aerobic exercise in men receiving radiation therapy for prostate cancer. *Journal of Clinical Oncology*, 27, 344–51.

Silver, J. K. and Baima, J. (2013) Cancer prehabilitation: an opportunity to decrease treatment-related morbidity, increase cancer treatment options, and improve physical and psychological health outcomes. *American Journal of Physical Medicine and Rehabilitation*, 92, 715–27.

Singh, F., Newton, R. U., Galvão, D. A., Spry, N. and Baker, M. K. (2013). A systematic review of pre-surgical exercise intervention studies with cancer patients. *Surgical Oncology*, 22, 92–104.

Speck, R. M., Courneya, K. S., Mässe, L. C., Duval, S. and Schmitz, K. H. (2010). An update of controlled physical activity trials in cancer survivors: a systematic review and meta-analysis. *Journal of Cancer Survivorship*, 4, 87–100.

Sprod, L. K., Hsieh, C. C., Hayward, R. and Schneider, C. M. (2010). Three versus six months of exercise training in breast cancer survivors. *Breast Cancer Research and Treatment*, 121, 413–19.

Stewart, B. W. and Wild, C. P. (2014). *World cancer report 2014*. Lyon: International Agency for Research on Cancer.

Strasser, B., Steindorf, K., Wiskemann, J. and Ulrich, C. M. (2013). Impact of resistance training in cancer survivors: a meta-analysis. *Medicine and Science in Sports and Exercise*, 45, 2080–90.

Sui, X., Lee, D. C., Matthews, C. E., Adams, S. A., Hébert, J. R., Church, T. S., Lee, C. D. and Blair, S. N. (2010). Influence of cardiorespiratory fitness on lung cancer mortality. *Medicine and Science in Sports Exercise*, 42, 872–8.

Valkenet, K., van de Port, I. G., Dronkers, J. J., de Vries, W. R., Lindeman, E., Backx, F. J. (2011). The effects of preoperative exercise therapy on postoperative outcome: a systematic review. *Clinical Rehabilitation*, 25, 99–111.

Winningham, M. L. and MacVicar, M. G. (1988). The effect of aerobic exercise on patient reports of nausea. *Oncology Nursing Forum*, 15, 447–50.

Winter, C., Müller, C., Hoffmann, C., Boos, J. and Rosenbaum, D. (2010). Physical activity and childhood cancer. *Pediatric Blood and Cancer*, 54, 501–10.

Winters-Stone, K. M., Schwartz, A. and Nail, L. M. (2010). A review of exercise interventions to improve bone health in adult cancer survivors. *Journal of Cancer Survivorship*, 4, 187–201.

Wiskemann, J. and Huber, G. (2008). Physical exercise as adjuvant therapy for patients undergoing hematopoietic stem cell transplantation. *Bone Marrow Transplantation*, 41, 321–9.

World Cancer Research Fund/American Institute for Cancer Research. (2007). *Food nutrition, physical activity, and the prevention of cancer: a global perspective*. Washington DC: AIRC.

Yamauchi, M., Lochhead, P., Imamura, Y., Kuchiba, A., Liao, X., Qian, Z. R., Nishihara, R., Morikawa, T., Shima, K., Wu, K., Giovannucci, E., Meyerhardt, J. A., Fuchs, C. S., Chan, A. T. and Ogino, S. (2013). Physical activity, tumor PTGS2 expression, and survival in patients with colorectal cancer. *Cancer Epidemiology Biomarkers and Prevention*, 22, 1142–52.

Yang, L., Klint, A., Lambe, M., Bellocco, R., Riman, T., Bergfeldt, K., Persson, I. and Weiderpass, E. (2008). Predictors of ovarian cancer survival: a population-based prospective study in Sweden. *International Journal of Cancer*, 123, 672–9.

Zeng, Y., Luo, T., Xie, H., Huang, M. and Cheng, A. S. (2014). Health benefits of qigong or tai chi for cancer patients: a systematic review and meta-analyses. *Complementary Therapies in Medicine*, 22, 173–86.

Chapter 7

Physical activity after stroke

Tom Balchin and Sarah Valkenborghs

Introduction

Stroke is defined by the World Health Organisation (WHO) as a clinical syndrome consisting of 'rapidly developing clinical signs of focal (at times global) disturbance of cerebral function, lasting more than 24 hours or leading to death with no apparent cause other than that of vascular origin' (WHO 2001). There are two main types of stroke:

1   Ischaemic stroke, which accounts for 85 per cent of strokes, result from a thrombosis or embolism which blocks or narrows a blood vessel that carries oxygenated blood to the brain;
2   Haemorrhagic stroke, which accounts for 15 per cent of strokes, carries a higher risk of fatality. This is when a blood vessel bursts, causing haemorrhaging into the brain tissue.

(Go et al. 2013)

The prevalence of risk factors for stroke is high. Almost all individuals who experience a stroke have at least one risk factor. Data from the South London Stroke Register indicates that 87.5 per cent of patients with first stroke have at least one modifiable risk factor (Redfern et al. 2002). Due to the similarities between coronary artery disease and ischaemic stroke, it is not surprising that many of the risk factors overlap. In particular, hypertension is the most important risk factor for both ischaemic and haemorrhagic stroke (Lawes et al. 2004), contributing to about 50 per cent of all strokes (World Health Federation 2015) (see Table 7.1).

Symptoms

The most common presentations of a stroke patient requiring rehabilitation are contralateral hemiparesis or hemiplegia. Other neurological manifestations vary depending upon the location of the stroke lesion (Teasell et al. 2014). Physical results of this damage include: reduced functional capacity, activity intolerance and fatigue, muscle wastage, partial paralysis, and residual gait deviations. Associated symptoms include memory loss, depression, anxiety, and, for some, an overwhelming sense of uncertainty. Several variables may influence the magnitude of the patient's deficits. These include lesion site, premorbid status, age, gender, deconditioning due to immobilisation, risk

Table 7.1 Modifiable risk factors for stroke (Salter et al. 2013)

Hypertension	Carotid stenosis
Diabetes	Congestive heart failure
Atrial fibrillation	Physical inactivity
Coronary artery disease	Hypercoagulable state
Smoking	Chronic infection
Dyslipidaemia	Peripheral vascular disease
Heavy alcohol use	Transient ischaemic attack

status, associated severity of neurological involvement, possibility of heart disease and the effect of conditions (e.g. diabetes, pulmonary disease, and osteoporosis), medications, time since the stroke, environmental support systems (including degree of social support), and compliance with a prescribed exercise and rehabilitation routine (if one has been provided).

Stroke in the UK

Every year, fifteen million people worldwide suffer a stroke, of which 152,000 are in the UK (Townsend et al. 2012). Stroke is ranked as the second biggest cause of death to occur at any age, but it has proven to be much more common in the elderly, with the death rate doubling every ten years between fifty five and eighty five (Feigin 2014). This is because the UK's population is living longer (Office for National Statistics 2014). Nearly a third (31 per cent) of all stroke victims are under the age of sixty five. However, the number of strokes affecting those aged between twenty and sixty five has leapt by 25 per cent over the last twenty years and is expected to double by 2030. More than 83,000 young people under the age of twenty die as the result of a stroke, equivalent to 125 people a day.

Stroke is far more disabling than it is fatal. 85 per cent of those who suffer a stroke survive the insult itself and the UK is experiencing the largest cohort of persons surviving brain injuries and strokes in history. Over the last decade, there has been a 30 per cent increase in the total number of stroke survivors. This has largely been due to improvements in medical technology, both in terms of the accuracy of diagnostic testing and in treatment options. Early detections of worsening neurological statuses have led to earlier interventions, decreased likelihoods of sicknesses, decreased resource consumption, and better outcomes. After treatment interventions, considerable spontaneous recovery may occur up to about six months (Cramer 2008). However, patients with a history of stroke are at risk of subsequent events (Table 7.2)

The proportion of patients achieving independence in self-care one year post-stroke ranges from 60–83 per cent (Appelros et al. 2003). This wide variation relates to whether care is community- or hospital-based, which activities are considered in estimating independence, and the methods used to rate ability.

Stroke causes a greater impact and range of disabilities than any other condition (Adamson et al. 2004). The resultant costs are substantial, with stroke care estimated to amount to more than 5 per cent of the UK's healthcare budget (Quinn et al. 2009). Of those who survive stroke, approximately 42 per cent will be independent, 22 per cent will

Table 7.2 The cumulative risk of recurrent stroke in the UK (Mohan et al. 2011)

Time after first stroke	Percentage risk rate of recurrence after first stroke
First 30 days	3%
At 1 year	11%
At 5 years	26%
At 10 years	39%

have mild disability, 14 per cent will have moderate disability, 10 per cent will have severe disability, and 12 per cent will have very severe disability (Royal College of Physicians 2011). Of the 1.1 million stroke survivors in the UK, half of them are dependent on others for help with everyday living (NICE 2008).

Current treatment pathway

Rehabilitation rather than exercise provision is recognised as a foundation of inpatient and outpatient multidisciplinary stroke care (Figure 7.1). Exercise after stroke is defined as structured and repetitive physical activity, whereas stroke rehabilitation is characterised by early initiated, intensive, and ongoing interventions, in which task and context specificity play an important role (Kwakkel et al. 2004).

National Institute for Health and Care Excellence stroke rehabilitation guidelines require in-patient assessment by all members of the multi-disciplinary team (MDT) within seventy two hours and to have agreed goals documented within five days (NICE 2013). Immediately after an acute stroke, the first goals relating to physical activity and exercise are aimed at preventing complications of prolonged inactivity, regaining voluntary movement, and recovering basic activities of daily living (ADLs). Evidence exists for early mobilisation (within twenty four hours) in-clinic (Billinger et al. 2014).

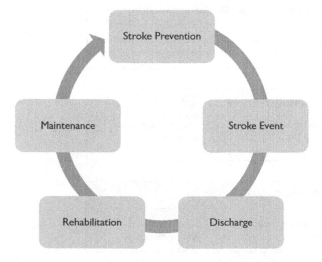

Figure 7.1 Rehabilitation rather than exercise provision as current clinical emphasis.

Early mobilisation at regular intervals can result in improved functional recovery of gait control (Cumming et al. 2011) and patients generally encounter no adverse effects by early mobilisation (Bernhardt et al. 2008a).

Stroke survivors who require on-going rehabilitation after acute care are usually relocated to a specialist stroke rehabilitation unit. Recovery of action control, speech, language, and cognitive function are then primary goals for patients, and ideally being referred to local commissioned services for exercise training and rehabilitation. Emerging evidence suggests that better outcomes are achieved if therapists provide advice regarding cardiorespiratory exercise in the community to patients (and families who may assist) who are approaching discharge date. Stroke survivors can refer quickly to the help of independent community exercise professionals who can come into their homes to train them, instead of undergoing a month or so of no physical activity. Action for Rehabilitation from Neurological Injury (ARNI) Instructors (Balchin 2013) carry out these activities, often sponsored by charities such as the UK Stroke Association (Poltawski et al 2013a). The stroke care pathway is shown in Figure 7.2.

Patients should undergo therapy appropriate to their rehabilitation goals, at a level that they are willing and able to tolerate, and in the early stages they should receive a minimum of forty five minutes of each therapy that is required for a minimum of five days per week (NICE 2013; Intercollegiate Stroke Working Party 2012). Whilst these guidelines ensure stroke survivors receive some rehabilitation, inpatient activity

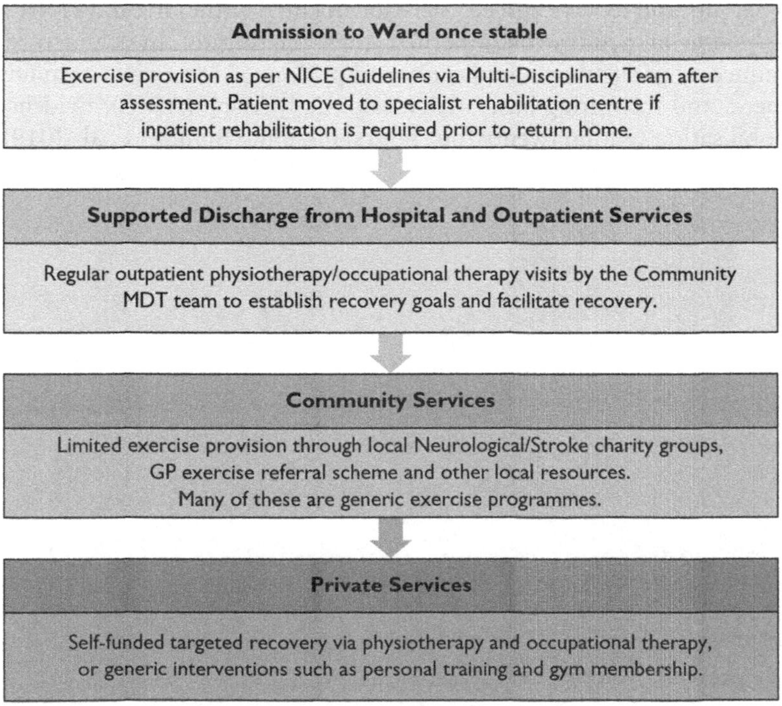

| **Admission to Ward once stable** |
| Exercise provision as per NICE Guidelines via Multi-Disciplinary Team after assessment. Patient moved to specialist rehabilitation centre if inpatient rehabilitation is required prior to return home. |

| **Supported Discharge from Hospital and Outpatient Services** |
| Regular outpatient physiotherapy/occupational therapy visits by the Community MDT team to establish recovery goals and facilitate recovery. |

| **Community Services** |
| Limited exercise provision through local Neurological/Stroke charity groups, GP exercise referral scheme and other local resources. Many of these are generic exercise programmes. |

| **Private Services** |
| Self-funded targeted recovery via physiotherapy and occupational therapy, or generic interventions such as personal training and gym membership. |

Figure 7.2 The UK stroke patient's care pathway from admission to discharge.

levels within stroke rehabilitation units are surprisingly low (Bernhardt et al. 2004). Early implementation of intensive stroke rehabilitation is associated with improved and faster progress in the performance of activities after stroke (Kwakkel et al. 1997; Langhorne et al. 1996).

Exercise after stroke

Chronic inactivity related to stroke has a multitude of physiological consequences that result in cardiovascular deconditioning, increased cardiovascular risk, and increased mortality and morbidity risk. Exercise training is a potent stimulus for improving cardiorespiratory fitness and associated physiological outcomes in stroke populations (Billinger et al. 2011).

> If we could put exercise into a drug, it would be one of the most effective medications to prevent vascular disease and treat patients with cardiovascular and cerebrovascular diseases including stroke.
>
> (Mead et al. 2012)

This statement is reinforced by the finding that exercise interventions are significantly more effective than drug treatments in both rehabilitation and reducing the odds of mortality among patients with stroke (Naci and Ioannidis 2013).

As reduced fitness levels often predate stroke, it cannot be inferred that low fitness is entirely a consequence of stroke. Nevertheless, physical fitness (inclusive of cardiorespiratory fitness and muscle strength and power) is low, and remains low for several years after stroke in comparison to age- and gender-matched controls (Billinger et al. 2012). Low fitness levels are not only indicators of risk of cardiovascular disease but also of degree of independence. A vicious circle exists in stroke survivors whereby chronic deficits limit physical activity and result in subsequent physical deconditioning and reduced fitness levels. This compromises functional mobility and propagates further disability, worsening the risk of other avoidable chronic conditions such as cardiovascular disease, diabetes, cancer, osteoporosis, and depression, with dramatic negative effects on the overall quality of life. Improving fitness has the potential to improve function and reduce secondary cardiovascular events (Billinger et al. 2012).

Secondary prevention

Optimal secondary prevention strategies can prevent as much as 80 per cent of all recurrent ischaemic strokes (Prabhakaran and Chong 2014). Although data about the association between physical activity and recurrent stroke are lacking, extrapolating the evidence that physical activity reduces the risk of a first-ever stroke by 27 per cent (Sanossian and Ovbiagele 2006), and conversely, that physical inactivity is associated with increased incidence of stroke (Lee et al. 2003), it is biologically plausible that physical activity after stroke may reduce the risk of recurrent stroke and other vascular events. Physical activity improves the profile of vascular risk factors through mechanisms including improved lipid profile, reduction in blood pressure, reduced plasma fibrinogen level and platelet aggregation, weight reduction and glucose metabolism (Gordon et al. 2004) (See Figure 7.3).

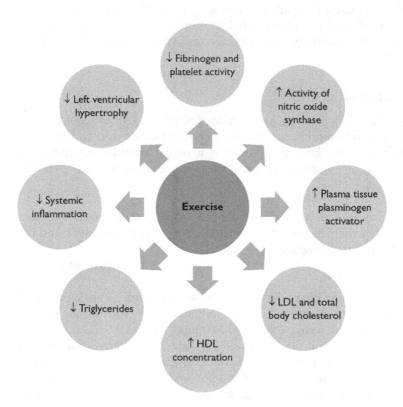

Figure 7.3 Putative pathophysiological benefits of exercise (reproduced with kind permission from Gallanagh et al. 2011).

There is growing evidence that exercise promotes brain neuroplasticity. Neuroplasticity mediates cognition and the relearning of motor skills and other skills after stroke. The potential mechanisms underlying the enhanced neurotrophic effects of exercise include increased noradrenergic activation (Ivy et al. 2003), improved brain oxygen saturation (Kramer et al. 1999), and enhanced upregulation of neurotrophic factors (Vaynman et al. 2004). Exercise induces angiogenesis and neurogenesis via a growth factor cascade involving, amongst others, vascular endothelial growth factor (VEGF), brain-derived neurotrophic factor (BDNF), and insulin-like growth factor (IGF-I). VEGF promotes angiogenesis in order to improve blood supply in areas where it is inadequate (Hoeben et al. 2004). Exercise is known to increase systemic blood flow and cerebral blood flow (Querido and Sheel 2007). After stroke, improved circulation is particularly important due to the amount of inactivity many stroke survivors experience (Bernhardt et al. 2008b; Askim et al. 2014). Exercise also strengthens the microvascular integrity after cerebral ischaemia and upregulates endothelial nitric oxide synthesis, which improves endothelial function by up regulating VEGF expression (Talwar et al. 2014). BDNF, found in the brain and periphery, supports and sustains brain health by playing a role in neurogenesis (Rossi et al. 2006), neuroregeneration (Ye and Houle 1997), and neuroprotection in the brain of humans (Jacobs et al. 2000). It has been reported to increase following exercise in humans (Knaepen et al. 2010). BDNF hinders neuron cell death, stimulates neuron cell survival, initiates neuroregeneration and synapse formation, and promotes and enhances plasticity, especially in motor and sensory neurons of the central and peripheral nervous system, which can contribute to memory and learning (Molteni et al. 2004; Alonso et al. 2002).

Quality of life

Although exercise has typically been used to enhance physical function post-stroke, evidence is emerging that exercise may also improve depression, health-related quality of life, and fatigue, which affects 39–72 per cent of stroke survivors (Colle et al. 2006; Zedlitz et al. 2012). Depression is identified as the strongest predictor of quality of life (Carod-Artal et al. 2000; Kim et al. 1999). There is a high incidence of clinical depression documented in people with stroke, with one third of survivors experiencing depression at some point after stroke (Hackett et al. 2005). In the general population, exercise is reported to be beneficial in the treatment of depression (Nabkasorn et al. 2006) and even as effective as psychotherapy, occupational therapy, and medication (Martinsen 2008). For stroke survivors, exercise is also linked with reduced depression and social isolation, even in the chronic stages of stroke (Stuart et al. 2009).

Group exercise classes seem to be the most promising approach, with positive influences on psychosocial outcomes including quality of life and confidence, as well as increased empowerment and motivation to take an active role in the recovery process (Carin-Levy et al. 2009). The success of group exercise classes may be partly attributable to the social capital that stroke survivors gain by participating in them. Social support is one of the key predictors of quality of life post-stroke (King 1996). This is confirmed by the fact that the most frequently reported perceived motivator to participate in group exercise classes post-stroke is the opportunity to meet other survivors, whom they subsequently do not want to let down by non-attendance, and this indirectly motivates increased physical activity (Nicholson et al. 2013). Classes also provide a purpose and structure to a stroke survivor's daily schedule, something which may be lost after stroke (Damush et al. 2007), and, although often overlooked, this is something that chronic disease sufferers value (Damush et al. 2005).

Community-based group exercise classes also improve and retain mobility, functional capacity, and balance, and result in a demonstrable impact upon the performance of activities and abilities that were considered meaningful to the subjects (Eng et al. 2003; Kilbride et al 2013). Stroke survivors report considerable levels of dissatisfaction with their quality of life one year after stroke, with the level of dissatisfaction correlated to the level of activity impairment (Hartman-Maeir et al. 2007). Fitness levels are not only important indicators of cardio- and cerebro-vascular disease but also of degree of independence. Loss of independence is associated with aerobic fitness levels below $18 \ mL \cdot kg^{-1} \cdot min^{-1}$ in men and $15 \ mL \cdot kg^{-1} \cdot min^{-1}$ in women (Shephard 2009). Physical fitness training after stroke results in various improved quality of life outcomes such as reduced dependence on others during ambulation, improved walking speed, and exercise tolerance (Brazzelli et al. 2011).

Whilst only a few studies have evaluated the efficacy of interventions to prevent falls in the stroke population, task-oriented exercise programmes are the most promising (Weerdesteyn et al. 2008). The diagram below describes the inter-relationship of quality of life with physical activity, fear of falling, and falls (Figure 7.4).

Reduced fall frequency should not be achieved through reduced physical activity, as this will lead to additional physical deconditioning, with reduced postural stability and quality of life. Instead, reduction in fall frequency, leading to better quality of life, should coincide with improved postural stability, decreased fear of falling, and increased physical activity. Since physical inactivity after stroke is common (Bernhardt et al. 2008b; Askim et al. 2014), and reduced physical activity is a component related to an increase in falls, it is no surprise that stroke is one of the biggest risk factors for falls in older adults.

Functional capacity

Around 40–70 per cent of stroke survivors will have at least one fall within a year of stroke (Weerdesteyn et al. 2008), and this population has over seven times the risk of experiencing a fracture compared to those without stroke (Kanis et al. 2001). Within the first year after stroke, the risk for a fragility fracture is 4 per cent, and this increases to 15 per cent at five years post-stroke (Ramnemark et al. 1998). The development of secondary osteoporosis (particularly on the paretic side) is linked to disuse and unloading. Weight-bearing and resistance exercise is well established as increasing bone mineral density and reducing the risk of osteoporosis (Howard 2011). As stroke is now a well-recognised risk factor for hip fracture, preventing the development of hemi-osteoporosis in stroke survivors is key to preventing fractures

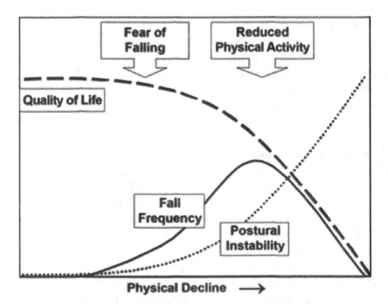

Figure 7.4 Inter-relationship of quality of life with physical activity, fear of falling, and falls. Reproduced with permission from Weerdesteyn et al. (2008).

and further injury (Poole et al. 2002). Physical activity can therefore serve a dual purpose in not only helping to prevent falls, but to reduce the risk of fracture when they do occur.

Reduced arm function limiting ability to perform ADLs has also been associated with repeat falling (Hyndman et al. 2002). Furthermore, motor impairment and limitations in the use of the upper limb have been highlighted as major contributors to poor wellbeing and quality of life amongst stroke survivors by impairing stabilisation of proximal arm segments, limiting reaching ability, confining hand usage, and affecting upper-limb control and coordination (Morris et al. 2013). These factors have a direct effect on the use of the paretic upper limb in daily activities, supporting the importance of paretic upper-limb strength (Harris and Eng 2007). Therefore, enhancing upper limb function is an essential component of rehabilitation.

Exercise intervention trials

Simply taking part in exercise training significantly improves physical function in participants (Mead et al. 2007). However, different types of physical activities work on different health-related components of physical fitness, and so may produce different outcomes. Therefore, in order to make an accurate exercise prescription, it is important to understand the aims of the intervention, the different types of exercise interventions, and the potential benefits associated with each of them.

Aerobic activity

Aerobic exercise is prolonged and rhythmical, and involves the use of large muscle groups. Examples of aerobic exercise include walking or jogging overground or on a treadmill (with or without support), cycling, recumbent stepping, swimming, circuit training, and chair-based exercise. Aerobic exercise is a therapeutic intervention that, despite the known benefits, is underutilised by clinicians during rehabilitation (Billinger et al. 2015). Even a single session of treadmill exercise improves grasping function in the hemiparetic hand for chronic stroke survivors (Ploughman et al. 2008). Treadmill training three times a week for six months not only improved cardiorespiratory fitness, but also ambulatory performance, and functional mobility compared to conventional care (Macko et al. 2005). Potentially long-lasting positive effects can also be achieved with treadmill training in terms of speed and endurance (Mehrholz et al. 2014).

Cycling is another beneficial form of aerobic exercise. Eight weeks of lower-extremity endurance cycling enhanced fine motor control of the upper extremity as well as cognitive function in chronic stroke survivors (Quaney et al. 2009). Even early and severely impaired stroke survivors may benefit from low-intensity bicycle ergometer training (Wang et al. 2014). This supports recommendations that exercise should be commenced early after stroke and carried out through the continuum of care (Billinger et al. 2015). The rationale is that it may sustain plasticity processes and extend the 'recovery window' for longer (Page et al. 2004), which may be important for patients who reach a plateau four to six weeks after stroke (Duncan et al. 1994). Patients judged to be already 'neurologically plateaued' in their rehabilitation saw improvement in a 'get up and go' task, as well as increased mean velocity and cadence following three months of low-intensity treadmill training for forty minutes three times a week (Silver et al. 2000).

Swimming can also be an effective exercise intervention post-stroke, particularly for those survivors with problems in balance or fear of falling. An eight-week programme of progressively intense training (up to 80 per cent of heart rate reserve for the last three weeks) improved cardiorespiratory fitness (Chu et al. 2004), which is associated with improved sensorimotor function (Gordon et al. 2004), and everyday activities were able to be carried out with less effort and for longer periods (Rimmer and Wang 2005). Generally, higher-intensity exercise promotes more effective and rapid physiological adaptations (Laurin and Pin-Barre 2014). A preliminary study examining the effects of three different exercise interventions found that thirty minutes of moderate-intensity aerobic exercise programme was more effective than programmes of sixty minutes of either lower-intensity aerobic exercise or non-aerobic therapeutic exercise in reducing blood pressure and blood lipid levels (Rimmer et al. 2009).

The use of aerobic exercise to improve cardiorespiratory fitness in post-stroke and general populations is well established; however, it may only yield additional functional benefits when the training is task-related (Saunders et al. 2010). An example of this is that task-specific training, such as treadmill exercise, improved walking outcomes as well as cardiorespiratory fitness (Billinger et al. 2015). Although task-oriented training can 'kick-start' motor functions that may have become dormant after stroke (Dobkin 2004), there is still a very large body of literature to support the use of aerobic exercise alone in motor control, cognitive function, and sensorimotor function (Gordon et al. 2004). Despite the variation in the types, intensities, and durations of aerobic exercise interventions outlined above, improvements are seen in all of the experimental groups in comparison to those undertaking programmes reflective of usual care. This suggests that, regardless of the specific activity, there is potential progress to be made in undertaking any form of aerobic exercise that is not observed in conventional rehabilitation programmes. The lack of consistency in terms of activity and frequency does pose problems, but there is a general consensus that better results can be seen from longer and more prolonged exercise periods (Dam et al. 1993; Ada et al. 2013), with one study identifying that a sixteen-hour programme is the minimum required to observe the positive effects of exercise (Kwakkel et al. 2004). Whatever the type or length of training, it does appear that any aerobic activity can have a beneficial rehabilitative effect following stroke (Pang et al. 2006a).

Muscle-strengthening activity

Strength training in stroke rehabilitation usually consists of progressive resistance exercises that aim to improve muscle strength. They can be provided by means of free weights, elastic bands, pneumatic machines, isokinetic machines, or body weight (Langhorne et al. 2011). Progressive resistance training (PRT) stimulates significant muscle hypertrophy and intramuscular fat reductions in disabled stroke survivors, who experience disproportionate muscle atrophy and other unfavourable changes in tissue composition on the paretic side (Ryan et al. 2011). Muscle weakness is one of the most prominent impairments for many stroke survivors, and may be an appropriate target for therapeutic interventions based on the relationship between muscle weakness and performance of functional activities. Several reviews have established that resistance training is effective in increasing strength in stroke survivors (Morris et al. 2004). An additional review concluded that it seems probable that strength training results in improvement in functional activities as well (Bohannon 2007).

Progressive resistance training with loads of 70 per cent or more of maximum strength is a safe and effective way to improve muscle strength post-stroke. Furthermore, the improvements in muscle strength enhance activity, gait performance, motor performance, balance, functional limitations, disability, and perceived participation without negative effects on muscle tone or spasticity (Lexell and Flansbjer 2008; Ada et al. 2006). However, strength training should be specific and tailored towards everyday activities (e.g. sit to stands, steps up, and impaired actions) (Bohannon 2007). For example, the Graded Repetitive Arm Supplementary Program (GRASP) is a functional programme of upper extremity strength training, fine motor tasks, and repetitive functional tasks that has been found to improve upper extremity assessment outcomes in two RCTs involving range of motion, weight-bearing, and trunk control (Pang et al. 2006b; Harris et al. 2009). Eccentric resistance training has also been found to be more effective than concentric resistance training in improving bilateral neuromuscular activation, strength, and walking speed in stroke survivors (Clark and Patten 2013).

Circuit training

The use of circuit or group exercise training is well researched and implemented, and is typically composed of a combination of aerobic and strength training activities to improve all round physical fitness and mobility (Langhorne et al. 2011), as well as vascular risk factors, gait, and gait-related activities (Wevers et al. 2009). This type of exercise is associated with increased aerobic fitness and mobility when compared to those undergoing routine therapy only (Galvin et al. 2011) and against a control group performing upper-body training in addition to routine provision (Pang et al. 2005). The advantage of this type of combined group exercise training is that it can be organised as a circuit of a series of workstations, providing opportunities for task-oriented training. Task-oriented group circuit training allows intense practice in a meaningful and progressive manner. It encourages peer support and social interaction through group dynamics, and represents a more time-efficient and cost-effective method of therapy in terms of staff-to-patient ratio (Wevers et al. 2009). Water-based group exercise programmes are also effective in stroke survivors (Chu et al. 2004), and use a combination of aerobic and resistance training. An RCT of a comprehensive therapeutic exercise programme utilising the full complement of all of the types of activities found that stroke survivors had improvements in balance, mobility, and endurance beyond those attributable to spontaneous recovery and usual care (Duncan et al. 2003).

Stretching activity

Stretching activities are movements applied by an external and/or internal force in order to increase muscle flexibility and/or joint range of motion. Stretching activities include static stretching, dynamic stretching, active stretching, slow movements, and proprioceptive neuromuscular facilitation (PNF). For upper limbs in particular, if the patient has spasticity, the velocity of the strength is a well-known factor for consideration. The evidence for task-related training is strong, and this is facilitated by passive stretching prior to tasks, as well as requiring the patient to stretch the paretic upper limb as much as they can themselves.

The majority of patients suffer balance impairment after stroke, caused by decreased muscle strength (Tinetti and Kumar 2010). 'Drop-foot', the uncontrolled plantar flexion and supination of the paretic foot, is one of the major problems survivors encounter. The first line of defence against unexpected destabilising forces, such as a collision, slip or trip, or self-induced movements, such as reaching or transferring, are postural reflexes (coordinated muscle activity). Older adult stroke survivors have delayed paretic limb postural reflex muscle onset latencies in comparison to age-matched healthy individuals (Di Fabio et al. 1986). Exercise programmes that incorporate stretching and weight-shifting exercises improve postural reflexes, mobility and functional balance, and subsequently may reduce the rate of falls in older adult stroke survivors (Marigold et al. 2005).

Preliminary data indicate that static stretching is most effective for improving torque relaxation, but both prolonged static and cyclic stretches can decrease ankle joint stiffness (Bressel and McNair 2002). Static stretching (constant-angle stretching and constant-torque stretching) and cyclic stretching are both effective for increasing range of motion and reducing the immediate viscoelastic components of hypertonic ankle joints in stroke survivors, but the constant-torque type of static stretching stimulates the most pronounced changes (Yeh et al. 2007). Ankle stiffness, walking speed, passive range of movement, and maximum voluntary contraction are all significantly improved by a feedback-controlled stretching device as an alternative intervention for patients with spasticity and/or contracture without the daily involvement of clinicians (Selles et al. 2005).

Neuromuscular activity

Neuromuscular activities involve the harmonious recruitment of both nervous and muscular tissue, and include balance, agility, and proprioceptive training. Neuromuscular activities are recommended as part of a comprehensive exercise programme, especially for older adults who are at increased risk of falling or have functional impairments (ACSM 2013). A wide range and variety of activities qualify as neuromuscular activity, including tai chi, yoga, active-play/interactive video gaming, and recreational activities using balls/paddles to stimulate hand-eye coordination (Billinger et al. 2014). The varied benefits of tai chi include decreased stress and anxiety, increased balance, decreased falls, improved gait, and increased muscle strength, which may help stroke survivors (Taylor-Piliae and Coull 2012). Not only can tai chi be practised in any place, at any time, without any special equipment; it is also a safe and effective exercise intervention for stroke survivors (Taylor-Piliae and Haskell 2007).

Research of recreational sports as rehabilitation interventions after stroke is sparse; however, one study assessed the use of a therapeutic golf programme (Shatil and Garland 2000). This comprehensive, task-oriented approach in a community-based leisure environment may foster balance, postural alignment and control, hand-eye coordination and the learning of a new motor skill, which can facilitate both an improvement in quality of life, and motivation to participate in such activities and therapies.

Moving towards more modern habits, active-play/interactive video gaming is a novel approach in stroke rehabilitation. Being a safe and feasible intervention in the stroke population, it is suggested as a suitable adjunct and/or alternative to conventional therapy (Joo 2010; Saposnik et al. 2010; Tsekleves et al. 2014). Such activity can enhance energy expenditure to a level that is sufficient to maintain or improve health post-stroke (Hurkmans et al. 2011), to significantly enhance motor function, which translates to improvements in ADLs post-stroke (Mouawad et al. 2011; Saposnik et al. 2010), and increase self-efficacy and self-awareness of one's ability to perform a task (Farrow and Reid 2004).

Standardised guidelines

The development of exercise recommendations for medical conditions such as stroke is comparable to the development of medications (Naci and Ioadinnidis, 2013). The FITT (frequency, intensity, time, and type) principle constitutes the dose needed to enhance health (Billinger et al. 2015). A safe and effective dose is recommended, based on consideration of exercise training principles alongside the patient's functional capacity and limitations, while simultaneously trying to optimise adherence and avoid over-/under-dosing. It is tempting to consider exercise as a simple, effective, and easily-prescribed intervention for stroke survivors; however, the evidence base is still limited and implementation is more complex. Drawing on the information in existing guidelines, based on evidence-based research, an outline of the content, process, and rationale for community-based exercise programmes for long-term stroke survivors has been constructed (Poltawski et al. 2013b).

Recommendations for content and process of programmes

Many of the guidelines recognise that there may be different requirements in acute, sub-acute, and chronic phases, but in some cases little or no such distinction is made (Poltawski et al. 2013b). A broad consensus suggests that programmes should contain endurance and muscle-strengthening exercises, with a focus on functional actions. In fact, making exercises functional or task-specific is regarded as essential by the majority of guidelines. A one-hour session at least three times a week meets the levels recommended by most of the guidelines, though there is variation in the suggested times allocated to each component of programmes, and a recognition that deconditioned participants may require shorter duration but more frequent sessions in the early stages of their programme. The benefits of exercise to stroke survivors are summarised in Table 7.3 along with proposed guidelines for prescription.

Because no single presentation of stroke or its impact is the same as another, the guidelines in Table 7.3 should be used as guidance only. However, stroke survivors who present with hemiplegia or hemiparesis will still be able to perform exercise in some form, whether it is weight-assisted, performed by the non-affected side only, or performed by both sides but at a lower capacity to that which the non-affected side can perform. As with any exercise prescription, suitability for the exercise programme must be assessed and the programme tailored to the functionality of the individual stroke survivor and their recovery goals. The ARNI Approach (Balchin 2011), used in the UK for the past fifteen years, adheres to the evidence-based principles

Table 7.3 Summary of exercise programming recommendations for stroke survivors

Type	Aims/Benefits	Intensity	Frequency/Time
Aerobic • Walking/jogging (or treadmill) • Stationary cycling • Seated stepper • Swimming.	• Increase independence in ADLs • Increase walking speed/efficiency • Improve tolerance for prolonged physical activity • Reduce risk of cardiovascular disease • Improve comorbid conditions e.g. hypertension hyperlipidemia, NIDD, depression etc.	40–70% Peak oxygen intake; 40–70% heart rate reserve; 50–80% maximal heart rate; RPE 11–14 (6–20 scale).	3–7 days/week 20–60min/session (or multiple 10min sessions).
Strength • Circuit training • Weight machines • Free weights • Isometric exercise • Core stability.	• Increase independence in ADLs • Maintain or increase muscular endurance • Increased grip strength • Reduce risk of falling	Body weight/ manual resistance Progressing to theraband gradations; 70% 1 rep. max; Unilateral resistance to cause failure between 10 to 15 repetitions.	2–3 days/week 1–3 sets of 10–15 repetitions of 8–10 exercises involving the major muscle groups; 3 days/week 2 sets of 20 repetitions
Stretching	• Increase ROM of involved extremities • Prevent contractures.		2–3 days/week (before or after aerobic or strength training) Hold each stretch for 10–30 seconds
Neuromuscular • Yoga • Tai Chi • Balance activities • Coordination activities.	• Improve level of safety during ADLs • Improved gait • Reduced fear of falling.		2–3 days/week (could be done on same day as strength activities).
Combined approach	• Improved coordination and ADL performance.	Body weight/manual resistance Progressing to theraband gradations.	2–3 days/week 90 mins (interval-based work and rest periods).

Adapted from Billinger et al. (2014) and Gordon et al. (2004)

of task-related training, adapted strength training, and self-management strategies, which can encourage independence and confidence, such as the hemiparetic patient learning how to get down and up from the floor autonomously.

Adaptations for exercise after stroke

General exercise programme considerations

The average stroke survivor is deconditioned and, consequently, blood flow is reduced; the functional range of motion at joints may be limited; the onset of fatigue may be quicker; and energy expenditure will be greater due to improper gait and increased concentration. Work and rest periods must allow for muscular and mental fatigue, as exercise requires periods of concentration. As with cardiac patients, warm-ups and cool-downs must take into account potentially reduced blood flow and cardiac output. Stroke survivors may require closer supervision than the average individual due to complications such as fatigue, risk of falls, and loss of grip on equipment; therefore, one-to-one or small group training is advisable. Furthermore, many stroke survivors present with muscular imbalances, due to spasticity, and/or hypertonicity, and reduced flexibility, which necessitate adapted exercises to reduce range of motion and regress exercises that require balance to be suitable for the exerciser.

Neuroplasticity is associated with repetition; therefore, applying lighter resistance to allow increased repetitions is conducive to neuroplastic change whilst minimising fatigue. Significant gains in voluntary strength and muscle activation on the deconditioned, more-affected side after stroke can be invoked through training the opposite limb (Dragert et al. 2013). Therefore even if one limb is weak, training the less-affected side is still worthwhile, and can bring about gains in the more-affected side.

Gait retraining has been used in non-stroke populations for rehabilitation after injury, posture correction during exercise, and visual feedback for correct exercise technique, and exercising in front of a mirror may promote gait correction in the stroke population (Cheng et al. 2001). The use of hip protectors to reduce the likelihood of fracture if a fall occurs is a worthwhile precaution, as is kinesiology-taping to help support a subluxed shoulder during exercise. When beginning an aerobic exercise programme, a body weight support system may be considered when using a treadmill. Recumbent steppers are a safe and easy device in this situation for transferring from a wheelchair, and they can also be used if upright posture, balance, or walking are causes for concern (Billinger et al. 2015).

Although we are still some way from understanding how best to foster participation in physical exercise activity amongst stroke survivors, the evidence for the benefits of exercise after stoke is sufficiently strong to justify the development of physical activity programmes for stroke survivors.

Contraindications, considerations, and barriers

Contraindications and considerations

Contraindications and considerations for exercise training in stroke populations include physiological and psychological factors, and also comorbidities and medication, which are proportionately correlated and often coexist (see Table 7.4).

Table 7.4 Contraindications and considerations for exercise training after stroke

Contraindications/considerations	Reason
Level of functional impairment	Functional impairment includes limb paralysis or paresis, muscular spasticity, subluxation of the shoulder, or sudden 'buckling' of affected knee/ankle are all factors that must be considered.
Level of cognitive impairment	Exercises can involve complex movements and can be difficult to understand and learn at first. For the safety of both stroke survivor and instructor, ensuring understanding of any exercise-related task and cooperating with the instructor is vital.
Level of deconditioning	Deconditioning is associated with fatigue, decreased bone mineral density, loss of strength, and poor endurance.
Impaired balance	Complex or compound movements, especially where resistance in the form of free weights or machines are involved, pose greater risks to a stroke survivor with impaired balance.
Comorbidities: • Atrial fibrillation/ arrhythmia • Hypertension • Fatigue • Chronic obstructive pulmonary disorder.	As with any exercise programme, adequate screening is required. Additional precautions may be required to ensure stroke survivors are able to exercise effectively whilst remaining as safe as possible.
Medication	Some post-stroke medications can cause systemic weakness, fatigue, dampened pain sensations, and other symptoms. Table 7.5 contains common classifications of medications taken by stroke survivors.
Depression/anxiety	The level of engagement and adherence to exercise prescription may alter depending on the level of depression and anxiety about falling or deviating from routine.
Anosodiaphoria/anosognosia	Whilst mainly present in the hyperacute stage, after six months, anosognosia may still be present (Vocat et al. 2010). Stroke survivors with anosognosia have a lack of awareness of motor, visual, or cognitive impairment (Berti et al. 1996), which means they may undertake potentially dangerous activities and may avoid appropriate safety measures (Hartman-Maeir et al. 2001). Anosognosia is predominantly prevalent in stroke populations with right hemispheric lesions (Coslett and Heilman 1989).
Visual field impairment/ Hemispatial neglect/ Proprioceptive loss	Visual field impairment or hemispatial neglect may pose safety issues as they can frequently misjudge gaps e.g. doorways, bump into objects or people on their affected side, and potentially injure the neglected side – in particular the appendages.
Aphasia (receptive or expressive)	Aphasic stroke survivors have poor communication skills and therefore may pose a safety risk if not adequately addressed.

(Poltawski et al. 2014)

The medications taken by stroke survivors can have side effects that affect exercise. Table 7.5 ranks medications in order of prevalence of use in the USA, which is similar to the UK.

Barriers

There are significant barriers that make the prescription and implementation of exercise for stroke survivors complex. Many stroke survivors have significant comorbidities, which decrease the feasibility of physical activity (Kwakkel et al. 2004). The nature and severity of neurological deficits vary individually, and this influences the range of activities suitable for each patient. Functional limitations due to stroke and environmental factors (e.g. stroke-related impairments, transportation access, and cost) are significant barriers to physical activity (Nicholson et al. 2013; Damush et al. 2007).

Perceived barriers in stroke survivors may differ considerably from the general population, due to the numerous long-term consequences of stroke. Lack of confidence in the ability to perform exercise and concerns about the excessive exertional demands and adverse effects are some of the barriers to participation perceived by stroke survivors (Nicholson et al. 2013). Stroke survivors may be unaware of the benefits of physical activity – a barrier which may be overcome via education from health professionals about the actual low risks associated with physical activity, and highlighting the benefits of participation (Nicholson et al. 2013).

Box 7.1 is an example of the effect of the limited availability of specialist stroke rehabilitation support in some communities.

Table 7.5 The prevalence of medication classifications prescribed for stroke survivors

Classification of medication	%
Antihypertensive	86.5
Antiplatelet	75.3
Antihyperlipidemia	59.8
Antidepressant	58.8
Antidiabetic	33.0
Antiseizure	25.8
Anticoagulant	22.7
Sedative	18.6
Laxative	17.5
Analgesic/anti-inflammatory	17.5
Antihistamine	14.4
Antibiotic	12.4
Antiarrhythmia	9.3
Antianxiety	8.2
Antianginal	7.2
Antipsychotic	6.2
Cardiotonic	6.2

Adapted from Ostwald et al. 2006

Box 7.1 Case study 1: no clear community-based referral pathway

Freddy suffered a haemorrhagic stroke on the left-side of his brain; his face was distorted, he lost his voice, and his right arm and leg were immobile. It took about two months of physiotherapy and occupational therapy to increase his mobility, plus speech therapy almost every day. He managed to progress from the bed to the armchair, then a wheelchair, and then being able to stand up with some minor assistance. The work done by the physiotherapists improved the mobility of his legs, while the occupational therapist devoted her time to working on his paralysed arm. The exercises on his arms and wrist consisted of:

a   Using plastic beakers to squeeze, push, hold, and lift off the tables and arrange into rows and on top of each other
b   Holding, pushing, lifting, and throwing bean bags
c   Holding, swinging, pressing, catching, and throwing with light plastic balls and Swiss balls – to them.
d   Hydro pool exercises
e   Swimming pool exercises with arm and legs alternately
f   Theraband exercises
g   Aerobic exercises using bicycle and rowing ergometry
h   Dumbbell exercises to train his wrist and arm.

Afterwards he went to a rehabilitation unit, which gave him stretching exercises to keep his limbs more relaxed and supple; however, he did not gain much from it. Despite his efforts thus far, he is still using a stick to get around and wears a plastic orthotic. He does not feel as though he is in charge of his own recovery but cannot pay for weekly rehabilitation. He cannot perform many vital functional tasks with his affected hand and does not feel like he has gained much in the last year. He has spent a great deal of money for little gain, plateauing with his exercises, and he also cannot find a comprehensive training source to help him; he will be trying BOTOX soon instead.

Box 7.2 is an example of a successful community-based specialist stroke rehabilitation support service.

Box 7.2 Case study 2: successful community-based exercise referral pathway

Six months post-stroke Diane began attending two exercise referral classes per week at her local leisure centre after being referred by her nurse and consultant as part of the Wales National Exercise Referral Scheme (NERS). The Functional Fitness Circuit Class is a group exercise class of approximately twenty participants that is fun and includes strength, balance, and mobility movements.

The Gym Circuit is a group exercise class of approximately twelve participants based in a fitness suite, which can include use of treadmills, bikes, rowing- and strength-based machines. 'The stroke I had affected my left side and balance. I found that the classes helped with both of these, with exercises adapted to build the strength back to my left arm and leg. I also found the classes a good way of getting back out and about, meeting people who may have had a similar experience' explains Diane. Participants receive a discount on the entry fees, which is also valid for three months after their prescribed classes finish, to encourage them to continue exercising.

Future research

Since exercise programmes comprise of numerous interacting content and process variables, and may produce a wide variety of outcomes, they constitute complex interventions (Campbell et al. 2007). Complex interventions should have a coherent rationale and be described fully so that they can be implemented properly, and evaluated and replicated by peers (Medical Research Council 2008). However, post-stroke exercise programmes are typically designed on the basis of empirical evidence of effectiveness, and consequently may lack a coherent and comprehensive theoretical basis. Descriptions of exercise programmes provided by trial reports often lack detail, and there is a need for more comprehensive accounts that describe all the components that may affect outcomes (DeJong et al. 2005; Marsden and Greenwood 2005). Although substantial ground has been gained in evidencing exercise as a therapeutic intervention post-stroke, there are still considerable gaps in our knowledge that need to be filled in order for exercise programmes to be based on as much evidence as possible.

An interesting new direction of research into the physiological benefits of exercise post-stroke is that motor learning may be better exploited if aerobic exercise is paired more closely in time with motor training (Mang et al. 2013; Ploughman et al. 2007). Recovery of the upper limb is enhanced by employing endurance exercise before a skilled forelimb task (Kwakkel et al. 2003; Jørgensen et al. 1999). Other recent studies have found that combining physical exercise training with cognitive training resulted in a mutual enhancement of both interventions (Hötting and Röder 2013). The theoretical rationale is that, through enhancing BDNF mechanisms, aerobic exercise may 'prime' the brain for the learning of subsequent tasks. However, the mechanisms underlying this 'priming' phenomenon and the optimum threshold required for these effects are currently not fully understood, so further investigation is warranted, especially into the use of combined exercise interventions. Furthermore, the consensus that the risk of recurrent stroke is reduced by physical activity is predominantly based on the effect of exercise on surrogate markers of stroke risk; however, the use of exercise in the secondary prevention of stroke needs further evidencing.

Additional studies are needed to determine the definite mechanisms of impaired cardiorespiratory fitness and longitudinal changes in stroke survivors, as it is unclear whether this is a consequence of stroke, a factor that predates stroke, and/or a combination of the two. Clearer recommendations on the optimum timing for, and physiological adaptations to, high-intensity aerobic exercise in stroke survivors are needed before it can become an integral component of rehabilitation. With regard to muscle-strengthening activities, even though progressive resistance training is demonstrated to be effective, more research is required to establish the most appropriate time to commence training after stroke and to identify the stroke survivors who can benefit most. Furthermore, no strong evidence is available for the efficacy of aerobic exercise during the acute stage of stroke recovery. In terms of neuromuscular activities, although results from the small amount of research on yoga after stroke suggest that it may be beneficial for survivors, further investigation is warranted to further examine and evidence its effects in this population. Other universal considerations include the fact that evidence for exercise after haemorrhagic stroke is lacking in comparison to ischaemic stroke, so specific trials in this stroke sub-population are essential.

Chapter summary

Stroke is the sudden death of brain cells in a localised area due to inadequate blood flow, resulting in deprivation of oxygen and nutrients. Contralateral hemiparesis/hemiplegia is the most common presentation of a stroke patient requiring rehabilitation. There is uncertainty about many aspects of physical activity prescription for rehabilitation after stroke; however, evidence for various benefits of exercise interventions is accumulating. Exercise promotes brain neuroplasticity, angiogenesis, and neurogenesis, and may reduce the risk of recurrent stroke and other vascular events through mechanisms including improved lipid profile, reduction in blood pressure, reduced plasma fibrinogen level and platelet aggregation, weight reduction, and glucose metabolism. Physical fitness training after stroke improves depression and fatigue, and also improves various quality-of-life outcomes such as reduced dependence on others during ambulation, improved walking speed and tolerance, and reduced fall frequency.

Exercise prescription for stroke survivors is rather complex. Many studies demonstrate benefits, but with so many methods used and no single presentation of stroke being the same as another, it is difficult to determine standardised guidelines for the prescription of exercise as a rehabilitation tool. Broad consensus exists that programmes should contain endurance and muscle strengthening exercises, with a focus on functional actions, but, as with any exercise prescription, suitability for the exercise programme must be assessed and the programme tailored to the functionality of the individual stroke survivor and their recovery goals.

Although substantial ground has been gained in evidencing exercise as a therapeutic intervention post-stroke, there are still considerable gaps in our knowledge. However, these knowledge gaps should not prevent implementation of what is known, and health professionals are urged to work with exercise professionals to develop pathways into exercise for stroke survivors.

Study tasks

1   Charlie is a sixty five-year-old stroke survivor living in the community, with upper limb impairment, having been discharged once achieving satisfactory ambulation in his rehabilitation programme. However, Charlie struggles to

carry out activities of daily living with his paretic arm, frequently becomes frustrated, and feels hopeless now that he no longer receives rehabilitative care. A friend has recommended exercise training. Charlie used to enjoy circuit training when he was in the military; however, he cannot imagine how he could do that intensity of exercise any more, and does not understand how joining the local walking group could help, since it is his hand and arm that are the problem;

    a   Based on methodologies of successful research interventions, make an outline of the types and intensity of exercises that usually form part of circuit class therapy for stroke survivors that you can give to Charlie.

    b   Write a list of the physiological mechanisms of how aerobic exercise (such as walking) could improve upper limb recovery after stroke, and summarise this in layman's terms that you can explain to Charlie.

    c   Drawing on research findings, give Charlie an overview of the additional benefits of exercise that can be obtained through training in a group environment.

2   You are the exercise specialist for a patient who has suffered a recent stroke and expressed an interest in exercise training to help them. Drawing on existing evidence, write a list of suitable exercise interventions for acute and sub-acute stroke survivors, detailing potential benefits, considerations and adaptations for each.

3   Emma is suffering with lower limb impairment following her stroke. Emma was making good progress in improving her locomotor function by going for short walks with the aid of a stick, and almost felt ready to try to walk unaided. Unfortunately, she had a fall last month. Since then her family will only let her go for a walk when one of them is around to accompany her, and are even discouraging her from getting up to do things around the house. Use current evidence to explain the vicious cycle of physical inactivity, falls, and quality of life in stroke survivors to Emma's family, and highlight the potential benefits and adaptations that she could use.

Further reading

Billinger, S. A., Boyne, P., Coughenour, E., Dunning, K. and Mattlage, A. (2015). Does aerobic exercise and the FITT principle fit into stroke recovery? *Current Neurology and Neuroscience Reports*, 15(2), 1–8.

Billinger, S., Arena, R., Bernhardt, J., Eng, J., Franklin, B., Johnson, C., MacKay-Lyons, M., Macko, R. F., Mead, G. E., Roth, E.J., Shaughnessy, M. and Tang, A. (2014). Physical activity and exercise recommendations for stroke survivors: a statement for healthcare professionals from the American Heart Association/American Stroke Association. *Stroke*, 45(8), 2532–53. doi: 10.1161/STR.0000000000000022.

Mead, G. and Van Wijk, F. (2012). *Exercise and fitness training after stroke: a handbook for evidence-based practice*. Oxford: Elsevier Health Sciences.

Saunders, D. H., Sanderson, M., Brazzelli, M., Greig, C. A. and Mead, G. E. (2013). Physical fitness training for stroke patients. *Cochrane Database of Systematic Reviews*, 10: CD003316. doi: 10.1002/14651858.CD003316.pub5.

References

Ada, L., Dean, C. M. and Lindley, R. (2013). Randomized trial of treadmill training to improve walking in community-dwelling people after stroke: the AMBULATE trial. *International Journal of Stroke*, 8(6), 436–44.

Ada, L., Dorsch, S. and Canning, C. G. (2006). Strengthening interventions increase strength and improve activity after stroke: a systematic review. *Australian Journal of Physiotherapy*, 52(4), 241–8.

Adamson, J., Beswick, A. and Ebrahim, S. (2004). *Reducing brain damage: faster access to better stroke care*. London: The Stationery Office Limited.

Alonso, M., Vianna, M. R., Depino, A. M., Mello e Souza, T., Pereira, P., Szapiro, G., Viola, H., Pitossi, F., Izquierdo, I. and Medina, J. H. (2002). BDNF-triggered events in the rat hippocampus are required for both short-and long-term memory formation. *Hippocampus*, 12(4), 551–60.

American College of Sports Medicine (ACSM) (2013). ACSM's guidelines for exercise testing and prescription. 9th ed. Baltimore: Lippincott Williams and Wilkins.

American Heart Association (AHA). (2003). *Heart disease and stroke statistics–2003 update*. Dallas, TX: American Heart Association.

Appelros, P., Nydevik, I. and Viitanen, M. (2003). Poor outcome after first-ever stroke predictors for death, dependency, and recurrent stroke within the first year. *Stroke*, 34(1), 122–6.

Askim, T., Bernhardt, J., Salvesen, Ø. and Indredavik, B. (2014). Physical activity early after stroke and its association to functional outcome 3 months later. *Journal of Stroke and Cerebrovascular Diseases*, 23(5), e305–12.

Balchin, T. (2011). *The successful stroke survivor: the new guide to functional recovery from stroke*. Tempe: Bagwyn Books.

Balchin, T. (2013). Neuroplasticity and the ARNI approach to functional recovery from stroke. In Sassoon, R. (ed.) *Understanding Stroke – for Patients, Carers and Health Professionals* (pp 105–16). Sussex: Book Guild Ltd.

Bernhardt, J., Chitravas, N., Meslo, I. L., Thrift, A. G. and Indredavik, B. (2008b). Not all stroke units are the same: a comparison of physical activity patterns in Melbourne, Australia, and Trondheim, Norway. *Stroke*, 39(7), 2059–65.

Bernhardt, J., Dewey, H., Thrift, A., Collier, J. and Donnan, G. (2008a). A very early rehabilitation trial for stroke (AVERT) phase II safety and feasibility. *Stroke*, 39(2), 390–6.

Bernhardt, J., Dewey, H., Thrift, A. and Donnan, G. (2004). Inactive and alone: physical activity within the first 14 days of acute stroke unit care. *Stroke*, 35(4), 1005–9.

Billinger, S. A., Boyne, P., Coughenour, E., Dunning, K. and Mattlage, A. (2015). Does aerobic exercise and the FITT principle fit into stroke recovery? *Current Neurology and Neuroscience Reports*, 15(2), 1–8.

Billinger, S. A., Coughenour, E., MacKay-Lyons, M. J. and Ivey, F. M. (2011). Reduced cardiorespiratory fitness after stroke: biological consequences and exercise-induced adaptations. *Stroke Research and Treatment*, 2012, 959120. doi: 10.1155/2012/959120.

Billinger, S. A., Taylor, J. M. and Quaney, B. M. (2012). Cardiopulmonary response to exercise testing in people with chronic stroke: a retrospective study. *Stroke Research and Treatment*, 2012, 987637. doi: 10.1155/2012/987637.

Billinger, S., Arena, R., Bernhardt, J., Eng, J., Franklin, B., Johnson, C., MacKay-Lyons, M., Macko, R. F., Mead, G. E., Roth, E.J., Shaughnessy, M. and Tang, A. (2014). Physical activity and exercise recommendations for stroke survivors: a statement for healthcare professionals from the American Heart Association/American Stroke Association. Stroke, 45(8), 2532–53. doi: 10.1161/STR.0000000000000022.

Bohannon, R. W. (2007). Muscle strength and muscle training after stroke. *Journal of Rehabilitation Medicine*, 39(1), 14–20.

Brainin, M., Teuschl, Y. and Kalra, L. (2007). Acute treatment and long-term management of stroke in developing countries. *The Lancet Neurology*, 6(6), 553–61.

Brazzelli, M., Saunders, D. H., Greig, C. A. and Mead, G. E. (2011). Physical fitness training for stroke patients. *Cochrane Database of Systematic Reviews*, 11:CD003316. doi: 10.1002/14651858.CD003316.pub4.

Bressel, E. and McNair, P. J. (2002). The effect of prolonged static and cyclic stretching on ankle joint stiffness, torque relaxation, and gait in people with stroke. *Physical Therapy*, 82(9), 880–7.

Broderick, J., Brott, T., Kothari, R., Miller, R., Khoury, J., Pancioli, A., Gebel, J., Mills, D., Minneci, L. and Shukla, R. (1998). The Greater Cincinnati/Northern Kentucky Stroke Study Preliminary first-ever and total incidence rates of stroke among blacks. *Stroke*, 29(2), 415–21.

Brosseau, L., Wells, G. A., Finestone, H. M., Egan, M., Dubouloz, C.-J., Graham, I., Casimiro, L., Robinson, V. A., Bilodeau, M., McGowan, J., Teasell, R., Desrosiers, J., Barreca, S., Laferriere, L., Fung, J., Corriveau, H., Gubitz, G., Sharma, M., Khadilkar, A., Phillips, K., Jean, N., Lamothe, C., Milne, S. and Sarnecka, J. (2006). Ottawa panel evidence-based clinical practice guidelines for post-stroke rehabilitation. *Top Stroke Rehabil*, 13(2), 1–269.

Campbell, N. C., Murray, E., Darbyshire, J., Emery, J., Farmer, A., Griffiths, F., Guthrie, B., Lester, H., Wilson, P. and Kinmonth, A. L. (2007). Designing and evaluating complex interventions to improve health care. *BMJ*, 334(7591), 455.

Carin-Levy, G., Kendall, M., Young, A. and Mead, G. (2009). The psychosocial effects of exercise and relaxation classes for persons surviving a stroke. *Canadian Journal of Occupational Therapy*, 76(2), 73–80.

Carod-Artal, J., Egido, J. A., González, J. L. and De Seijas, E. V. (2000). Quality of life among stroke survivors evaluated 1 year after stroke experience of a stroke unit. *Stroke*, 31(12), 2995–3000.

Chen, M.-D. and Rimmer, J. H. (2011). Effects of exercise on quality of life in stroke survivors a meta-analysis. *Stroke*, 42(3), 832–7.

Cheng, P.-T., Wu, S.-H., Liaw, M.-Y., Wong, A. M. and Tang, F.-T. (2001). Symmetrical body-weight distribution training in stroke patients and its effect on fall prevention. *Archives of Physical Medicine and Rehabilitation*, 82(12), 1650–4.

Chu, K. S., Eng, J. J., Dawson, A. S., Harris, J. E., Ozkaplan, A. and Gylfadóttir, S. (2004). Water-based exercise for cardiovascular fitness in people with chronic stroke: a randomized controlled trial. *Archives of Physical Medicine and Rehabilitation*, 85(6), 870–4.

Clark, D. J. and Patten, C. (2013). Eccentric versus concentric resistance training to enhance neuromuscular activation and walking speed following stroke. *Neurorehabilitation and Neural Repair*, 27(4), 335–44.

Colle, F., Bonan, I., Gellez Leman, M., Bradai, N. and Yelnik, A. (2006). Fatigue after stroke. *Ann Readapt Med Phys*, 49(6), 272–6, 361–4.

Coslett, H. B. and Heilman, K. M. (1989). Hemihypokinesia after right hemisphere stroke. *Brain and Cognition*, 9(2), 267–78.

Cramer, S. C. (2008). Repairing the human brain after stroke: I. Mechanisms of spontaneous recovery. *Annals of Neurology*, 63(3), 272–87.

Cumming, T. B., Thrift, A. G., Collier, J. M., Churilov, L., Dewey, H. M., Donnan, G. A. and Bernhardt, J. (2011). Very early mobilization after stroke fast-tracks return to walking: further results from the phase II AVERT randomized controlled trial. *Stroke*, 42(1), 153–8.

Dam, M., Tonin, P., Casson, S., Ermani, M., Pizzolato, G., Iaia, V. and Battistin, L. (1993). The effects of long-term rehabilitation therapy on poststroke hemiplegic patients. *Stroke*, 24(8), 1186–91.

Damush, T. M., Perkins, S. M., Mikesky, A. E., Roberts, M. and O'Dea, J. (2005). Motivational factors influencing older adults diagnosed with knee osteoarthritis to join and maintain an exercise program. *J Aging Phys Act*, 13(1), 45–60.

Damush, T. M., Plue, L., Bakas, T., Schmid, A. and Williams, L. S. (2007). Barriers and facilitators to exercise among stroke survivors. *Rehabilitation Nursing*, 32(6), 253–62.

Dean, C. M., Richards, C. L. and Malouin, F. (2000). Task-related circuit training improves performance of locomotor tasks in chronic stroke: a randomized, controlled pilot trial. *Archives of Physical Medicine and Rehabilitation*, 81(4), 409–17.

DeJong, G., Horn, S. D., Conroy, B., Nichols, D. and Healton, E. B. (2005). Opening the black box of poststroke rehabilitation: stroke rehabilitation patients, processes, and outcomes. *Archives of Physical Medicine and Rehabilitation*, 86(12), 1–7.

Di Fabio, R. P., Badke, M. B. and Duncan, P. W. (1986). Adapting human postural reflexes following localized cerebrovascular lesion: analysis of bilateral long latency responses. *Brain Research*, 363(2), 257–64.

Dobkin, B. H. (2004). Strategies for stroke rehabilitation. *The Lancet Neurology*, 3(9), 528–36.

Dragert, K. and Zehr, E. P. (2013). High-intensity unilateral dorsiflexor resistance training results in bilateral neuromuscular plasticity after stroke. *Experimental Brain Research*, 225(1), 93–104.

Duncan, P., Studenski, S., Richards, L., Gollub, S., Lai, S. M., Reker, D., Perera, S., Yates, J., Koch, V., Rigler, S. and Johnson, D.. (2003). Randomized clinical trial of therapeutic exercise in subacute stroke. *Stroke*, 34(9), 2173–80.

Duncan, P. W., Goldstein, L. B., Horner, R. D., Landsman, P. B., Samsa, G. P. and Matchar, D. B. (1994). Similar motor recovery of upper and lower extremities after stroke. *Stroke*, 25(6), 1181–8.

Elkins, J. S. and Johnston, S. C. (2003). Thirty-year projections for deaths from ischemic stroke in the United States. *Stroke*, 34(9), 2109–12.

Eng, J. J. (2010). Fitness and Mobility Exercise (FAME) program for stroke. *Topics in Geriatric Rehabilitation*, 26(4), 310.

Eng, J. J., Chu, K. S., Kim, C. M., Dawson, A. S., Carswell, A. and Hepburn, K. E. (2003). A community-based group exercise program for persons with chronic stroke. *Medicine and Science in Sports and Exercise*, 35(8), 1271.

European Stroke Organization (ESO) (2008). Guidelines for management of ischaemic stroke and transient ischaemic attack. *Cerebrovascular Diseases*, 25, 457–507.

Farrow, S. and Reid, D. (2004). Stroke survivors' perceptions of a leisure-based virtual reality program. *Technology and Disability*, 16(2), 69–81.

Feigin, V. L., Forouzanfar, M. H., Krishnamurthi, R., Mensah, G. A., Connor, M., Bennett, D. A., Moran, A. E., Sacco, R. L., Anderson, L., Truelsen, T., O'Donnell, M., Venketasubramanian, N., Barker-Collo, S., Lawes, C. M., Wang, W., Shinohara, Y., Witt, E., Ezzati, M., Naghavi, M., Murray, C. (2014). Global and regional burden of stroke during 1990–2010: findings from the Global Burden of Disease Study 2010. *Lancet*, 383(9913), 245–54.

French, B., Thomas, L. H., Leathley, M. J., Sutton, C. J., McAdam, J., Forster, A., Langhorne, P., Price, C. I., Walker, A. and Watkins, C. L. (2009). Repetitive task training for improving functional ability after stroke. *Stroke*, 40(4), e98–9.

Fujitani, J., Ishikawa, T., Akai, M. and Kakurai, S. (1999). Influence of daily activity on changes in physical fitness for people with post-stroke hemiplegia. *American Journal of Physical Medicine and Rehabilitation*, 78(6), 540–4.

Gallanagh, S., Quinn, T. J., Alexander, J. and Walters, M. R. (2011). Physical activity in the prevention and treatment of stroke. *International Scholarly Research Notices*, 2011. doi:10.5402/2011/953818.

Galvin, R., Cusack, T., O'Grady, E., Murphy, T. B. and Stokes, E. (2011). Family-Mediated Exercise Intervention (FAME): evaluation of a novel form of exercise delivery after stroke. *Stroke*, 42(3), 681–6.

Go, A. S., Mozaffarian, D., Roger, V. L., Benjamin, E. J., Berry, Borden, W. B., Bravata, D. M., Dai, S., Ford, E. S., Fox, C. S., Franco, S., Fullerton, H. J., Gillespie, C., Hailpern, S. M.,

Heit, J. A., Howard, V. J., Huffman, M. D., Kissela, B. M., Kittner, S. J., Lackland, D. T., Lichtman, J. H., Lisabeth, L. D., Magid, D., Marcus, G. M., Marelli, A., Matchar, D. B., McGuire, D. K., Mohler, E. R., Moy, C. S., Mussolino, M. E., Nichol, G., Paynter, N. P., Schreiner, P. J., Sorlie, P. D., Stein, J., Turan, T. N., Virani, S. S., Wong, N. D., Woo, D. and Turner, M. B. (2013). Heart disease and stroke statistics–2013 update: a report from the American Heart Association. *Circulation*, 127(1), e6.

Gordon, N. F., Gulanick, M., Costa, F., Fletcher, G., Franklin, B. A., Roth, E. J. and Shephard, T. (2004). Physical activity and exercise recommendations for stroke survivors: an American heart association scientific statement from the council on clinical cardiology, subcommittee on exercise, cardiac rehabilitation, and prevention; the council on cardiovascular nursing; the council on nutrition, physical activity, and metabolism; and the stroke council. *Stroke*, 35(5), 1230–40.

Hackam, D. G. and J. D. Spence (2007). Combining multiple approaches for the secondary prevention of vascular events after stroke a quantitative modeling study. *Stroke* 38(6), 1881–5.

Hacke, W., Donnan, G., Fieschi, C., Kaste, M., von Kummer, R., Broderick, J.P., Brott, T., Frankel, M., Grotta, J. C., Haley, E. C. Jr, Kwiatkowski, T., Levine, S. R., Lewandowski, C., Lu, M., Lyden, P., Marler, J. R., Patel, S., Tilley, B. C., Albers, G., Bluhmki, E., Wilhelm, M. and Hamilton, S. (2004). Association of outcome with early stroke treatment: pooled analysis of ATLANTIS, ECASS, and NINDS rt-PA stroke trials. *The Lancet*, 363(9411), 768–74.

Hackett, M. L., Yapa, C., Parag, V. and Anderson, C. S. (2005). Frequency of depression after stroke: a systematic review of observational studies. *Stroke*, 36(6), 1330–40.

Hankey, G. J. and Warlow, C. P. (1999). Treatment and secondary prevention of stroke: evidence, costs, and effects on individuals and populations. *The Lancet*, 354(9188), 1457–63.

Harris, J. E. and Eng, J. J. (2007). Paretic upper-limb strength best explains arm activity in people with stroke. *Physical Therapy*, 87(1), 88–97.

Harris, J. E., Eng, J. J., Miller, W. C. and Dawson, A. S. (2009). A self-administered graded repetitive arm supplementary program (GRASP) improves arm function during inpatient stroke rehabilitation a multi-site randomized controlled trial. *Stroke*, 40(6), 2123–8.

Hartman-Maeir, A., Soroker, N. and Katz, N. (2001). Anosognosia for hemiplegia in stroke rehabilitation. *Neurorehabilitation and Neural Repair*, 15(3), 213–22.

Hartman-Maeir, A., Soroker, N., Ring, H., Avni, N. and Katz, N. (2007). Activities, participation and satisfaction one-year post stroke. *Disability and Rehabilitation*, 29(7), 559–66.

Hoeben, A., Landuyt, B., Highley, M. S., Wildiers, H., Van Oosterom, A. T. and De Bruijn, E. A. (2004). Vascular endothelial growth factor and angiogenesis. *Pharmacological Reviews*, 56(4), 549–80.

Hötting, K. and Röder, B. (2013). Beneficial effects of physical exercise on neuroplasticity and cognition. *Neuroscience and Biobehavioral Reviews*, 37(9), 2243–57.

Howard, A. (2011). Coding for bone diseases. *For the Record*, 23(9) 27. Available at: http://www.fortherecordmag.com/archives/050911p27.shtml.

Huber, K. M., Sawtell, N. B. and Bear, M. F. (1998). Brain-derived neurotrophic factor alters the synaptic modification threshold in visual cortex. *Neuropharmacology*, 37(4), 571–9.

Hurkmans, H. L., Ribbers, G. M., Streur-Kranenburg, M. F., Stam, H. J. and Van Den Berg-Emons, R. J. (2011). Energy expenditure in chronic stroke patients playing Wii Sports: a pilot study. *J Neuroeng Rehabil*, 8(38), 1–7.

Hyndman, D., Ashburn, A. and Stack, E. (2002). Fall events among people with stroke living in the community: circumstances of falls and characteristics of fallers. *Archives of Physical Medicine and Rehabilitation*, 83(2), 165–70.

Intercollegiate Stroke Working Party. (2012) *National clinical guidelines for stroke*. 4th ed. London: Royal College of Physicians. National Institute for Health and Clinical Excellence. Available at: http://www.rcplondon.ac.uk/sites/default/files/national-clinical-guidelines-for-stroke-fourth-edition.pdf.

Ivey, F., Macko, R., Ryan, A. and Hafer-Macko, C. (2005). Cardiovascular health and fitness after stroke. *Top Stroke Rehabil*, 12(1), 1–16.

Ivy, A., Rodriguez, F., Garcia, C., Chen, M. and Russo-Neustadt, A. (2003). Noradrenergic and serotonergic blockade inhibits BDNF mRNA activation following exercise and antidepressant. *Pharmacology Biochemistry and Behavior*, 75(1), 81–8.

Jacobs, B., Van Praag, H. and Gage, F. (2000). Adult brain neurogenesis and psychiatry: a novel theory of depression. *Molecular Psychiatry*, 5, 262–9.

Jones, A. Y., Dean, E. and Scudds, R. J. (2005). Effectiveness of a community-based tai chi program and implications for public health initiatives. *Archives of Physical Medicine and Rehabilitation*, 86(4), 619–25.

Joo, L. Y., Yin, T. S., Xu, D., Thia, E., Chia, P. F., Kuah, C. W. K. and He, K. K. (2010). A feasibility study using interactive commercial off-the-shelf computer gaming in upper limb rehabilitation in patients after stroke. *Journal of Rehabilitation Medicine*, 42(5), 437–41.

Jørgensen, H. S., Reith, J., Nakayama, H., Kammersgaard, L. P., Raaschou, H. O. and Olsen, T. S. (1999). What determines good recovery in patients with the most severe strokes? The Copenhagen Stroke Study. *Stroke*, 30(10), 2008–12.

Kanis, J., Oden, A. and Johnell, O. (2001). Acute and long-term increase in fracture risk after hospitalization for stroke. *Stroke*, 32(3), 702–6.

Kilbride, C., Norris, M., Theis, N. and Mohagheghi, A. A. (2013). Action for Rehabilitation from Neurological Injury (ARNI): a pragmatic study of functional training for stroke survivors. *Open Journal of Therapy and Rehabilitation*, 1(2), 40–51. doi: 10.4236/ojtr.2013.12008.

Kim, P., Warren, S., Madill, H. and Hadley, M. (1999). Quality of life of stroke survivors. *Quality of Life Research*, 8(4), 293–301.

King, R. B. (1996). Quality of life after stroke. *Stroke*, 27(9), 1467–72.

Knaepen, K., Goekint, M., Heyman, E. M. and Meeusen, R. (2010). Neuroplasticity: Exercise-induced response of peripheral brain-derived neurotrophic factor. *Sports Medicine*, 40(9), 765–801.

Kramer, A. F., Hahn, S., Cohen, N. J., Banich, M. T., McAuley, E., Harrison, C. R., Chason, J., Vakil, E., Bardell, L., Boileau, R. A. and Colcombe, A. (1999). Ageing, fitness and neurocognitive function. *Nature*, 400(6743), 418–19.

Kwakkel, G., Kollen, B. J., van der Grond, J. and Prevo, A. J. (2003). Probability of regaining dexterity in the flaccid upper limb impact of severity of paresis and time since onset in acute stroke. *Stroke*, 34(9), 2181–6.

Kwakkel, G., van Peppen, R., Wagenaar, R. C., Dauphinee, S. W., Richards, C., Ashburn, A., Miller, K., Lincoln, N., Partridge, C., Wellwood, I. and Langhorne, P. (2004). Effects of augmented exercise therapy time after stroke: a meta-analysis. *Stroke*, 35(11), 2529–39.

Kwakkel, G., Wagenaar, R. C., Koelman, T. W., Lankhorst, G. J. and Koetsier, J. C. (1997). Effects of intensity of rehabilitation after stroke: a research synthesis. *Stroke*, 28(8), 1550–6.

Langhorne, P., Bernhardt, J. and Kwakkel, G. (2011). Stroke rehabilitation. *The Lancet*, 377(9778), 1693–1702.

Langhorne, P., Coupar, F. and Pollock, A. (2009). Motor recovery after stroke: a systematic review. *The Lancet Neurology*, 8(8), 741–54.

Langhorne, P. and Duncan, P. (2001). Does the organization of postacute stroke care really matter? *Stroke*, 32(1), 268–74.

Langhorne, P., Wagenaar, R. and Partridge, C. (1996). Physiotherapy after stroke: more is better? *Physiotherapy Research International*, 1(2), 75–88.

Laurin, J. and Pin-Barre, C. (2014). Physiological adaptations following endurance exercises after stroke: focus on the plausible role of high-intensity interval training. *International Journal of Physical Medicine and Rehabilitation*, S3:006. doi: 10.4172/2329-9096.S3-006.

Lawes, C. M., Bennett, D. A., Feigin, V. L. and Rodgers, A. (2004). Blood pressure and stroke: an overview of published reviews. *Stroke*, 35(3), 776–85.

Lee, C. D., Folsom, A. R. and Blair, S. N. (2003). Physical activity and stroke risk: a meta-analysis. *Stroke*, 34(10), 2475–81.

Lexell, J. and Flansbjer, U.-B. (2008). Muscle strength training, gait performance and physiotherapy after stroke. *Minerva Medica*, 99(4), 353–68.

Lezak, M. D. (2004). *Neuropsychological assessment*: Oxford: Oxford University Press.

Macko, R., DeSouza, C., Tretter, L., Silver, K., Smith, G., Anderson, P., Tomoyasu, N., Gorman, P. and Dengel, D. (1997). Treadmill aerobic exercise training reduces the energy expenditure and cardiovascular demands of hemiparetic gait in chronic stroke patients: a preliminary report. *Stroke*, 28(2), 326–30.

Macko, R. F., Ivey, F. M., Forrester, L. W., Hanley, D., Sorkin, J. D., Katzel, L. I., Silver, K. H. and Goldberg, A. P. (2005). Treadmill exercise rehabilitation improves ambulatory function and cardiovascular fitness in patients with chronic stroke: a randomized, controlled trial. *Stroke*, 36(10), 2206–11.

Mang, C. S., Campbell, K. L., Ross, C. J. and Boyd, L. A. (2013). Promoting neuroplasticity for motor rehabilitation after stroke: considering the effects of aerobic exercise and genetic variation on brain-derived neurotrophic factor. *Physical Therapy*, 93(12), 1707–16.

Marigold, D. S., Eng, J. J., Dawson, A. S., Inglis, J. T., Harris, J. E. and Gylfadóttir, S. (2005). Exercise leads to faster postural reflexes, improved balance and mobility, and fewer falls in older persons with chronic stroke. *Journal of the American Geriatrics Society*, 53(3), 416–23.

Marsden, J. and Greenwood, R. (2005). Physiotherapy after stroke: define, divide and conquer. *Journal of Neurology, Neurosurgery and Psychiatry*, 76(4), 465–6.

Martin, J., Meltzer, H. and Elliot, D. (1988). *The prevalence of disability among adults*. London: HMSO Books.

Martinsen, E. W. (2008). Physical activity in the prevention and treatment of anxiety and depression. *Nordic Journal of Psychiatry*, 62(S47), 25–9.

Mead, G. and Bernhardt, J. (2011). Physical fitness training after stroke, time to implement what we know: more research is needed. *International Journal of Stroke*, 6(6), 506–8.

Mead, G., Bernhardt, J. and Kwakkel, G. (2012). Stroke: physical fitness, exercise, and fatigue. *Stroke research and treatment*, 2012, 632531. doi: 10.1155/2012/632531.

Mead, G. E., Greig, C. A., Cunningham, I., Lewis, S. J., Dinan, S., Saunders, D. H., Fitzsimons, C. and Young, A. (2007). Stroke: a randomized trial of exercise or relaxation. *Journal of the American Geriatrics Society*, 55(6), 892–9.

Medical Research Council. (2008). *Developing and evaluating complex interventions: new guidance*. Medical Research Council: London.

Mehrholz, J., Pohl, M. and Elsner, B. (2014). Treadmill training and body weight support for walking after stroke. *Cochrane Database of Systematic Rev*, 1: CD002840. doi: 10.1002/14651858.CD002840.pub3.

Miller, E. L., Murray, L., Richards, L., Zorowitz, R. D., Bakas, T., Clark, P. and Billinger, S. A. (2010). Comprehensive overview of nursing and interdisciplinary rehabilitation care of the stroke patient: a scientific statement from the American Heart Association. *Stroke*, 41(10), 2402–48.

Mohan, K. M., Wolfe, C. D., Rudd, A. G., Heuschmann, P. U., Kolominsky-Rabas, P. L. and Grieve, A. P. (2011). Risk and cumulative risk of stroke recurrence: a systematic review and meta-analysis. *Stroke*, 42(5), 1489–94.

Molteni, R., Zheng, J.-Q., Ying, Z., Gómez-Pinilla, F. and Twiss, J. L. (2004). Voluntary exercise increases axonal regeneration from sensory neurons. *Proceedings of the National Academy of Sciences of the United States of America*, 101(22), 8473–8.

Morris, J. H., van Wijck, F., Joice, S. and Donaghy, M. (2013). Predicting health related quality of life 6 months after stroke: the role of anxiety and upper limb dysfunction. *Disability and Rehabilitation*, 35(4), 291–9.

Morris, S. L., Dodd, K. J. and Morris, M. E. (2004). Outcomes of progressive resistance strength training following stroke: a systematic review. *Clinical Rehabilitation*, 18(1), 27–39.

Mouawad, M. R., Doust, C. G., Max, M. D. and McNulty, P. A. (2011). Wii-based movement therapy to promote improved upper extremity function post-stroke: a pilot study. *Journal of Rehabilitation Medicine*, 43(6), 527–33.

Murray, C. J. L. and Lopez, A. D. (1996). *The global burden of disease: a comprehensive assessment of mortality and disability from diseases, injuries,and risk factors in 1990 and projected to 2020*. Cambridge, MA: Harvard School of Public Health.

Nabkasorn, C., Miyai, N., Sootmongkol, A., Junprasert, S., Yamamoto, H., Arita, M. and Miyashita, K. (2006). Effects of physical exercise on depression, neuroendocrine stress hormones and physiological fitness in adolescent females with depressive symptoms. *European Journal of Public Health*, 16(2), 179–84.

Naci, H. and Ioannidis, J. (2013). Comparative effectiveness of exercise and drug interventions on mortality outcomes: metaepidemiological study. *BMJ*, 347, f5577. doi: 10.1136/bmj.f5577.

National Institute for Health and Care Excellence (NICE). (2008). *Stroke: diagnosis and initial management of acute stroke and transient ischaemic attack (TIA) (clinical guideline CG68)*. Available at: http://www.nice.org.uk/guidance/CG68.

National Institute for Health and Care Excellence (NICE). (2013). *Stroke rehabilitation: long-term rehabilitation after stroke (clinical guideline CG162)*. Available at: http://guidance.nice.org.uk/CG162.

Nicholson, S., Sniehotta, F. F., Wijck, F., Greig, C. A., Johnston, M., McMurdo, M. E., Dennis, M. and Mead, G. E. (2013). A systematic review of perceived barriers and motivators to physical activity after stroke. *International Journal of Stroke*, 8(5), 357–64.

Office for National Statistics. (2014). *Life expectancy at birth and at age 65 by local areas in the United Kingdom, 2006–08 to 2010–12*. Available at: http://www.ons.gov.uk/ons/rel/subnational-health4/life-expec-at-birth-age-65/2006-08-to-2010-12/stb-life-expectancy-at-birth-2006-08-to-2010-12.html.

Ostwald, S. K., Wasserman, J. and Davis, S. (2006). Medications, comorbidities, and medical complications in stroke survivors: the CAReS study. *Rehabilitation Nursing*, 31(1), 10–14.

Ouellette, M. M., LeBrasseur, N. K., Bean, J. F., Phillips, E., Stein, J., Frontera, W. R. and Fielding, R. A. (2004). High-intensity resistance training improves muscle strength, self-reported function, and disability in long-term stroke survivors. *Stroke*, 35(6), 1404–9.

Page, S. J., Gater, D. R. and Bach-y-Rita, P. (2004). Reconsidering the motor recovery plateau in stroke rehabilitation. *Archives of Physical Medicine and Rehabilitation*, 85(8), 1377–81.

Palmer, A. J., Valentine, W. J., Roze, S., Lammert, M., Spiesser, J. and Gabriel, S. (2004). Overview of costs of stroke from published, incidence-based studies spanning 16 industrialized countries. *Current Medical Research and Opinion*, 21(1), 19–26.

Pang, M. Y., Eng, J. J., Dawson, A. S. and Gylfadóttir, S. (2006a). The use of aerobic exercise training in improving aerobic capacity in individuals with stroke: a meta-analysis. *Clinical Rehabilitation*, 20(2), 97–111.

Pang, M. Y., Eng, J. J., Dawson, A. S., McKay, H. A. and Harris, J. E. (2006b). A community-based fitness and mobility exercise program for older adults with chronic stroke: a randomized, controlled trial. *Journal of the American Geriatrics Society*, 53(10), 1667–74.

Pang, M. Y., Harris, J. E. and Eng, J. J. (2005). A community-based upper-extremity group exercise program improves motor function and performance of functional activities in chronic stroke: a randomized controlled trial. *Archives of Physical Medicine and Rehabilitation*, 87(1), 1–9.

Ploughman, M., Attwood, Z., White, N., Doré, J. J. and Corbett, D. (2007). Endurance exercise facilitates relearning of forelimb motor skill after focal ischemia. *European Journal of Neuroscience*, 25(11), 3453–60.

Ploughman, M., McCarthy, J., Bossé, M., Sullivan, H. J. and Corbett, D. (2008). Does treadmill exercise improve performance of cognitive or upper-extremity tasks in people with chronic stroke? A randomized cross-over trial. *Archives of Physical Medicine and Rehabilitation*, 89(11), 2041–7.

Poltawski, L., Abraham, C., Forster, A., Goodwin, V. A., Kilbride, C., Taylor, R. S. and Dean, S. (2013b). Synthesising practice guidelines for the development of community-based exercise programmes after stroke. *Implementation Science*, 8(1), 115.

Poltawski, L., Boddy, K., Forster, A., Goodwin, V. A., Pavey, A. C. and Dean, S. (2014). Motivators for uptake and maintenance of exercise: perceptions of long-term stroke survivors and implications for design of exercise programmes. *Disability and Rehabilitation*, 37(9), 795–801. doi: 10.3109/09638288.2014.946154.

Poltawski, L., Briggs, J., Forster, A., Goodwin, V. A., James, M., Taylor, R. S. and Dean, S. (2013a). Informing the design of a randomised controlled trial of an exercise-based programme for long term stroke survivors: lessons from a before-and-after case series study. *BMC Research Notes*, 6(1), 324.

Poole, K. E., Reeve, J. and Warburton, E. A. (2002). Falls, fractures, and osteoporosis after stroke: time to think about protection? *Stroke*, 33(5), 1432–6.

Potempa, K., Lopez, M., Braun, L. T., Szidon, J. P., Fogg, L. and Tincknell, T. (1995). Physiological outcomes of aerobic exercise training in hemiparetic stroke patients. *Stroke*, 26(1), 101–5.

Prabhakaran, S. and Chong, J. Y. (2014). Risk factor management for stroke prevention. *Continuum*, 20(2 Cerebrovascular Disease), 296–308.

Quaney, B. M., Boyd, L. A., McDowd, J. M., Zahner, L. H., He, J., Mayo, M. S. and Macko, R. F. (2009). Aerobic exercise improves cognition and motor function post-stroke. *Neurorehabilitation and Neural Repair*, 23(9), 879–85. doi: 10.1177/1545968309 338193.

Querido, J. S. and Sheel, A. W. (2007). Regulation of cerebral blood flow during exercise. *Sports Medicine*, 37(9), 765–82.

Quinn, T. J., Paolucci, S., Sunnerhagen, K. S., Sivenius, J., Walker, M. F., Toni, D. and Lees, K. R. (2009). Evidence-based stroke rehabilitation: an expanded guidance document from the European Stroke Organisation (ESO) guidelines for management of ischaemic stroke and transient ischaemic attack 2008. *Journal of Rehabilitation Medicine*, 41(2), 99–111.

Ramnemark, A., Nyberg, L., Borssén, B., Olsson, T. and Gustafson, Y. (1998). Fractures after stroke. *Osteoporosis International*, 8(1), 92–5.

Redfern, J., McKevitt, C., Rudd, A. G. and Wolfe, C. D. (2002). Health care follow-up after stroke: opportunities for secondary prevention. *Family Practice*, 19(4), 378–82.

Rimmer, J. H., Rauworth, A. E., Wang, E. C., Nicola, T. L. and Hill, B. (2009). A preliminary study to examine the effects of aerobic and therapeutic (nonaerobic) exercise on cardiorespiratory fitness and coronary risk reduction in stroke survivors. *Archives of Physical Medicine and Rehabilitation*, 90(3), 407–12.

Rimmer, J. H. and Wang, E. (2005). Aerobic exercise training in stroke survivors. *Top Stroke Rehabil*, 12(1), 17–30.

Rossi, C., Angelucci, A., Costantin, L., Braschi, C., Mazzantini, M., Babbini, F., Fabbri, M. E., Tessarollo, L., Maffei, L., Berardi, N. and Caleo M.. (2006). Brain-derived neurotrophic factor (BDNF) is required for the enhancement of hippocampal neurogenesis following environmental enrichment. *European Journal of Neuroscience*, 24(7), 1850–6.

Royal College of Physicians. (2011). National Sentinel Stroke Clinical Audit 2010 Round 7 Public report for England, Wales and Northern Ireland. Prepared on behalf of the Intercollegiate Stroke Working Party. Available at: https://www.rcplondon.ac.uk/sites/default/files/documents/national_sentinel_stroke_clinical_audit_round_7_-_supplementary_report_on_therapy_intensity_march_2012.pdf.

Ryan, A. S., Ivey, F. M., Prior, S., Li, G. and Hafer-Macko, C. (2011). Skeletal muscle hypertrophy and muscle myostatin reduction after resistive training in stroke survivors. *Stroke*, 42(2), 416–20.

Salter K., Teasell, R., Foley, N., Bhogal, S., Speechley, M. and Madady, M. (2013). *Secondary prevention of stroke. Section 8.1 and 8.2 – introduction and risk factor management.* Available at: http://www.ebrsr.com/sites/default/files/chapter-8_secon-prev_final_omnibus_16ed_001. pdf.

Sanossian, N. and Ovbiagele, B. (2006). Multimodality stroke prevention. *The Neurologist*, 12(1), 14–31.

Saposnik, G., Teasell, R., Mamdani, M., Hall, J., McIlroy, W., Cheung, D., Thorpe, K. E., Cohen, L. G. and Bayley, M. (2010). Effectiveness of virtual reality using Wii gaming technology in stroke rehabilitation: a pilot randomized clinical trial and proof of principle. *Stroke*, 41(7), 1477–84.

Saunders, D. H., Greig, C. A., Young, A. and Mead, G. E. (2010). Physical fitness training for patients with stroke: an updated review. *Stroke*, 41(3), 160–1.

Schäbitz, W.-R., Schwab, S., Spranger, M. and Hacke, W. (1997). Intraventricular brain-derived neurotrophic factor size after focal cerebral ischemia in rats. *Journal of Cerebral Blood Flow and Metabolism*, 17(5), 500–6.

Schäbitz, W.-R., Berger, C., Kollmar, R., Seitz, M., Tanay, E., Kiessling, M., Schwab, S. and Sommer, C. (2004). Effect of brain-derived neurotrophic factor treatment and forced arm use on functional motor recovery after small cortical ischemia. *Stroke*, 35(4), 992–7.

Selles, R. W., Li, X., Lin, F., Chung, S. G., Roth, E. J. and Zhang, L.-Q. (2005). Feedback-controlled and programmed stretching of the ankle plantarflexors and dorsiflexors in stroke: effects of a 4-week intervention program. *Archives of Physical Medicine and Rehabilitation*, 86(12), 2330–6.

Shatil, S. and Garland, S. J. (2000). Strengthening in a therapeutic golf program for individuals following stroke. *Topics in Geriatric Rehabilitation*, 15(3), 83–94.

Shephard, R. J. (2009). Maximal oxygen intake and independence in old age. *British Journal of Sports Medicine*, 43(5), 342–6.

Silver, K. H., Macko, R. F., Forrester, L. W., Goldberg, A. P. and Smith, G. V. (2000). Effects of aerobic treadmill training on gait velocity, cadence, and gait symmetry in chronic hemiparetic stroke: a preliminary report. *Neurorehabilitation and Neural Repair*, 14(1), 65–71.

SkillsActive. (2013) *Design and agree and adapt a physical activity programme with adults after stroke (unit D516).* Available at: http://www.skillsactive.com/PDF/mapping_toolkits/CPD %20Mapping %20Toolkit-Stroke %20(D516).doc.

Stroke Association. (2015). *State of the nation stroke statistics – January 2015.* Available at: http://www.stroke.org.uk/sites/default/files/State %20of %20the %20Nation_2015.pdf.

Stroke Unit Trialists Collaboration (2002). Organised inpatient (stroke unit) care for stroke. *Cochrane Database Syst Rev* 2002; 1: CD000197.

Stuart, M., Benvenuti, F., Macko, R., Taviani, A., Segenni, L., Mayer, F., Sorkin, J. D., Stanhope, S. J., Macellari, V. and Weinrich, M. (2009). Community-based adaptive physical activity program for chronic stroke: feasibility, safety, and efficacy of the Empoli model. *Neurorehabilitation and Neural Repair*, 23(7), 726–34. doi: 10.1177/1545968309 332734.

Talwar, T. and Srivastava, M. V. P. (2014). Role of vascular endothelial growth factor and other growth factors in post-stroke recovery. *Annals of Indian Academy of Neurology*, 17(1), 1.

Taylor-Piliae, R. E. and Coull, B. M. (2012). Community-based Yang-style Tai Chi is safe and feasible in chronic stroke: a pilot study. *Clinical Rehabilitation*, 26(2), 121–31. doi: 10.1177/0269215511419381.

Taylor-Piliae, R. E. and Haskell, W. L. (2007). Tai chi exercise and stroke rehabilitation. *Top Stroke Rehabil*, 14(4), 9–22.

Teasell, R., Hussein, N., Viana, R., Donaldson, S. and Madady, M. (2014). Clinical consequences of stroke. *Stroke Rehabilitation Clinician Handbook*. Available at: http://www.ebrsr.com/sites/default/files/Chapter %201_Clinical %20Consequences_June %2018 %202014.pdf.

Tinetti, M. E. and Kumar, C. (2010). The patient who falls: 'It's always a trade-off'. *JAMA*, 303(3), 258–66.

Townsend, N., Wickramasinghe, K., Bhatnagar, P., Smolina, K., Nichols, M., Leal, J., Luengo-Frenandez, R. and Rayner, M. (2012). *Coronary heart disease statistics 2012 edition*. London: British Heart Foundation.

Tsekleves, E., Paraskevopoulos, I. T., Warland, A. and Kilbride, C. (2014). Development and preliminary evaluation of a novel low cost VR-based upper limb stroke rehabilitation platform using Wii technology. *Disabil Rehabil Assist Technol*, 13, 1–10.

Turton, A. J., Cunningham, P., Heron, E., van Wijck, F., Sackley, C., Rogers, C., Wheatley, K., Jowett, S., Wolf, S. L. and van Vliet, P. (2013). Home-based reach-to-grasp training for people after stroke: study protocol for a feasibility randomized controlled trial. *Trials*, 14(1), 109.

van de Port, I. G., Wood-Dauphinee, S., Lindeman, E., and Kwakkel, G. (2007). Effects of exercise training programs on walking competency after stroke: a systematic review. *American Journal of Physical Medicine and Rehabilitation*, 86(11), 935–51.

Van Peppen, R. P., Kwakkel, G., Wood-Dauphinee, S., Hendriks, H. J., Van der Wees, P. J. and Dekker, J. (2004). The impact of physical therapy on functional outcomes after stroke: what's the evidence? *Clinical Rehabilitation*, 18(8), 833–62.

Vaynman, S., Ying, Z. and Gomez-Pinilla, F. (2004). Hippocampal BDNF mediates the efficacy of exercise on synaptic plasticity and cognition. *European Journal of Neuroscience*, 20(10), 2580–90.

Veerbeek, J. M., Koolstra, M., Ket, J. C., van Wegen, E. E. and Kwakkel, G. (2011). Effects of augmented exercise therapy on outcome of gait and gait-related activities in the first 6 months after stroke: a meta-analysis. *Stroke*, 42(11), 3311–15.

Veerbeek, J. M., van Wegen, E., van Peppen, R., van der Wees, P. J., Hendriks, E., Rietberg, M. and Kwakkel, G. (2014). What is the evidence for physical therapy poststroke? A systematic review and meta-analysis. *PLOS ONE*, 9(2), e87987.

Vicario-Abejón, C., Collin, C., McKay, R. D. and Segal, M. (1998). Neurotrophins induce formation of functional excitatory and inhibitory synapses between cultured hippocampal neurons. *The Journal of Neuroscience*, 18(18), 7256–71.

Vocat, R., Staub, F., Stroppini, T. and Vuilleumier, P. (2010). Anosognosia for hemiplegia: a clinical-anatomical prospective study. *Brain*, 133(12), 3578–97.

Wang, Z., Wang, L., Fan, H., Jiang, W., Wang, S., Gu, Z. and Wang, T. (2014). Adapted low intensity ergometer aerobic training for early and severely impaired stroke survivors: a pilot randomized controlled trial to explore its feasibility and efficacy. *Journal of Physical Therapy Science*, 26(9), 1449.

Weerdesteyn, V., de Niet, M., van Duijnhoven, H. J. and Geurts, M. (2008). Falls in individuals with stroke. *J Rehabil Res Dev*. 45(8), 1195–213.

Wevers, L., van de Port, I., Vermue, M., Mead, G. and Kwakkel, G. (2009). Effects of task-oriented circuit class training on walking competency after stroke: a systematic review. *Stroke*, 40(7), 2450–9.

World Health Federation. (2015). *Stroke: stroke and hypertension*. Available at: http://www.world-heart-federation.org/cardiovascular-health/stroke/stroke-and-hypertension/.

World Health Organization (WHO) (2001). *International classification of functioning disability and health (ICF)*. Geneva: WHO.

WHO (2002). *Towards a common language for functioning, disability and health (ICF)*. Geneva: WHO.

Ye, J.-H. and Houle, J. D. (1997). Treatment of the chronically injured spinal cord with neurotrophic factors can promote axonal regeneration from supraspinal neurons. *Experimental Neurology*, 143(1), 70–81.

Yeh, C.-Y., Chen, J.-J. J. and Tsai, K.-H. (2007). Quantifying the effectiveness of the sustained muscle stretching treatments in stroke patients with ankle hypertonia. *Journal of Electromyography and Kinesiology*, 17(4), 453–61.

Yeh, G. Y., Roberts, D. H., Wayne, P. M., Davis, R. B., Quilty, M. T. and Phillips, R. S. (2010). Tai chi exercise for patients with chronic obstructive pulmonary disease: a pilot study. *Respiratory Care*, 55(11), 1475–82.

Zedlitz, A. M., Rietveld, T. C., Geurts, A. C. and Fasotti, L. (2012). Cognitive and graded activity training can alleviate persistent fatigue after stroke a randomized, controlled trial. *Stroke*, 43(4), 1046–51.

Chapter 8

Physical activity for long term neurological conditions

Multiple sclerosis and Huntington's disease

Jonathan Collett, Helen Dawes, and James Bateman

Introduction

Over three million people in the UK and an estimated one billion people worldwide are affected by neurological disorders, according to the World Health Organization (WHO) (WHO, 2006). Neurological disorders are diseases of the central and peripheral nervous system: the brain, spinal cord, cranial nerves, peripheral nerves, nerve roots, autonomic nervous system, neuromuscular junction, and muscles. These disorders include epilepsy, Alzheimer's disease (and other dementias), cerebrovascular diseases (including stroke), migraine, multiple sclerosis, Parkinson's disease, neuroinfections, brain tumours, traumatic disorders of the nervous system such as (traumatic brain injury), and neurological disorders as a result of malnutrition (WHO 2014). The term 'long term neurological condition' (LTNC) is used to classify any of this diverse group of neurological conditions, which result from injury or disease, that will affect an individual for the rest of their lives (Royal College of Physicians, 2008). Conditions may have the following presentations:

- Sudden onset: such as spinal cord injury, stroke, and traumatic brain injury
- Intermittent: such as epilepsy
- Progressive: such as multiple sclerosis, Huntington's disease, motor neurone disease, and Parkinson's disease
- Stable: with/without age-related degeneration, such as polio or cerebral palsy.

These conditions have a growing human, societal, and economic cost as the elderly population increases worldwide. Indeed, there is evidence that pinpoints neurological disorders as one of the greatest threats to public health (WHO, 2006). The burden of these LTNC is largely due to the disability caused. Symptoms are diverse, and many patients have complex disabilities which include cognitive, behavioural, and communication problems, as well as physical deficits (Royal College of Physicians, 2008). Typical problems caused by LTNC include those affecting:

- Motor performance: such as muscle weakness (paresis), increased muscle tone (spasticity contracture), and coordination problems (including ataxia)
- Cognition, communication and behaviour: such as problems with decision making (executive function), attention, memory, and speaking (aphasia)
- Mood: such as anxiety or depression

- Fatigue
- Pain and sensation (dysesthesia): such as numbness and tingling
- Autonomic function: such as bladder and sexual problems, and problems with regulating of temperature and blood pressure.

Symptom severity affects how well a person can perform functional tasks and participate in daily activities. The WHO's International Classification of Functioning, Disability and Health (ICF) provides a framework to describe the health of people with LTNCs by relating problems caused by the condition to the effect these may have on a person's ability to engage in meaningful life roles and activities (WHO, 2002).

Participation in regular exercise provides health and social benefits for all, and the evidence for the benefits of physical activity in the general population is now overwhelming. The ICF model can be applied to physical activity participation for people with LTNC. Impairments to body functions, such as muscle weakness, fatigue, or bladder control problems, might limit the types of physical activity someone can do, and restrict their participation in certain physical activities; this can be further affected by environmental issues (e.g. location and accessibility of facilities), and personal factors (motivation or money). Certainly, LTNC often have low levels of participation in leisure-time physical activities, perceive themselves as isolated, and have high rates of secondary complications from inactivity. Some people may receive short periods of hospital-based rehabilitation, but there is minimal initiation or maintenance of community activity. For people with LTNC, who may find themselves in a negative spiral of condition-related impairments that limit activities, which in turn will lead to deconditioning, the evidence suggests that attaining a physically-active lifestyle can benefit mobility, health, and wellbeing, and reduce the impact of disease and health care costs (Life Group, 2010). Importantly, even small increases in activity levels can make an impact on both health and wellbeing for many.

It is not feasible to cover all LTNC in this chapter; physical activity after stroke is covered in Chapter 7, and many of the considerations for exercise in stroke can be

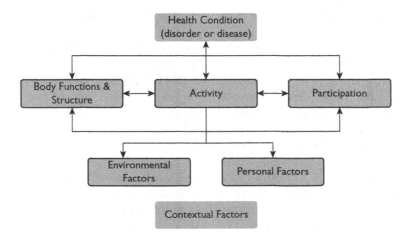

Figure 8.1 The ICF Model: interaction between ICF components (WHO, 2002).

applied to other sudden onset brain conditions, such as traumatic brain injury. This chapter will use multiple sclerosis (MS), and Huntington's disease (HD) to illustrate exercise prescription for LTNC. Whilst these conditions are both progressive, incurable, and share some symptoms, each presents issues to consider for exercise delivery, and the body of evidence to support physical activity in people with MS (pwMS) is far more advanced.

Multiple sclerosis

MS is an inflammatory neurodegenerative disease and the most common chronic neurological condition affecting young adults worldwide (WHO 2008). It is characterised by focal areas of demyelination in the central nervous system and a disease course that is variable in both presentation of symptoms and progression. It affects more women than men (approximately 3:1), with the estimated UK lifetime risk from birth of receiving an MS diagnosis of 285.8 per 100,000 in women and 113.1 per 100,000 in men. There are approximately 126,669 individuals living with MS in the UK, and peak incidence is at forty years of age in women and forty five years of age in men (Mackenzie et al., 2014). Therefore, for many individuals, diagnosis of the disease occurs at the peak of their career and family development. The early onset, high disability levels, and normal life span of pwMS increase the impact and cost of the disease on individuals, families, the health care system, and society. Indeed, large resources are needed to help pwMS. Total cost per patient is estimated at £17,000 per year in the UK. Informal care accounts for 26 per cent of this total, and direct medical cost only 16 per cent. A cost of approximately £3,400 per patient per year falls on the National Health Service, and the remainder is borne by patients, their families, and careers (Naci et al., 2010).

Pathophysiology

Despite relatively recent research indicating grey matter involvement (Peterson et al., 2001), the disease is primarily associated with demyelination. Indeed, the term 'multiple sclerosis' refers to the multifocal (multiple) white matter plaques (sclerosis) that occur in various parts of the central nervous system including the cerebrum, cerebellum, brainstem, and optic nerve. The exact pathophysiology is not known; however, it seems to involve two overlapping disease processes: inflammation and degeneration. The autoimmune process is believed to start with the triggering of T-lymphocytes, possibly by infection, which penetrate the blood-brain barrier. The T-cells produce pro-inflammatory cytokines and attract macrophages that 'attack' the myelin surrounding the axon. The degeneration is understood to result from the loss of myelin, which disrupts the axon membrane potential and, combined with the cytotoxicity of the inflammatory process, results in axon damage and loss (Mallucci et al., 2015).

Disease progression

The severity of symptoms and the rate at which they progress is unpredictable and unique to the individual. However, the disease course has been broadly classified into three types:

- Relapsing remitting: this is the most common presentation, and approximately 80 per cent of people are initially diagnosed with this disease type. It is associated with the most inflammatory activity, and, as the name suggests, it is characterised by unpredictable, acute inflammatory events where symptoms worsen (relapses or exacerbations). These attacks evolve over days or weeks and can last several weeks or months. Between relapses there are periods where symptoms recover and the disease remains stable. Active disease is defined by two clinically-significant relapses in the previous two years (NHS England, 2014).
- Secondary progressive: approximately 65 per cent of those initially diagnosed with relapsing remitting MS will have developed secondary progressive MS after fifteen years. During this stage of the disease it is believed that a combination of ongoing chronic low-level inflammation with degenerative processes is occurring. Individuals may still experience exacerbations but there will now generally be a gradual worsening of symptoms over time.
- Primary progressive: this is when the disease is manifested by a primarily degenerative process without the relapsing remitting stage. This is the least prevalent form of MS, although it is more common in those who develop the disease in later life.

Symptoms

Typically, health professionals classify MS symptoms in order to better understand the impact of the condition on activities. To do this, professionals commonly use the Expanded Disability Status Scale (EDSS), an MS-specific scale used to quantify and monitor the level of disability. The scale ranges from 0 to 10 (in 0.5 unit increments), with higher scores representing greater symptom severity. The scale considers eight 'functional systems': 1) weakness in limbs (pyramindal); 2) coordination (cerebellar); 3) speech, swallowing, and nystagmus (brainstem); 4) sensory; 5) bowel and bladder function; 6) visual function; 7) cognitive function (cerebral); and 8) other. The ICF as they might be applied to an individual with MS are as follows:

Body Functions

- Fatigue and fatigability
- Speech
- Vision (nystagmus)
- Bladder and bowel
- Heat sensitivity
- Cognitive
- Behavioural/emotional
- Movement
- Spasticity
- Muscle weakness
- Autonomic dysfunction
- Balance and coordination
- Tremor.

Activity

* Reduced walking, balance, and mobility
* Difficulty communicating.

Participation

* Reduced participation in work, social, and physical related activities.

Secondary

* Detraining all elements of fitness
* Non-communicable disease associated with inactivity (later on).

Currently there is no cure for MS, however, a number of disease-modifying drug therapies are licensed in the UK (Beta-interferon, Glatiramer Acetate, Natalizumb and Fingolimod). These drugs essentially target the inflammatory process, and therefore are only indicated for people with relapsing remitting MS or secondary progressive MS when relapses are the predominant cause of disability (NHS England, 2014). Whilst these drugs arc effective in slowing relapse rate, it is not known whether they slow disease progression in the longer term. Exercise is now seen as a valuable treatment option to relieve symptoms in pwMS (NICE, 2014).

Exercise guidelines

Exercise is recommended for pwMS, and healthcare professionals are encouraged to advise people that regular exercise may have a beneficial effect on their MS (NICE, 2014). The evidence supporting the beneficial effects of exercise for pwMS is compelling, and exercise may accrue benefits across the ICF framework. Systematic reviews demonstrate that there is good evidence to support that exercise improves aerobic fitness, muscle power (body functions), and mobility-related activities (activity). They also demonstrate that there is moderate evidence indicating that exercise may have the potential to improve mood and fatigue (body function) and health-related quality of life (participation) (Rietberg et al., 2005; Ensari et al., 2014; Latimer-Cheung et al., 2013b). In addition there is interest developing in the possibility that exercise may influence immunoregulation, neuroprotection, and neuroplasticity in MS. However, evidence to support the role of exercise in MS pathogenesis is limited and inconsistent (Motl and Pilutti, 2012).

Current guidelines

Physical activity guidelines for people with MS were established in 2013 for the MS society of Canada (Latimer-Cheung et al., 2013a), based on a systematic review of studies which examined the effects of exercise on fitness, mobility, fatigue, and health-related quality of life. The review included randomised and non-randomised controlled trials and all type of MS, with no age or disability level excluded (Latimer-Cheung et al., 2013b). The guidelines were also informed by expert consensus and stake holder refinement, and are deemed appropriate for adults with minimal to moderate MS. The guidelines refer to the minimal exercise dose required to accrue benefits, and consider both aerobic and strength training exercise. The guidelines state pwMS need at least:

- 30 min moderate intensity aerobic activity two times per week, and
- Strength training exercises for major muscle groups two times per week.

Aerobic and strength training can be done on the same day, and one day of rest between strength training sessions is recommended.

- Aerobic training moderate intensity guide: a rating of perceived exertion of five to six on a Borg category-ratio 0–10 scale.
- Strength training guide: progress towards two sets of 10–15 repetitions, with 1–2 minutes rest between sets. Resistance should be set so that 10–15 repetitions can be barely but safely finished.

Supporting evidence for guideline

Aerobic training: this recommendation is based on the results of eleven studies, including seven randomised controlled trials (RCTs), which indicated that to increase $\dot{V}O_{2peak}$ aerobic training at 60 per cent–80 per cent maximum work rate or 60 per cent $\dot{V}O_{2max}$ is required two to three times a week for thirty to sixty minutes (Latimer-Cheung et al., 2013b).

Strength training: this recommendation is primarily based on positive results of five studies (four RCTs) of supervised progressive resistance training (Latimer-Cheung et al., 2013b). Studies included exercise doses of ten to twelve repetitions at ~ 70–80 per cent of one repetition maximum, performed two to three times a week. A home-based programme was also considered, which found resistance bands effective at increasing upper limb strength and lower limb muscular endurance.

Considerations

Approximately half of the studies included in the review to inform the guidance were of low quality (e.g. quasi-experimental pre-post designs); however, the evidence informing aerobic and strength training was primarily from good quality RCTs. It is also important to consider the duration of the studies included. The guidelines are based on evidence from studies with a mean duration of 10.25 (±5.98) weeks. Therefore, whilst this evidence informs effective exercise doses over the short term, it may not indicate optimal exercise for sustaining such benefits and participation rates. Furthermore, the reporting of adherence and dropout is generally poor in MS exercise trials. A systematic review (Pilutti et al., 2014) found that only 65 per cent of the studies reported participant flow using a CONSORT flow diagram (Altman, 1996) (a reporting requirement for clinical trials). Given the barriers pwMS face to participate in physical activity and the progressive nature of the disease, sustainability of exercise for maintenance and slowing progression may be a valuable outcome to evaluate exercise interventions over the longer term.

The evaluation of the evidence for exercise, and the development of guidelines, have been primarily concerned with outcomes that address specific problems or deficits associated with MS, such as improving aerobic fitness, muscle strength, mobility, fatigue, and health-related quality of life. It is also important to consider the general health benefits of increased physical activity. Recent evidence suggests increasing physical activity in those who are inactive by even a small amount, such as twenty minutes of brisk walking, may benefit public health (Ekelund et al., 2015). This, combined with the results of a systemic review which demonstrated that exercise training in MS is not associated with an increase in relapse rate and the occurrence of adverse events, is similar to that in the general populations (Pilutti et al., 2014). This suggests that even modest amounts of participation in exercise, or increases in physical activity, should be in encouraged, as the benefits are likely to outweigh any harms. The preamble of the guidelines reflects this, and recommends that

> For those who are currently inactive, activities performed at a lower intensity, frequency and duration than recommended may bring some benefit. It is appropriate for inactive adults to gradually increase duration, frequency and intensity as a progression towards meeting guidelines.
>
> (Latimer-Cheung et al., 2013a)

Putting into practice

When prescribing and delivering exercise for pwMS, a personal profile should be created. The guidelines above pertain to a minimal amount, and the ability of an individual will ultimately determine if the guidelines are currently achievable, or indeed not challenging enough. Standard contraindications and risk stratification should be considered, and it is also important to consider specific MS symptoms. These factors will inform the exact form of prescribed exercises, specifically FITT (frequency, duration, intensity, and timing of sessions, and mode of exercise). Exercises may have to be modified in order to account for symptoms such as mobility and balance problems, and spasticity. However, other problems may not be as immediately apparent, and may also require consideration. Some common problems, such as bladder symptoms, heat sensitivity, and fatigue are discussed below.

Bladder symptoms

The majority of pwMS will suffer bladder dysfunction during the course of their disease, resulting in continence problems and affecting quality of life (Khan et al., 2009). Bladder dysfunction in MS is complex and includes detrusor and sphincter disorders that result in a variable combination of irritative (urgency, urinary frequency, and/or urge incontinence) and obstructive symptoms. Bladder dysfunction can be an early symptom, and the severity of detrusor overactivity is consistent with the extent of pyramidal damage and the general disability level. The issue of bladder symptoms may be sensitive for some with MS to discuss, especially men, who are reported to have fewer coping strategies for bladder continence than women (Shaw, 2001). Therefore, a safe assumption is that an individual has urgency and frequency symptoms, so it is important to consider toilet location and accessibility in the exercise environment.

It may be that an individual has a urinary catheter and certain exercises may need to be modified to accommodate the location of the bag. A general consensus for MS bladder management in the UK recommends that one to two litres of fluid be consumed a day, but it is acknowledged that pwMS may reduce fluid intake to manage symptoms (Fowler et al., 2009), and it may be that some pwMS become dehydrated (Collett et al., 2011a). The possibility of under-hydration in an individual should be considered, as it may affect their ability to participate in exercise, especially in a hot environment.

Heat sensitivity

Between 60–80 per cent of pwMS will be sensitive to increases in body temperature and experience Uhthoff's phenomenon. Uhthoff's phenomenon occurs when increases in body temperature lead to a transient intensification of MS symptoms. The influence that body temperature has on nerve conduction may account for heat sensitivity, as Uhthoff's phenomenon occurs in people with central conduction slowing who are also particularly vulnerable to develop temperature-dependent central motor conduction block (Humm et al., 2004). It is therefore important to consider the temperature of the exercise environment when delivering exercise in pwMS with heat sensitivity. Further consideration might also be given to employing strategies to reduce body temperature and selecting appropriate types of exercise on hot days. Cooling strategies such as wearing cooling suits or cooling the head or hand pre- or during exercise has shown to be effective at improving exercise tolerance and symptoms of fatigue (Grahn et al., 2008, Flensner and Lindencrona, 2002), and there is some evidence to suggest that heat-sensitive pwMS may be more tolerant to resistance exercise than endurance exercise (Skjerbaek et al., 2013).

Fatigue

Fatigue is a chronic, pervasive, and disabling symptom that effects mobility and participation in work, and social activities for the majority of pwMS (Wood et al., 2012); and being too tired is the main barrier to exercise pwMS give (Asano et al., 2013). This chronic neurological fatigue seen in MS is notoriously difficult to define. The exact mechanism is complex and not fully understood, but is thought to be influenced by immune and endocrine processes, as well as altered signal transmissions and activations in the central nervous system. Fatigue symptoms can be both physical and cognitive, and include feelings of exhaustion, a lack of energy, low motivation, and physical tiredness that is not relieved by sleep. The effect that exercise has on fatigue is inconsistent in the literature, with some studies showing no effect and others, particularly those with a resistance training component, showing a positive effect (Latimer-Cheung et al., 2013b). A meta-analysis of fatigue management interventions in MS found exercise had an overall positive effect on fatigue when data was pooled, with an effect size of 0.57 (95 per cent CI: 0.10–1.04, $P = 0.02$), and was more effective than pharmacological interventions (Asano and Finlayson, 2014). Therefore, the evidence suggests that exercise, at least, does not have a negative impact on fatigue and may have a positive effect.

Whilst exercise should not be avoided through fears of exacerbating general fatigue levels, it is important to consider the impact that an exercise session may have on an individual's day. PwMS with fatigue are advised to prioritise and plan daily activities in order to include time for rest and recuperation. A recent study found an altered perceptual response in pwMS during recovery after a maximal aerobic exercise test, with pwMS perceiving higher levels of leg fatigue than healthy controls (Dawes et al., 2014). Furthermore, the increase in perception of leg fatigue after exercise was greatest in those pwMS with higher levels of general chronic fatigue (Dawes et al., 2014). It is therefore important to consider recovery from exercise and how the exercise can be incorporated within other daily responsibilities.

Case study

Background

Height: 1.68m (5ft 6 in)
Weight: 52 kg (115 lbs)
BMI: 18.6 kg·m²
RHR: 76 bpm
BP: 122/82 mmHg.

The client was a fifty six-year-old female with a four-year history of primary progressive multiple sclerosis (PPMS). She presented with no other comorbidities and was considered low risk in cardiovascular risk stratification, with the only risk factor being her age. She was clinically stable with full support from her GP. There was only a slight concern of lower back pain which she felt was postural and due to core weakness.

The EDSS score was provided by her neurologist, and the score was 4.0–4.5. Whilst this translated to having 'Significant Disability' with some limitation of full activity and requiring 'minimal assistance', she was self-sufficient, able to walk without aid or rest for 500m, was up and about most of the day, and able to work a full day.

The client's most disabling symptom was impaired gait with severe right-sided muscle weakness, with loss of ability to flex the hip and dorsiflex at the ankle. Whilst she felt 'groggy' when it was very warm and humid, she generally did not experience heat sensitivity. She was urinary continent and mentioned she had had the occasional accident but her medication had been very successful.

Medication was 10mg Citalopram daily for depression and 5mg Solifenacin for bladder control. The client was referred to a community-based wellness programme for exercise.

Exercise programme

Exercise programme goals:

- To increase quadriceps power in the right leg
- Improve the 6 minute walk test by 25 per cent
- Improve footdrop in the right leg and gait by increasing ankle flexibility.

Progression

Over the four weeks progression was achieved by manipulating the intensity on relevant exercise machines to maintain an estimated aerobic work load of between

Table 8.1 The client attended a four week community-based exercise programme

Mode	Frequency	Intensity	Time
Aerobic-arm ergometer, recumbent bike, treadmill (with assistance).	Two days/week.	60–80% $\dot{V}O_{2peak}$ RPE 5–6 (1–10 scale).	30 minutes.
Strength/resistance training	Two days/week.	10–15 repetitions set.	Two sets of 10–15 repetitions, with 1–2 min rest between sets.
Flexibility.	Daily.	Take until the point of stretch.	2–4 repetitions holding for 30–60 seconds.
Warm up/cool-down.	At the beginning and end of every session.	50–70% $\dot{V}O_{2peak}$ RPE 3–5 (1–10 scale).	5–10 minutes.

60–80 per cent of $\dot{V}O_{2peak}$. This work-train zone was indicated by using heart rate and RPE. At the beginning the person worked largely at the lower end of the training zone, but towards the four-week point the client was achieving segments that equated to an estimated 80 per cent of $\dot{V}O_{2peak}$. Resistance training progression was achieved by working at a lower repetition range of around ten until the client could manage fifteen repetitions with a given weight. When the volume of repetitions and sets could be achieved, the repetitions were again dropped and more resistance was added until again she could achieve the higher volume of work.

Outcome

Functional Tests at baseline:

6 minute walk (Total distance walked in 6 minutes): 168.5 m
Time up and go test (TUG – time taken to stand from a chair walk 3m, go around a cone and return to the chair and sit): 13.72 seconds
Sit to stands: eight reps

Follow up

After four weeks of a structured exercise programme the 6 minute walk test increased to 180m. Both the TUG test and sit-to-stand also improved, by a reduction of 1.06 seconds for the TUG test and seven extra repetitions performed on the sit-to-stand test. The client had increased confidence after the four weeks, feeling less tired compared to before the start of the programme, and felt happier managing their MS by adhering to a frequent exercise regime.

Future research

One exciting area for future research is to confirm and translate findings from basic science, other populations, and the early promising work in MS on the potential influence that exercise has on MS pathogenesis. That aside, the current body of evidence informing MS exercise guidelines has limitations. Generally, the reporting of studies has been poor, and, in particular, the lack of reporting on occurrence of adverse event, and adherence to the intervention, may have important implications for prescription. Results from an RCT of different exercise intensities found that, despite data indicating that high-intensity exercise may elicit greater mobility benefits, it was less well tolerated in terms of attendance at sessions and withdrawing from the intervention (Collett et al., 2011b). Optimal dose in terms of performance gains may, therefore, not be the equivalent to optimal dose in terms of adherence. These issues are compounded by the short follow-up periods in many studies, and thus there is a lack of evidence to inform exercise that is sustainable over the longer-term. This information, alongside building on research into pragmatic delivery systems and cost effectiveness, is required in order to the provide evidence relevant to those who commission services (Tosh et al., 2014; Life Group, 2010; Elsworth et al., 2011). However, one of the main challenges of research into exercise for people with MS is obtaining the funding required to perform large multi-centre trials, in order to provide robust, ecologically-valid evidence, and detect modest but important effect sizes (Asano et al., 2009). A further area for future research to address is the questions that remain concerning the beneficial effects that exercise may have on fatigue. In addition, a better understanding of how exercise prescription is delivered alongside daily activities and responsibilities and fatigue management is required. Furthermore, the majority of current research is on pwMS with mild to moderate disability, and research is required to inform exercise in those who are not ambulatory.

Further reading

Systematic reviews on the benefits of exercise in MS and subsequent guidelines:

Latimer-Cheung, A. E., Martin Ginis, K. A., Hicks, A. L., Motl, R. W., Pilutti, L. A., Duggan, M., Wheeler, G., Persad, R. and Smith, K. M. (2013a). Development of evidence-informed physical activity guidelines for adults with multiple sclerosis. *Arch Phys Med Rehabil*, 94, 1829–36: e7.
Latimer-Cheung, A. E., Pilutti, L. A., Hicks, A. L., Martin Ginis, K. A., Fenuta, A. M., MacKibbon, K. A. and Motl, R. W. (2013b). Effects of exercise training on fitness, mobility, fatigue, and health-related quality of life among adults with multiple sclerosis: a systematic review to inform guideline development. *Arch Phys Med Rehabil*, 94, 1800–28: e3.

A systematic review on the safety of exercise in MS that also considers the reporting of adherence in trials:

Pilutti, L. A., Platta, M. E., Motl, R. W. and Latimer-Cheung, A. E. (2014). The safety of exercise training in multiple sclerosis: a systematic review. *J Neurol Sci*, 343, 3–7.

A study that investigated leg fatigue following exercise and found that these symptoms took longer to recover in pwMS than controls, and longer still in pwMS with fatigue:

Dawes, H., Collett, J., Meaney, A., Duda, J., Sackley, C., Wade, D., Barker, K. and Izadi, H. (2014). Delayed recovery of leg fatigue symptoms following a maximal exercise session in people with multiple sclerosis. *Neurorehabil Neural Repair*, 28, 139–48.

A study that investigated exercise type in heat-sensitive people with MS and found that resistance exercise may be better tolerated than endurance:

Skjerbaek, A. G., Møller, A. B., Jensen, E., Vissing, K., Sørensen, H., Nybo, L., Stenager, E. and Dalgas, U. (2013). Heat sensitive persons with multiple sclerosis are more tolerant to resistance exercise than to endurance exercise. *Mult Scler*, 19, 932–40.

Huntington's disease

Huntington's Disease (HD) is a genetic progressive neurodegenerative condition caused by a cytosine-adenine-guanine (CAG) repeat mutation in the gene that codes for the protein huntingtin. The mutation gives the protein an abnormally long polyglutamine repeat, affecting its function. The disease is characterised by the abnormal involuntary movements that gave rise to the name Huntington's chorea (*choriea* meaning a dance). HD is rare, with a prevalence of 2.71 per 100,000 worldwide, although it is more common in those of European descent. The prevalence in Europe, North America, and Australia is reported at 5.70 per 100,000 compared to 0.40 per 100,000 in Asia (Pringsheim et al., 2012).

Pathophysiology

Inheritance is autosomal dominant, whereby only one abnormal gene is required in order to develop the disease. The protein huntingtin is found in many tissues but is in the highest levels in the brain. Whilst the exact function of huntingtin is not fully understood, it is involved in signalling, transporting, and binding within the cell, prevents apoptosis, appears to be important for normal neuron functioning, and is essential for normal brain development. The mutant protein predominantly causes dysfunction and death of the medium spiny striatal projection neurons in the basal ganglia. Mitochondrial defects that affect cellular energy metabolism are also implicated in the aetiology of HD, with defects found in mitochondrial function in the central nervous system and peripheral tissues of HD patients (Ciammola et al., 2011; Ross et al., 2014).

Disease progression

The number of CAG repeat mutations determine whether some will develop the disease and the potential risk to offspring (Ross et al., 2014):

- 28 or less CAG repeats: normal range
- 29–34 CAG repeats: someone will not develop HD but their children are at greater risk
- 35–39 CAG repeats: some individuals will develop HD and children at a greater risk
- 40 or greater CAG repeats: an individual will develop HD.

HD has a long premanifest stage where individuals carrying the gene have no symptoms, with a mean age of clinical onset ~ 45 years. The age of onset is highly variable and is strongly related to the number of the CAG repeat mutations. A disease burden score can be calculated from the number of CAG repeats an individual has and their age (CAG repeats − 35.5 × age). This score has also shown to partially predict the rate of disease progression, which is inexorable and will eventual lead to death over a period of fifteen to twenty years (Ross and Tabrizi, 2011).

Symptoms

Whilst HD is considered a movement disorder, impairing voluntary movements (bradykinesia and rigidity) and causing involuntary ones (chorea), it also affects cognition and behaviour (Papoutsi et al., 2014). Clinical features of HD can be quantified using the Unified Huntington's Disease Rating Scale (UDHRS). The UHDRS comprises a series of clinical scales to assess motor function, cognitive function, behavioural abnormalities, and functional capacity (Reilmann et al., 2012). Typically, the symptom progression can be classified within the following stages:

Early stage: subtle changes in mood, movement, and cognition. The person with HD may still be able to drive and hold down their job, but might require support.

Mid stage: people with HD generally lose the ability to work and drive, and need help with activities of daily living. The movement disorder will lead to difficulties with balance, swallowing, and voluntary motor tasks. Individuals will have increased difficulty organising and prioritising information. The behavioural symptoms will affect everyone differently, but irritability, aggression, depression, and apathy at this stage can lead to personal and family issues.

Late Stage: people require help in all activities of daily living. During this time, the person with HD may lose the ability to speak and respond, but is still able to comprehend what is happening around them. Chorea can be severe or may be replaced by other movement symptoms, including rigidity, dystonia, and bradykinesia. During this stage, most people are in long-term care. The ICF as applied to a person with early HD is outlined below:

Body functions

- Fatigue and fatigability
- Depression, irritability, and disinhibition, hypersexuality
- Cognitive (difficulty thinking through difficult tasks and problem solving, speed of thinking)
- Behavioural/emotional: apathy and loss of interest in activities
- Movement and coordination
- Involuntary movements – chorea
- Bradykinesia
- Rigidity
- Muscle weakness
- Autonomic dysfunction
- Balance and falls
- Speaking, swallowing and weight loss.

Activity

- Reduced walking, balance, and mobility
- Loss of ability to drive
- Difficulty communicating.

Participation

- Affected physical, social, and work commitments
- Relationships.

Secondary

- Detraining all elements of fitness (strength, speed, power, endurance, balance, and flexibility).

Currently, there is no cure for HD, but, unlike MS, there are also no disease-modifying treatments currently available. However, advances in understanding of the pathogenesis of the disease have led to a number of targets for drug treatment, and therapeutic trials of potential disease-modifying therapies are currently under development (Wild and Tabrizi, 2014).

Exercise guidelines

In contrast to MS, there has been little research investigating exercise for people with HD. Therefore, guidelines based on a specific evidence base are not yet possible. Evidence from exercise studies in animals (Zuccato and Cattaneo, 2007), healthy people (Winter et al., 2007), and people with other neurological conditions (White and Castellano, 2008) suggests that exercise can improve mobility and function, benefit health and wellbeing, and possibly slow disease progression in people with progressive neurological conditions, including those with HD (Zinzi et al., 2007).

Current guidelines

Due to the lack of HD-specific evidence, prescription is informed using general exercise principles. Studies have shown prescribing aerobic and anaerobic exercises in this way is safe, feasible, and effective in individuals with HD (Meaney et al., 2009; Khalil et al., 2012; Khalil et al., 2013). However, information about the physiological response during exercise, and as a result of training, in people with HD is limited. People with symptomatic HD have reduced work capacity and muscle strength (Busse et al, 2009, Ciammola et al., 2011). A normal cardiopulmonary response, with normal cardiac output and ventilation, during maximal exercise testing has been reported, but a reduced ability to perform aerobic exercise has also been shown (Ciammola et al., 2011). Individuals may have chorea movements that may require modifications to equipment, and activities should consider balance requirements (Quinn and Busse, 2012). With this in mind, following the American College of Sports Medicine (ACSM) Guidelines (ACSM, 2013), people with HD should aim to do at least:

- 30 minutes of moderate intensity aerobic activity three times per week, and
- Strength training exercise for all major muscle groups two times per week
- Flexibility training.

If a person is unable to do thirty minutes of continuous exercise, then fifteen minutes five times per week is recommended.

Aerobic training moderate intensity guide: exercising hard enough to be breathing fast and feeling warm. Aerobic exercise, such a cycling on a stationary bicycle, has been found to be feasible and safe in people with early-mid stage HD, and may provide some benefits (Dawes et al., 2015).

Considerations

Barriers and facilitators: people with early and mid-stage HD may benefit from support to engage with sport and exercise. Many individuals may participate with family or carers, who will also benefit from support. Approaches based on self-determination theory for both carers and patients may help individuals to build the skills, confidence, and connections to engage and maintain participation. Knowledge and understanding of the condition and symptoms can help fitness professionals to build participants' confidence and enjoyment of exercise sessions.

Physiological: mitochondrial deficiency is implicated in the pathogenesis of HD, causing abnormal metabolites and oxidative stress (Ross and Tabrizi, 2011). People with HD also show signs of reduced metabolic activity in the striatum, and a prominent symptom of the disease is weight loss. This dysfunction may result in an altered response to aerobic exercise training in some people with HD. During maximal exercise testing, people with HD have been observed to have an early increase in blood lactate and low lactate/anaerobic threshold (AT) (~ 60 per cent maximum heart rate) (Ciammola et al., 2011). An altered blood glucose response to maximal exercise has been observed in pwHD and further investigation in the R6/2 mouse model suggests that this is due to reduced liver gluconeogenesis (Josefsen et al., 2010). People with HD do not reach steady state heart rate within three minutes when starting low-intensity exercise, and individuals may generate energy anaerobically even during low-intensity (aerobic) physical activities such as walking or cycling (Dawes et al., 2015). Therefore, standard ACSM guidelines (ACSM, 2013) may not be appropriate for all individuals in this patient group, and some may need to exercise within the lower percentages of HR zones. However, to date, the exercise response during lower-intensity aerobic activities has not been explored. It is also important that the exercise practitioner monitors the body mass of pwHD. Weight loss is common in HD and is more associated with the number of CAG repeats than with motor, cognitive, or behavioural problems (Aziz et al., 2008). It appears that the weight loss is due to a hypermetabolic state and therefore increased energy expenditure brought about by exercise needs to be adequately compensated by more calories in the diet.

Putting into practice

Any person who is considering participation in an exercise programme should have a personalised fitness profile created that considers their medical presentation and health, social circumstances and goals, and fitness. These factors will inform the exact form of prescribed exercises, specifically FITT (frequency, duration, intensity, and timing of sessions, and mode of exercise). The European EHDN has provided clinical tips for physical activity and exercise in HD (Dawes et al., 2013). It is important to consider long-term delivery issues when supporting people with HD to exercise, particularly as exercise prescription in this population may be further complicated by apathy or other behavioural issues. Specific considerations should be given to the most appropriate setting (i.e. in a gym or clinic or home-based) and structure (i.e. group-based vs. individual) for an exercise programme. Gym staff or class instructors/ coaches may often not be able to meet the needs of the person with HD, who may not be aware of when to progress exercise, when to request help, or is unaware of poor technique. Careful instruction of exercises is therefore often required to ensure safety. And individualised support may be required. In some cases, the mode of delivery may need to be completely altered where impairments such as cognitive, behavioural, or motor issues prevent the current mode of delivery, such as the timing of an exercise session during the day and the content of the session. Training of functional activities such as squats/sit-to-stand may have both physiological and functional utility for patients (Quinn et al., 2014).

Case study

Background

Height: 1.73m. (5ft 8 in)
Weight: 60 kg (132 lbs)
BMI: 20.1 kg·m²
RHR: 80 bpm
BP: 125/85 mmHg.

The client was a fifty four-year-old female with fifty three CAG repeat mutations on the huntingtin gene, and diagnosis of symptomatic Huntington's disease. She presented with no other comorbidities and was considered low risk in cardiovascular risk stratification. She was clinically stable with full support from her GP.

Disease severity was assessed using the UHDRS, and she had a Total UHDRS Motor Score (TMS) of fifty, and a chair sit-to-stand test of eight. She was fully able to walk without aid or rest.

Medication was Amitriptyline 10mg daily and Tetrabenazine 12.5mg weekly (for chorea).

Exercise programme

Exercise programme goals:

- Improve walking efficiency/endurance
- Improve chair sit-to-stand test
- To maintain weight.

Table 8.2 The client attended an eight week community-based exercise programme

Mode	Frequency	Intensity	Time
Aerobic-predictable and rhythmical-bike ergometer.	Three days/week.	Moderate, 65–80% HR max.	30 minutes.
Strength/resistance training.	Two days/week.	40–50% 1RM.	20 minutes.
Flexibility.	Daily.	Point of stretch. Be careful of uncontrolled movements (chorea).	30–60 seconds per stretch.
Warm up/cool-down	At the beginning and end of every session.	50–70% of HR max.	5–10 minutes.

The client enrolled onto an eight-week supervised community training programme that was supported by an exercise professional, who also gave dietary advice to increase calorie intake, in order to maintain weight.

Progression

Progression over the eight weeks was achieved by manipulating the intensity on relevant exercise machines to maintain an aerobic work load between a moderate range of 65 to 85 per cent of HR max using heart rate and RPE. At the beginning the person worked at the lower end of the range until time could be achieved then they were adjusted up towards 80 per cent HR max accordingly. Resistance training progression was achieved by working at a lower repetition range of around ten until the client could manage fifteen repetitions with a given weight. When the volume of repetitions and sets could be achieved, the repetitions were again dropped and more resistance was added until, again, they could achieve the higher volume of work.

Outcome

Functional Tests at baseline:

Chair sit-to-stand: ten repetitions
Daily step counts: 3596 steps.

Follow-up

After eight weeks of the structured exercise programme the client reported that they were able to walk further daily. This was reflected in their step count of 5355 steps per day at the end of the eight weeks. Sit to stand repetitions had increased to fifteen. Weight had been maintained throughout the programme, fluctuating between 58.5 and 61.3kg, and was 59.2kg at eight weeks.

Future research

Essentially, exercise research in HD is in its infancy; thus, there are many questions to be answered, from mechanism to pragmatic delivery. It is unclear how the mitochondrial and metabolic dysfunction found in HD affects responses and adaptations to exercise. Data from animal models of HD (Potter et al., 2010) and myopathy found in a marathon runner with the HD gene (Kosinski et al., 2007) even suggested that excessive exercise training might accelerate onset of some symptoms. Therefore, there is a pressing need for studies to investigate the physiological response to exercise and adaptation mechanisms specific to HD. For exercise prescription, whilst studies have shown that it is feasible to deliver exercise for pwHD (Busse et al., 2013; Khalil et al., 2013), there is not yet an evidence base that has assessed the effectiveness of exercise interventions. Therefore, there is a need for trials, including appropriate sample sizes, that are designed to assess if exercise is beneficial, what outcomes improve, and what constitutes effective or optimal doses.

Further reading/resources

This RCT investigated whether it was feasible to deliver gym-based exercise for pwHD. The study demonstrated that the combined aerobic and resistance exercise programme was feasible and well-tolerated, and the effect size on clinical outcomes supports a trial to assess effectiveness:

Busse, M., Quinn, L., Debono, K., Jones, K., Collett, J., Playle, R., Kelly, M., Simpson, S., Backx, K., Wasley, D., Dawes, H. and Rosser, A. (2013). A randomized feasibility study of a 12-week community-based exercise program for people with Huntington's disease. *J Neurol Phys Ther*, 37, 149–58.

This paper provided a further analysis of the exercise response of pwMS from the study above. They found pwHD had higher blood lactate, respiratory exchange ratio, and perceived exertion during submaximal exercise than a healthy comparator group, and did not achieve steady state heart rate. No change in the exercise response was observed after the training intervention:

Dawes, H., Collett, J., Debono, K., Quinn, L., Jones, K., Kelson, M. J., Simpson, S. A., Playle, R., Backx, K., Wasley, D., Nemeth, A. H., Rosser, A., Izardi, H. and Busse, M. (2015). Exercise testing and training in people with Huntington's disease. *Clin Rehabil*, 29, 196–206.

This study investigated metabolic response to exercise in pwMS and used the R6/2 mouse model of HD to derive further insight. They found that, following exercise, pwHD metabolised lactate more slowly than control participants and the post-exercise blood glucose spike was absent in pwHD. The mouse model revealed reduced liver gluconeogenesis:

Josefsen, K., Nielsen, S. M., Campos, A., Seifert, T., Hasholt, L., Nielsen, J. E., Nørremølle, A., Skotte, N. H., Secher, N. H. and Quistorff, B. (2010). Reduced gluconeogenesis and lactate clearance in Huntington's disease. *Neurobiol Dis*, 40, 656–62.

Below is a link to the Europeans Huntingdon's Disease Network (EHDN) physiotherapy working group. The working group has produced the EHDN guidelines for physiotherapists. The document informs the management of pwHD by physiotherapy and includes advice on assessment and training for balance, co-ordination, gait and exercise:

http://www.euro-hd.net/html/network/groups/physio.

Study tasks

1   The term 'long term neurological condition' classifies a diverse group of neurological conditions, which can result from injury or disease, that will affect an individual for the rest of their lives. This chapter has focused on two *progressive* conditions, but use the ICF model to classify the problems caused by a *sudden onset* condition of your choice, and think about how these might affect the person's ability to engage in meaningful life roles and activities, including participation in exercise.

2   Jenifer is a thirty-eight-year-old woman with relapsing remitting MS, and suffers with fatigue. She works part time at as a court clerk and has a two sons aged six and nine. She has heard about the potential benefits of exercise, but is concerned that exercise may exacerbate her fatigue. How might existing evidence be used to a) alleviate her concerns regarding fatigue; b) inform an exercise programme that considers her work and family responsibilities?

3   Steven is a sixty-five-year-old overweight man with secondary progressive MS; he is able to get around his home using the furniture and a walking stick, but uses a wheelchair outside his home. What further information would you deem a) essential before starting an exercise programme, b) helpful to inform an exercise programme?

Chapter summary

The term 'neurological conditions' covers a range of disorders and should not be treated as a single condition; and hence only two such conditions could be considered in this chapter. Therefore, people with such conditions should not be assumed to be a homogenous group, since the considerations and adaptations for safe and effective exercise will also vary. Common aspects include carefully providing an aerobic training stimulus to maintain or enhance cardiovascular fitness and provide progressive muscular strength and balance exercises to limit declines in neuromuscular function, thus reducing the risk of falling and maintaining independence.

References

ACSM (2013). *ACSM's guildines for exercise testing and prescription.* 9th ed. Baltimore, MD: Wolters Kluwer Lippincott Williams and Wilkins.

Altman, D. G. (1996). Better reporting of randomised controlled trials: the CONSORT statement. *BMJ*, 313, 570–1.

Asano, M., Dawes, D. J., Arafah, A., Moriello, C. and Mayo, N. E. (2009). What does a structured review of the effectiveness of exercise interventions for persons with multiple sclerosis tell us about the challenges of designing trials? *Mult Scler*, 15, 412–21.

Asano, M., Duquette, P., Andersen, R., Lapierre, Y. and Mayo, N. E. (2013). Exercise barriers and preferences among women and men with multiple sclerosis. *Disabil Rehabil*, 35, 353–61.

Asano, M. and Finlayson, M. L. (2014). Meta-analysis of three different types of fatigue management interventions for people with multiple sclerosis: exercise, education, and medication. *Mult Scler Int*, 2014, 798285.

Aziz, N. A., van der Burg, J. M., Landwehrmeyer, G. B., Brundin, P., Stijnen, T., Group, E. S. and Roos, R. A. (2008). Weight loss in Huntington disease increases with higher CAG repeat number. *Neurology*, 71, 1506–13.

Busse, M., Hughes G., Wiles C. M. and Rosser A. E. (2009). Use of hand-held dynamometry in the evaluation of lower limb muscle strength in people with Huntington's Disease. *J Neurol*, 225, 1534–40.

Busse, M., Quinn, L., Debono, K., Jones, K., Collett, J., Playle, R., Kelly, M., Simpson, S., Backx, K., Wasley, D., Dawes, H., Rosser, A. and members of the Comet HD Management Group. (2013). A randomized feasibility study of a 12-week community-based exercise program for people with Huntington's disease. *J Neurol Phys Ther*, 37, 149–58.

Ciammola, A., Sassone, J., Sciacco, M., Mencacci, N. E., Ripolone, M., Bizzi, C., Colciago, C., Moggio, M., Parati, G., Silani, V. and Malfatto, G. (2011). Low anaerobic threshold and increased skeletal muscle lactate production in subjects with Huntington's disease. *Mov Disord*, 26, 130–7.

Collett, J., Dawes, H., Cavey, A., Meaney, A., Sackley, C., Wade, D. and Howells, K. (2011a). Hydration and independence in activities of daily living in people with multiple sclerosis: a pilot investigation. *Disabil Rehabil*. 33(19–20), 1822–5.

Collett, J., Dawes, H., Meaney, A., Sackley, C., Barker, K., Wade, D., Izardi, H., Bateman, J., Duda, J. and Buckingham, E. (2011b). Exercise for multiple sclerosis: a single-blind randomized trial comparing three exercise intensities. *Mult Scler*, 17, 594–603.

Dawes, H., Collett, J., Debono, K., Quinn, L., Jones, K., Kelson, M. J., Simpson, S. A., Playle, R., Backx, K., Wasley, D., Nemeth, A. H., Rosser, A., Izardi, H. and Busse, M. (2015). Exercise testing and training in people with Huntington's disease. *Clin Rehabil*, 29, 196–206.

Dawes, H., Collett, J., Meaney, A., Duda, J., Sackley, C., Wade, D., Barker, K. and Izadi, H. (2014). Delayed recovery of leg fatigue symptoms following a maximal exercise session in people with multiple sclerosis. *Neurorehabil Neural Repair*, 28, 139–48.

Dawes, H., Khalil, H., Busse, M., Quinn, L., On behalf of the European Huntington's Disease Network Physiotherapy Working Group. (2013). *HD clinical tips: physical activity and exercise*. European Huntington's Disease Network. Available at: https://healthcarestudies.cf.ac.uk/ActiveHD/clinical-tips-for-physiotherapists/.

Ekelund, U., Ward, H. A., Norat, T., Luan, J., May, A. M., Weiderpass, E., Sharp, S. J., Overvad, K., Ostergaard, J. N., Tjonneland, A., Johnsen, N. F., Mesrine, S., Fournier, A., Fagherazzi, G., Trichopoulou, A., Lagiou, P., Trichopoulos, D., Li, K., Kaaks, R., Ferrari, P., Licaj, I., Jenab, M., Bergmann, M., Boeing, H., Palli, D., Sieri, S., Panico, S., Tumino, R., Vineis, P., Peeters, P. H., Monnikhof, E., Bueno-De-Mesquita, H. B., Quiros, J. R., Agudo, A., Sanchez, M. J., Huerta, J. M., Ardanaz, E., Arriola, L., Hedblad, B., Wirfalt, E., Sund, M., Johansson, M., Key, T. J., Travis, R. C., Khaw, K. T., Brage, S., Wareham, N. J. and Riboli, E. (2015). Physical activity and all-cause mortality across levels of overall and abdominal adiposity in European men and women: the European Prospective Investigation into Cancer and Nutrition Study (EPIC). *Am J Clin Nutr*, 101, 613–21.

Elsworth, C., Winward, C., Sackley, C., Meek, C., Freebody, J., Esser, P., Izadi, H., Soundy, A., Barker, K., Hilton-jones, D., Lowe, C. M., Paget, S., Tims, M., Parnell, R., Patel, S., Wade, D. and Dawes, H. (2011). Supported community exercise in people with long-term neurological conditions: a phase II randomized controlled trial. *Clin Rehabil*, 25, 588–98.

Ensari, I., Motl, R. W. and Pilutti, L. A. (2014). Exercise training improves depressive symptoms in people with multiple sclerosis: results of a meta-analysis. *J Psychosom Res*, 76, 465–71.

Flensner, G. and Lindencrona, C. (2002). The cooling-suit: case studies of its influence on fatigue among eight individuals with multiple sclerosis. *J Adv Nurs*, 37, 541–50.

Fowler, C. J., Panicker, J. N., Drake, M., Harris, C., Harrison, S. C., Kirby, M., Lucas, M., Macleod, N., Mangnall, J., North, A., Porter, B., Reid, S., Russell, N., Watkiss, K. and Wells, M. (2009). A UK consensus on the management of the bladder in multiple sclerosis. *J Neurol Neurosurg Psychiatry*, 80, 470–7.

Grahn, D. A., Murray, J. V. and Heller, H. C. (2008). Cooling via one hand improves physical performance in heat-sensitive individuals with multiple sclerosis: a preliminary study. *BMC Neurol*, 8, 14.

Humm, A. M., Beer, S., Kool, J., Magistris, M. R., Kesselring, J. and Rosler, K. M. (2004). Quantification of Uhthoff's phenomenon in multiple sclerosis: a magnetic stimulation study. *Clin Neurophysiol*, 115, 2493–501.

Josefsen, K., Nielsen, S. M., Campos, A., Seifert, T., Hasholt, L., Nielsen, J. E., Norremolle, A., Skotte, N. H., Secher, N. H. and Quistorff, B. (2010). Reduced gluconeogenesis and lactate clearance in Huntington's disease. *Neurobiol Dis*, 40, 656–62.

Khalil, H., Quinn, L., Van Deursen, R., Dawes, H., Playle, R., Rosser, A. and Busse, M. (2012). A pilot study of an exercise intervention to improve motor function in people with Huntington's disease. *Journal of Neurology, Neurosurgery and Psychiatry*, 83, A59.

Khalil, H., Quinn, L., Van Deursen, R., Dawes, H., Playle, R., Rosser, A. and Busse, M. (2013). What effect does a structured home-based exercise programme have on people with Huntington's disease? A randomized, controlled pilot study. *Clin Rehabil*, 27, 646–58.

Khan, F., Pallent, J., Shea, T. and Whishaw, M. (2009). Multiple sclerosis: prevalence and factors impacting bladder and bowel function in an Australian community cohort. *Disabil Rehabil*, 31, 1567–76.

Kosinski, C. M., Schlangen, C., Gellerich, F. N., Gizatullina, Z., Deschauer, M., Schiefer, J., Young, A. B., Landwehrmeyer, G. B., Toyka, K. V., Sellhaus, B. and Lindenberg, K. S. (2007). Myopathy as a first symptom of Huntington's disease in a marathon runner. *Mov Disord*, 22, 1637–40.

Latimer-Cheung, A. E., Martin ginis, K. A., Hicks, A. L., Motl, R. W., Pilutti, L. A., Duggan, M., Wheeler, G., Persad, R. and Smith, K. M. (2013a). Development of evidence-informed physical activity guidelines for adults with multiple sclerosis. *Arch Phys Med Rehabil*, 94, 1829–36 e7.

Latimer-Cheung, A. E., Pilutti, L. A., Hicks, A. L., Martin Ginis, K. A., Fenuta, A. M., Mackibbon, K. A. and Motl, R. W. (2013b). Effects of exercise training on fitness, mobility, fatigue, and health-related quality of life among adults with multiple sclerosis: a systematic review to inform guideline development. *Arch Phys Med Rehabil*, 94, 1800–28 e3.

Life Group, (2010). *Long-term Individual Fitness Enablement (LIFE) study*. London: Department of Health.

Mackenzie, I. S., Morant, S. V., Bloomfield, G. A., Macdonald, T. M. and O'Riordan, J. (2014). Incidence and prevalence of multiple sclerosis in the UK 1990–2010: a descriptive study in the General Practice Research Database. *J Neurol Neurosurg Psychiatry*, 85, 76–84.

Mallucci, G., Peruzzotti-Jametti, L., Bernstock, J. D. and Pluchino, S. (2015). The role of immune cells, glia and neurons in white and gray matter pathology in multiple sclerosis. *Prog Neurobiol*. In Press.

Meaney, A., Busse M. E., Dawes H., and Rosser, A. (2009). Response to a structured exercise programme for Huntington's disease: a single case study. *Journal of Sport Sciences*, 124.

Motl, R. W. and Pilutti, L. A. (2012). The benefits of exercise training in multiple sclerosis. *Nat Rev Neurol*, 8, 487–97.

Naci, H., Fleurence, R., Birt, J. and Duhig, A. (2010). Economic burden of multiple sclerosis: a systematic review of the literature. *Pharmacoeconomics*, 28, 363–79.

NHS England. (2014). *Clinical commissioning policy: disease modifying therapies for patients with multiple sclerosis (MS)*. NHS England Clinical Reference Group for Neurosciences.

NICE (2014). *Multiple sclerosis: management of multiple sclerosis in primary and secondary care*. National Institute for Health and Care Excellence. Available at: https://www.nice.org.uk/guidance/cg8.

Papoutsi, M., Labuschagne, I., Tabrizi, S. J. and Stout, J. C. (2014). The cognitive burden in Huntington's disease: pathology, phenotype, and mechanisms of compensation. *Mov Disord*, 29, 673–83.

Peterson, J. W., Bo, L., Mork, S., Chang, A. and Trapp, B. D. (2001). Transected neurites, apoptotic neurons, and reduced inflammation in cortical multiple sclerosis lesions. *Ann Neurol*, 50, 389–400.

Pilutti, L. A., Platta, M. E., Motl, R. W. and Latimer-Cheung, A. E. (2014). The safety of exercise training in multiple sclerosis: a systematic review. *J Neurol Sci*, 343, 3–7.

Potter, M. C., Yuan, C., Ottenritter, C., Mughal, M. and Van Praag, H. (2010). Exercise is not beneficial and may accelerate symptom onset in a mouse model of Huntington's disease. *PLOS Curr*, 2, RRN1201.

Pringsheim, T., Wiltshire, K., Day, L., Dykeman, J., Steeves, T. and Jette, N. (2012). The incidence and prevalence of Huntington's disease: a systematic review and meta-analysis. *Mov Disord*, 27, 1083–91.

Quinn, L. and Busse, M., On behalf of the European Huntington's Disease Network Physiotherapy Working Group. (2012). Physiotherapy clinical guidelines for Huntington's disease. Special report. *Neurodegen. Dis. Manage*, 2(1), 21–31.

Quinn, L., Debono, K., Dawes, H., Rosser, A. E., Nemeth, A. H., Rickards, H., Tabrizi, S. J., Quarrell, O., Trender-Gerhard, I., Kelson, M. J., Townson, J., Busse, M. and Members of the TRAIN HD project group. (2014). Task-specific training in Huntington disease: a randomized controlled feasibility trial. *Phys Ther*, 94, 1555–68.

Reilmann, R., Rumpf, S., Beckmann, H., Koch, R., Ringelstein, E. B. and Lange, H. W. (2012). Huntington's disease: objective assessment of posture – a link between motor and functional deficits. *Mov Disord*, 27, 555–9.

Rietberg, M. B., Brooks, D., Uitdehaag, B. M. and Kwakkel, G. (2005). Exercise therapy for multiple sclerosis. *Cochrane Database Syst Rev*, CD003980.

Ross, C. A., Aylward, E. H., Wild, E. J., Langbehn, D. R., Long, J. D., Warner, J. H., Scahill, R. I., Leavitt, B. R., Stout, J. C., Paulsen, J. S., Reilmann, R., Unschuld, P. G., Wexler, A., Margolis, R. L. and Tabrizi, S. J. (2014). Huntington disease: natural history, biomarkers and prospects for therapeutics. *Nat Rev Neurol*, 10, 204–16.

Ross, C. A. and Tabrizi, S. J. (2011). Huntington's disease: from molecular pathogenesis to clinical treatment. *Lancet Neurol*, 10, 83–98.

Royal College of Physicians, National Council for Palliative Care, British Society of Rehabilitation Medicine. (2008). *Long-term neurological conditions: management at the interface between neurology, rehabilitation and palliative care*. Concise Guidance to Good Practice series, No. 10. London: RCP.

Shaw, C. (2001). A review of the psychosocial predictors of help-seeking behaviour and impact on quality of life in people with urinary incontinence. *J Clin Nurs*, 10, 15–24.

Skjerbaek, A. G., Moller, A. B., Jensen, E., Vissing, K., Sorensen, H., Nybo, L., Stenager, E. and Dalgas, U. (2013). Heat sensitive persons with multiple sclerosis are more tolerant to resistance exercise than to endurance exercise. *Mult Scler*, 19, 932–40.

Tosh, J., Dixon, S., Carter, A., Daley, A., Petty, J., Roalfe, A., Sharrack, B. and Saxton, J. (2014). Cost effectiveness of a pragmatic exercise intervention (EXIMS) for people with multiple sclerosis: economic evaluation of a randomised controlled trial. *Mult Scler*, 20, 1123–30.

White, L. J. and Castellano, V. (2008). Exercise and brain health – implications for multiple sclerosis: Part 1 – neuronal growth factors. *Sports Med*, 38, 91–100.

WHO (2002). *Towards a common language for functioning, disability and health ICF*. Geneva: World Health Organization.

WHO (2006). *Neurological disorders: public health challenges*. Geneva: World Health Organization.

WHO (2008). *Atlas: multiple sclerosis resources in the world 2008*. Geneva: World Health Organization.

WHO (2014). *Neurology* [Online]. WHO. Available at: http://www.who.int/topics/neurology/en/

Wild, E. J. and Tabrizi, S. J. (2014). Targets for future clinical trials in Huntington's disease: what's in the pipeline? *Mov Disord*, 29, 1434–45.

Winter, B., Breitenstein, C., Mooren, F. C., Voelker, K., Fobker, M., Lechtermann, A., Krueger, K., Fromme, A., Korsukewitz, C., Floel, A. and Knecht, S. (2007). High impact running improves learning. *Neurobiol Learn Mem*, 87, 597–609.

Wood, B., Van Der Mei, I., Ponsonby, A. L., Pittas, F., Quinn, S., Dwyer, T., Lucas, R. and Taylor, B. (2012). Prevalence and concurrence of anxiety, depression and fatigue over time in multiple sclerosis. *Mult Scler*, 19(2), 217–24.

Zinzi, P., Salmaso, D., De Grandis, R., Graziani, G., Maceroni, S., Bentivoglio, A., Zappata, P., Frontali, M. and Jacopini, G. (2007). Effects of an intensive rehabilitation programme on patients with Huntington's disease: a pilot study. *Clin Rehabil* 21(7), 603–13.

Zuccato, C. and Cattaneo, E. (2007). Role of brain-derived neurotrophic factor in Huntington's disease. *Prog Neurobiol*, 81, 294–330.

Chapter 9

Physical activity for osteoarthritis

Gladys Onambélé-Pearson and Neil Reeves

Introduction

Osteoarthritis is a metabolically active, dynamic process that involves all joint tissues. Generally, it tends to affect the hand, knee, hip, spine, and foot joints, where its pathology (i.e. the detected biochemical and physiological abnormalities) involves new bone formation (osteophyte) at the joint margins and results in the degeneration of the hyaline cartilage (the capsule), synovial fluid and soft tissues (i.e. ligaments and muscle) of the affected joints. The combination of reduced tissue loss and increased new tissue synthesis in osteoarthritis supports the view that it is the repair process of synovial joints that is most responsible for the condition.

In fact, a variety of joint traumas may trigger the need to repair, but, once initiated, all the joint tissues take part, showing increased cell activity and new tissue production. Thus, initially, the factors involved in osteoarthritis are a slow but efficient repair process, which often compensates for the initial physical/physiological trauma, resulting in a structurally-altered but symptom-free joint. Where the insult is prolonged and/or extensive, this overwhelms the repair process, resulting essentially in overcompensation, and, ultimately, presentation with symptomatic osteoarthritis or 'joint failure'. Genetic and evolutionary factors (a hypothesis suggests that some joints are biomechanically under-designed, and hence more prone to osteoarthritic failure), as well as the extensive nature of the insult, modulate the propensity for the initial repair mechanism's ability to cope, thereby explaining the extreme variability in clinical presentation and outcome, both between individuals and at different joint sites.

Osteoarthritis statistics

Arthritis and, in particular, osteoarthritis, is generally recognised as the leading cause of disability among ageing adults (Covinsky, 2006; Covinsky et al., 2008; Dunlop et al., 1997; Dunlop et al., 2001; Felson et al., 2000). In fact, frequently described as 'wear and tear', the propensity of osteoarthritis in persons aged 80+ is nearly universal, as evidenced through radiographic scans (van Saase et al. 1989). It should nevertheless be noted that concordance between symptoms and radiographic osteoarthritis only seem reliable in cases demonstrating advanced structural damage (Peat et al., 2006). Verbrugge et al. estimated that, in the over-fifty five-year-olds in the US, 32.7 per cent of males and 47.1 per cent of females have osteoarthritis (Verbrugge et al., 1991). In the UK, more than six million people have painful osteoarthritis in one or both knees, more than 650,000 have painful osteoarthritis in one or both hips, a further 1.5 million have X-ray evidence of hip osteoarthritis (but may not have any symptoms), and, finally, almost 8.5 million people have X-ray evidence of osteoarthritis of the spine (Arthritis Research, 2008). To emphasise the point, knee joint osteoarthritis is one of the most prevalent forms of this degenerative joint disease (Felson, 1988).

In spite of the widespread prevalence of the condition, the scientific evidence for the principal contributors to osteoarthritis and ensuing decreased functional ability (increased disability) is yet to be complete, therefore making it an excellent topic for a clinical guideline. It is clear, however, that osteoarthritis is a common complex disorder, in which the progression of disability is slow (Mallen et al., 2007; Roos et al., 2008; Sharma et al., 2003; van Dijk et al., 2006) and characterised by varying degrees of functional limitations and reduced quality of life.

Osteoarthritis aetiology

It is now becoming increasingly apparent that biomechanical factors play a key role in the development and progression of osteoarthritis, especially osteoarthritis affecting the lower limbs (Block and Shakoor, 2010; Englund, 2010; Shakoor and Moisio, 2004). The medial tibio-femoral compartment of the knee is most commonly affected by osteoarthritis (Felson and Radin, 1994), and this particular compartment is a good example of how biomechanical factors are now known to play a key role in the development of osteoarthritis. The high prevalence of medial knee osteoarthritis stems from the type of biomechanical loading experienced during everyday activities such as walking and using stairs. While the foot is in contact with the ground during walking, an external knee adduction moment acts around the knee joint in the frontal plane. The external knee adduction moment tends to cause a rotational moment of the tibia medially in relation to the femur (Hurwitz et al., 1998).

The external knee adduction moment causes compression of the medial tibio-femoral compartment of the knee, compressing the meniscus and hyaline cartilage. The external knee adduction moment can therefore be considered as a surrogate measure for medial knee compression, and this moment is primarily caused by a medially-acting ground reaction force present during walking and other locomotor paradigms such as stair negotiation (Hamel et al., 2005; Reeves et al., 2009). The knee adduction moment has been shown as a strong predictor of osteoarthritis progression in the medial knee compartment (Miyazaki et al., 2002). In this study, over 100 patients were assessed at baseline and followed up six years later. After the six-year follow-up, a sub-group of these patients had shown disease progression (based upon radiographic evaluation) and these patients had displayed significantly higher knee adduction moments and greater pain compared to the sub-group not showing any evidence of disease progression. The level of joint space narrowing in the group showing evidence of progression was also correlated with an increasing varus angle at the knee. The varus angle has also been identified by other studies as one of the best predictors of the knee adduction moment magnitude (Barrios et al., 2009); this is intuitive, as it will increase the moment arm of the ground reaction force acting around the knee joint.

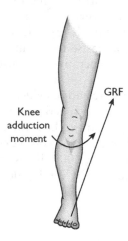

Figure 9.1 Illustration of how the ground reaction force (GRF) acts medially to the knee joint during walking and other daily activities, causing an external knee adduction moment to act around the knee in the frontal plane. The external knee adduction moment will cause compression of the medial knee compartment. (Produced by Sarah Reeves of RedRockingBird Designs).

The knee varus angle has been reported as the best predictor of the knee adduction moment in osteoarthritis patients, with correlation coefficients of R = 0.751 (Hurwitz et al., 2002). Whilst the majority of research investigating biomechanical loading and knee osteoarthritis has assessed and compared peaks in the knee adduction moment profile, some patients with the most severe osteoarthritis symptoms may show a 'flatter' knee adduction moment profile, with the peaks less clearly evident. Such a joint moment profile may suggest that the knee is not alleviated from the loading during walking as the moment remains relatively high throughout. This can be quantified by measuring the entire area under the curve, known as the knee adduction moment-time integral or the knee adduction angular impulse. This measure (the knee adduction moment time-integral) has been shown to identify differences between knee osteoarthritis patients of varying severity when, otherwise, no differences were evident, simply from examination of the peak knee adduction moments (Thorp et al., 2006).

Interestingly, there is a disassociation between osteoarthritis pathology and the speed and intensity of the decreased functional ability (increased disability), so much so that there is wide variation in symptoms for those with radiographic evidence of joint degeneration changes, and many with radiographic changes report from minimal to severe pain and stiffness (Lawrence et al., 1966). This therefore suggests a large number of potential pharmaceutical and non-pharmaceutical treatment avenues, which can be used to disrupt the pathway that links the pathology and the development of disability.

With variability in the type and intensity of symptoms in osteoarthritis comes increased complexity in summarising the literature for its characteristics. Whilst clinical diagnosis is often made on the basis of both radiographic signs and joint symptoms, the fact that the former may only develop at the later stages of the disease means

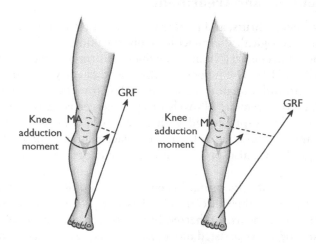

Figure 9.2 Illustration of how an increased varus angle at the knee can increase the external knee adduction angle. The left illustration shows a neutrally-aligned knee joint, whereas the right illustration shows a knee with an increased varus angle. An increased varus angle causes the ground reaction force (GRF) to act further away from the knee joint centre, thereby increasing the moment arm (MA – dashed line) around the knee. For the same ground reaction force magnitude and direction, a larger frontal plane moment arm at the knee as illustrated, will cause a greater knee adduction moment. (Produced by Sarah Reeves of RedRockingBird Designs).

that a more reliable framework, which would apply to all stages of the pathology, needs to be adopted. To this end, researchers have used the Disablement Model developed by Verbrugge and Jette, based on the seminal work by Nagi (Nagi, 1965; Nagi, 1979; Verbrugge and Jette, 1994). This proposes both intrinsic and extrinsic factors (though not making a jump between association and causality) to the development of disability in osteoarthritis.

Briefly, it is proposed that the main intrinsic modulators include genetic factors (i.e. 40–60 per cent heritability), constitutional factors (i.e. age, body mass index, obesity, female sex, high bone density, lack of exercise, comorbid conditions, depression, and depressive symptoms), and biomechanical risk factors (e.g. joint injury, occupational/ recreational usage, reduced muscle strength, joint laxity, joint mal-alignment). The main extrinsic factors, on the other hand, include decreased physical independence, as well as decreased access to transportation (McDonough and Jette, 2010). In the presence of these, pathologic physiologic signs are as described above, specifically the development of sclerotic changes in subchondral bone tissue, osteophyte growth, and synovial tissue proliferation. Linked to these, impairment to the joints is translated through visible joint swelling, deformity or mal-alignment, decreased strength, limitations in range of motion or stiffness, abnormalities of gait, and joint pain. At the whole body level, to the individual, the decreased functional ability, or increased disability would tend to be experienced as restrictions in walking, picking up items from the floor, stair ascent/descent, dressing, doing household chores, and, ultimately, participating in social activities or family events.

Osteoarthritis management and treatment

There is currently no cure for osteoarthritis, and treatment options may be pharmaco-logical, surgical, or non-pharmacological. Pharmacologically speaking, the National Institute for Health and Clinical Excellence (NICE) guidelines confirm paracetamol in early pain management (NICE, 2014). The guidelines also suggests early considera-tion of topical non-steroidal anti-inflammatory drugs (NSAIDs) for knee and hand arthritis, and suggest that wherever systemic NSAIDs or cyclooxygenase-2 (COX-2) inhibitors are used, they should be co-prescribed with cover from a proton pump inhibitor (PPI). Surgically speaking, total knee or hip joint replacement is common for advanced disease, whilst the guidelines also provide restricted support for the use of acupuncture.

Interestingly, non-care management options have been used, including rest, relaxa-tion, and pacing, though evidence for their effectiveness has not proved conclusive. The guidelines, however, do promote the use of thermotherapy (i.e. local heat or cold), and manual therapy (i.e. passive or active assisted movement techniques that use man-ual force to improve the mobility of restricted joints, connective tissue, or skeletal mus-cles), as adjuncts to core treatment. Notably, the positive role of exercise is emphasised, in contrast to the natural inclination some might have to rest when a joint is affected by osteoarthritis (National Collaborating Centre for Chronic Conditions, 2008). In fact, the guidelines also promote positive behavioural changes such as exercise, weight loss, use of suitable footwear, and pacing, in the self-management of osteoarthritis.

A number of management strategies can be used to prevent, arrest, or slow the progression of osteoarthritis based upon modifying certain biomechanical factors. Many of these are well-established for knee osteoarthritis, and have shown efficacy in clinical trials (for a review see Reeves and Bowling, 2011). In terms of prevention, wearing high-heeled shoes in women without knee osteoarthritis has been shown to significantly increase the knee adduction moment (Kerrigan et al., 2001; Kerrigan et al., 1998). Over time, the use of high-heeled shoes may, therefore, lead to the devel-opment of knee osteoarthritis through compression of the medial knee compartment. Wearing appropriate footwear, which would substantially lower the loading on the knee joint, can prevent this. Furthermore, in terms of footwear, it has been shown that shoes with a thin, flexible sole can reduce the loading on the knee joint compared with more inflexible shoes with thicker soles (Shakoor et al., 2010). Although thicker-soled shoes may attenuate the loading on the sole of the foot, they may also conceal the transfer of loads up to the knee, which could contribute to the development and progression of knee osteoarthritis. Lateral wedge insoles have been used as a method for reducing the loading on the knee and slowing the progression of knee osteoarthri-tis. However, they are only effective for patients with early-stage knee osteoarthritis, and not for those patients with a more advanced stage of the disease (Sasaki and Yasuda, 1987). Lateral wedge insoles are suggested to exert an effect on knee load-ing via shifting the centre of pressure under the foot and altering the direction of the ground reaction force around the knee, thereby altering the knee adduction moment (Kakihana et al., 2005). Walking with a 'toe-out gait' i.e. the foot externally rotated relative to the direction of walking, has been shown to reduce the knee adduction moment in patients with knee osteoarthritis (Guo et al., 2007). This strategy changes the axis of the knee joint and also the direction of the ground reaction force in relation to the knee. Patients with knee osteoarthritis could spontaneously adopt this walking strategy to reduce the loading on their knees. In a study of knee osteoarthritis patients with an eighteen-month follow-up period, a greater toe-out angle was associated with reduced likelihood of disease progression (Chang et al., 2007). In theory, this could be a walking strategy that is taught to patients in an attempt to potentially reduce knee loading and minimise disease progression. Knee bracing may be used for osteoarthritis affecting the patello-femoral or tibio-femoral compartments. Valgus bracing is used for patients with medial tibio-femoral osteoarthritis, and functions by applying a valgus moment to the knee joint that unloads the medial knee compartment. Valgus knee braces have been shown to reduce the net knee adduction moment in patients with knee osteoarthritis (Pollo et al., 2002), and have also been shown to reduce pain and improve function in patients wearing the brace for between six and twelve months (Kirkley et al., 1999; van Raaij et al., 2010). Despite their clinical effectiveness, on the practical side, valgus knee braces are bulky and sometimes uncomfortable, and, as a result, they may not be worn on a daily basis by many patients who could benefit from their use.

Evidence for exercise

Physical activity and/or exercise is generally adopted and recognised by health professionals and patients, not least owing to the perceived ease of application and comparatively low costs. Physical activity can be targeted to specific joint(s) to improve general mobility, function, and reduce pain (Fransen et al., 2002). More intensive exercise can strengthen muscles around the affected joint. However, it is not uncommon for patients to be unclear over the benefits of exercise, particularly where exercise is not only perceived as an activity that 'wears out' joints, but it may also seem to exacerbate pain. In addition, patients may also be under the impression that resting seems to ease their pain. Research in fact shows that while a limited number of individuals may indeed experience increased intensity in osteoarthritis symptoms upon taking up exercise, an appropriately-targeted and paced exercise programme will not cause any adverse reaction in the vast majority of people, including those significantly affected by the condition (Hurley et al., 2007). Indeed, even patients with severe osteoarthritis can ride a bicycle, go swimming, or exercise at a gym, even if analgesia is required to help.

The following section looks at the research evidence for different types of exercise for the joints usually affected by osteoarthritis. Specifically, only trials (and reviews) on the manipulation of exercise (i.e. not exercise combined with other therapies such as pharmaceuticals, diet, physiotherapy etc.), nor combined exercise programmes, are explored.

Osteoarthritis and aerobic exercise

The American Geriatrics Society has developed general guidelines for training parameters in people with osteoarthritis pain. The guidelines stipulate that aerobic exercises should be carried out two to five times a week at 40–60 per cent of VO_{2max}/HR_{max}, (i.e. moderate aerobic activity, where HR_{max} is age-predicted heart rate maximum and VO_{2max} is maximal aerobic capacity) progressing from twenty to thirty minutes each session, with each contraction being held for one to six seconds (as capacity increases) (AGS, 2001). The dosages in these guidelines are somewhat less than those recommended by the American Heart Association and the American College of Sports Medicine for healthy older adults (Nelson et al., 2007), where recommendations are for up to 150 minutes of moderate-intensity aerobic activity per week. Hence, it would seem that adhering to the AHA or ACSM exercise recommendations would also fit with the exercise needs of osteoarthritis sufferers.

The spectrum of aerobic exercises that patients with osteoarthritis can partake in is as varied as the imagination, with the only restrictions being to preferentially avoid high-impact exercise, given the potentially deleterious effects of high joint load as shown in animal studies (Radin et al., 1978; Radin et al., 1984). Aerobic exercise may include activities such as walking, cycling, dancing, or chair-based exercise, so long as the patient is comfortable, outcomes are attainable, and the routine is likely to minimise boredom whilst maximising patient's adherence. It is notable that other forms of exercise such as stretching, range of motion, and postural/dynamic balance may be incorporated to achieve specific goals based on individual patients' assessments.

One school of thought (e.g. Osteoarthritis Research Society International) recommends that if obesity is an issue, then accumulating greater volumes of weekly exercise is desirable, not least to help reduce excessive body weight. However, whether losing weight *per se* leads to improved prognosis for people with osteoarthritis, particularly in the lower limb joints, is still an ongoing research topic.

Osteoarthritis and resistance exercise

Clinical trials of strengthening exercise have spanned isometric, isotonic, isokinetic, concentric, concentric/eccentric, and dynamic modalities, but there is little evidence that the type of strengthening exercise influences outcome (Bennell and Hinman, 2011). Nonetheless, the American Geriatrics Society has developed general guidelines for training parameters in people with Osteoarthritis pain, whereby isometric strengthening exercises should be carried out on a daily basis at 40–60 per cent of maximal contractile capacity, progressing from one to ten submaximal contractions for each exercised muscle group, with each contraction being held for one to six seconds (as capacity increases). The society also stipulates that where isotonic training is taken up, it should be carried out two to three times weekly, so that 40 per cent, 40–60 per cent, or > 60 per cent of maximal contractile capacity should employ ten to fifteen, eight to ten, or six to eight repetitions respectively (AGS, 2001). It should be noted that, whilst moderate exercise is highlighted here, where a direct comparison has been made between high- versus low-intensity resistance exercise in a research study, the effectiveness of the two training intensities was, in fact, matched, with no greater incidence of pain sensation in the high-intensity training (Jan et al., 2008). In fact, with the latter, since sessions were relatively short (twenty minutes shorter, in fact), it is possible that adherence to a training programme may be enhanced.

Notably, also, a recent meta-analysis points to a combination of resistance exercise plus manual therapy as being optimal for reducing the pain association with osteoarthritis (Jansen et al., 2011). By analysing data from twelve studies, these authors demonstrated that the effect size on pain is 0.38 (95 per cent CI 0.23 to 0.54) for strength training, 0.34 (95 per cent CI 0.19 to 0.49) for combined 'resistance,

Table 9.1 Sample of studies favouring aerobic exercise against osteoarthritis

Positive outcome	Reference	Intervention and study duration	Outcome specifics
Decreased pain	1 MA (Roddy et al., 2005), 4 RCTs (N = 449)	Aerobic walking vs. no-exercise control interventions (8 weeks to 2 years)	Pain
	1 RCT (Messier et al., 1997) (N = 103)	Aerobic training exercise groups vs. health education (18 months follow-up)	Transfer pain intensity and frequency (getting in and out of bed, chair, car etc.)
Decreased disability	1 MA (Roddy et al., 2005) 2 RCTs (N = 385)	Aerobic walking vs. no-exercise control interventions (8 weeks to 2 years)	Self-reported disability
	1 RCT (Penninx et al., 2001) (N = 250)	Aerobic exercise vs. attention control (18 months follow-up)	Risk of activities of daily living (ADL) disability (30-item questionnaire); risk of moving from a non-ADL disabled to an ADL-disabled state over this period
Increased muscular strength	1 RCT (Messier et al., 1997) (N = 103)	Aerobic exercise vs. health education control (18 months follow-up)	Knee mean angular velocity
	1 RCT (Messier et al., 1997) (N = 103)	Aerobic exercise vs. education control (18 months of follow-up)	Walking velocity; absolute and relative stride length
	1 RCT (Messier et al., 1997) (N = 103)	Aerobic exercise groups vs. health education (18 months follow-up)	Double legged, eyes closed, postural balance
Improved quality of life	1 RCT (Penninx et al., 2002) (N = 439)	Aerobic exercise vs. education (18 months follow-up)	Lower depression scores (CES-D scale) over time

NB. MA is a meta-analysis; RCT is a randomised control trial, N is the study sample size.

ROM plus aerobic' exercise, and 0.69 (95 per cent CI 0.42 to 0.96) for exercise plus manual mobilisation (Jansen et al., 2011). Another meta-analysis, which included 433 knee osteoarthritis patients, corroborates with the conclusion that resistance exercise positively impacts osteoarthritis through increased muscle strength, reduced pain, and improved functional ability (Kristensen and Franklyn-Miller, 2012).

Muscle groups which could be said to be key to physical independence, arguably including the quadriceps, hip abductors, hip extensors, hamstrings, and calf muscles and as such, should be particularly targeted for local strengthening workout.

Based on the research evidence, it would appear that resistance training has the edge where osteoarthritis symptom amelioration is concerned. To expand further on the

Table 9.2 Sample of studies favouring resistance exercise against osteoarthritis

Positive outcome	Reference	Intervention	Outcome specifics
Decreased pain	1 MA (Roddy et al., 2005), 8 RCTs (N = 2004)	Home-based quadriceps strengthening vs. no-exercise control interventions (Eight weeks to two years)	Pain
	1 RCT (Huang et al., 2003) (N = 132)	Isokinetic, isotonic, and isometric exercise vs. no exercise (One year follow-up)	VAS score
	1 RCT (Tak et al., 2005) (N = 94)	Exercise (strength training and home exercises) vs. no treatment (three months follow-up)	Self-reported pain (VAS score), Observed pain (HHS pain scale)
	1 RCT (Messier et al., 1997) (N = 103)	Weight training exercise groups vs. health education (Eighteen months follow-up)	Transfer pain intensity and frequency (getting in and out of bed, chair, car etc)
	1 RCT (Brismee et al., 2007) (N = 41)	Tai chi exercise vs. attention control (Nine to twelve weeks)	Mean overall and maximal knee pain (VAS)
Decreased disability	1 MA (Roddy et al., 2005), 8 RCTs (N = 2004)	Home-based quadriceps strengthening vs. no-exercise control interventions (8 weeks-2 years)	Self-reported disability
	1 RCT (Huang et al., 2003) (N = 132)	Isokinetic, isotonic, and isometric exercise groups vs. no exercise (One year follow-up)	Self-reported disability (LI 17 questionnaire)
	1 RCT (Penninx et al., 2001) (N = 250)	Resistance exercise vs. attention control (18 months follow-up)	Risk of activities of daily living (ADL) disability (30-item questionnaire); risk of moving from a non-ADL disabled to an ADL-disabled state over this period
	1 RCT (Fransen et al., 2007) (N = 152)	Tai chi exercise vs. attention control (Twelve weeks)	WOMAC function
	1 RCT (Brismee et al., 2007) (N = 41)	Tai chi exercise vs. attention control (Nine weeks)	WOMAC overall score

	Study	Intervention	Outcome measure
	1 RCT(Borjesson et al., 1996) (N = 68)	Strengthening exercise vs. control groups (three months)	Step-down ability
	1 RCT (Fransen et al., 2007) (N = 152)	Tai chi vs. attention control (twelve weeks)	Stair climb (seconds)
Increased muscular strength	1 RCT (Huang et al., 2003) (N = 132)	Exercise (isokinetic, isotonic, and isometric exercise) vs. no exercise (One-year follow-up)	Mean peak torque values for knee extensor and flexor muscles at 60 and 180 degrees
	1 RCT (Keefe et al., 2004) (N = 72)	Exercise (strength plus endurance training) vs. no-treatment (twelve weeks)	Improvements in muscle strength for leg extensions; leg flexions; bicep curls
	1 RCT (Borjesson et al., 1996) (N = 68)	Strengthening exercise vs. control (3 months)	Mean peak torque values for knee extensor and flexor muscles
	1 RCT (Huang et al., 2003) (N = 132)	Exercise (isokinetic, isotonic, and isometric groups) vs. control (One year follow-up)	Improvement in walking speed
	1 RCT (Messier et al., 1997) (N = 103)	Weight-training vs. education control (eighteen months of follow-up)	Walking velocity; absolute and relative stride length
	1 RCT (Messier et al., 1997) (N = 103)	Weight-training exercise groups vs. health education (eighteen months follow-up)	Double legged, eyes closed, postural balance
	1 RCT (Tak et al., 2005) (N = 94)	Exercise (strength training and home exercises) vs. no treatment (Three months follow-up)	Timed up-and-go performance
	1 RCT (Fransen et al., 2007) (N = 152)	Tai chi vs. attention control (Twelve weeks)	Timed up-and-go performance
	1 RCT (Song et al., 2003) (N = 43)	Tai chi vs. control (twelve weeks)	Balance and abdominal muscle strength
Improved quality of life	1 RCT (Thorstensson et al., 2005) (N = 61)	Weight-bearing exercise vs. no treatment (Six months)	Improvement in quality of life scores (KOOS subscale)
	1 RCT (Tak et al., 2005) (N = 94)	Exercise (strength training and home exercises) vs. no treatment (Three months follow-up)	Improvement in health status (Sickness Impact Profile)
	1 RCT (Fransen et al., 2007) (N = 152)	Tai chi vs. attention control (Two weeks)	SF-12 version 2, physical component

MA: meta-analysis; RCT: randomised control trial; N: study sample size.

studies listed in Table 2, it is notable that resistance training for general strengthening of the quadriceps muscle group has been advocated in the management of knee osteo-arthritis (Roddy et al, 2005; Zhang et al., 2007). A longitudinal study has shown how higher quadriceps strength is associated with a lower incidence of developing symp-tomatic knee osteoarthritis (Segal et al., 2009), suggesting that knee extensor resist-ance training may be a useful prophylactic measure. However, some caution should be advocated here when specific compartments are affected and joint deformities are very pronounced. A twelve-week quadriceps resistance training programme in patients with knee osteoarthritis failed to influence the external knee adduction moment (which would unload the medial knee compartment), and only relieved pain in patients with a fairly neutral knee alignment (Lim et al., 2008). This resistance training programme had no effect on pain in patients with a valgus knee alignment, suggesting that the degree of joint deformity should be taken into account in designing resistance train-ing programs. In patients affected by medial compartment knee osteoarthritis, there is a rationale for targeting of the hip abductor muscles with resistance training, since this may help to stabilise the pelvis and exert an internal valgus moment, which will oppose the external knee adduction moment that acts to compress the medial knee compartment. A small pilot study employing four weeks of hip abductor resistance training in patients with medial knee osteoarthritis reported significant reductions in the external knee adduction moment and marked reduction in pain (Thorp et al., 2010). A much larger, randomised, controlled trial consisting of hip abductor and adductor resistance training reported reductions in pain but no changes in the knee adduction moment (Bennell et al., 2010).

Potential mechanisms of exercise

What is the physiological pathway underlying the effects of exercise? Joint cartilage has outstanding tensile strength, with the loading sustained during normal high-intensity exercise (e.g. running, jumping, and throwing, and hence torsional strains) only approximately 1/3 of the tensile capacity of the cartilage capacity (Bellucci and Seedhom, 2001; Fukubayashi and Kurosawa, 1980). However, the effect of chronic low-level loading of the joint cartilage is unclear. It may be that there is a decreased ability to adapt to joint loading in already unhealthy, previously-injured cartilage, or cartilage in a mal-aligned or excessively lax or taut (knee) joint, thereby rendering the joint more susceptible to chronic deleterious changes.

Where exercise is used therapeutically, it enhances the diffusion of substances through synovial fluid, and thus increases the rate and magnitude of nourishment to the mature cartilage cells (Hall et al., 1991). Indeed, cartilage loading in the form of regular, moderate exercise enhances glycosaminoglycan content in knee cartilage (Roos and Dahlberg, 2005). The cartilaginous matrix adapts to loading stresses by enhanced crosslinking analogous to osteoblastic activity in bones under moderate duress. What is not known is if a loading threshold exists, above which injury out-weighs benefit. Of particular note is the fact that exercise is often associated with reactive oxygen species (ROS), molecules that are involved in normal metabolism. Certainly, the in-vitro evidence appears to link exercise with release of reactive oxy-gen species from osteoblast-like cells (Yamamoto et al., 2005). In the case of bone, and, in fact, cartilage homeostasis, the impact of reducing levels of ROS is thought to be beneficial (Beecher et al., 2007). Whilst metadata is not yet available to support the idea of the exact threshold of exercise intensity to minimise potential deleterious results, the research on ROS suggests that the combination of exercise and nutritional interventions may be a promising therapeutic avenue.

Evidence for exercise and diet in osteoarthritis

Given the low side-effect profile for the great majority of nutritional supplements, identifying disease-modifying dietary components capable of not only preventing, but also minimising the progress of osteoarthritis, should remain an important paradigm in the management of this condition. This approach, coined nutraceutics, has principally concentrated in dietary fortification with the long-chain ω-3 essential fatty acids, eicosapentaenoic acid and docosahexaenoic acid, functional ω-6 fatty acid, γ-linolenic acid, as well as the macronutrient composition of background diet. The take-home message here seems to be that a high-fibre diet, with a high ω-3:ω-6 ratio, would appear to be advantageous in the management of osteoarthritis (Lopez, 2012a). Diet additives such as glucosamine, chondroitin sulfate, antioxidants, and green-lipped mussel may also have some benefit in managing osteoarthritis. In fact, the idea of 'rational polysupplementation' is coined, whereby a number of nutritional agents may be simultaneously used in a concerted effort to improve osteoarthritis prognosis (Lopez, 2012b). Such polysupplementation would ideally include vitamins (C, E [mixed isomers], D_3, K_2), minerals (Selenium, Zinc, Manganese, and Boron), probiotics (lactate-producing bacteria of the Bifidobacterium and Lactobaccilli genus), and prebiotics (select nondigested oligosaccharide fibers composed of inulin, fructooligosaccharides, and/or galactooligosaccharides), as well as phytofavonoids/polyphenols (present in a variety of fruits, berries, teas, spices, nuts, wine, cocoa, and vegetables).

A special mention of the evidence-based clinical practice guideline on the use of physical activity and diet for the management of osteoarthritis in overweight or obese adults (body mass index ≥ 25 kg/m^2) should be made as decreased functional ability/mobility, often seen with osteoarthritis, leads to weight gain (even where weight was not initially an issue). Obesity is frequently present among physically-inactive people with osteoarthritis (Veenhof et al., 2012). It increases the risk of development and progression of lower-limb osteoarthritis, and increases the risk of knee osteoarthritis by four times compared to people with a body mass index (BMI) of < 30 kg/m^2 (Anderson and Felson, 1988). Not only this, but the increased joint loading and the inflammation associated with high BMI will compound the impact on the joints. Systematic reviews confirm a positive impact of exercise to pain and functional ability in populations with a BMI > 30 kg/m^2 (Brosseau et al., 2011).

Future research

This chapter illustrates that clinical guidelines for the recommendations of exercise in the treatment of osteoarthritis are justified. Specifically, the evidence for both weight-bearing (e.g. aerobic and/or strengthening) and water-based exercises as beneficial is strong, as these tend to improve a number of markers of pain and function in people with osteoarthritis.

It is also clear that whilst the beneficial impact of exercise can be seen across the range of disease severities, optimising type, dosage, and periodisation is yet to be determined. It may be that the principal outcomes, desired by the patient and/or their therapist, may be the only way to individualise the approach to exercise prescription. Indeed, specifying the criteria for exercise therapy to be described as ultimately successful is not universal and has to be aligned with the patient's principal health issue (is it pain? Weakness? Joint mobility?). In terms of approach to exercise, many factors such as degree/site of impairments, comorbidities, socio-economic factors (e.g. affordability/accessibility), exercise prescription format (e.g. class-based vs. home-based, weekly-supervised vs. intermittent supervisions with spaced-out refresher sessions), as well as patient predisposition to sensitivity to pain/discomfort/disability (Tsai, 2005; Wade et al., 2011), may all interplay to modulate adherence to exercise prescription.

It is notable that the effect sizes of exercise have been shown to be similar to those effects achieved from simple analgesia and non-steroidal anti-inflammatory drugs, but with far fewer side-effects (Bennell and Hinman, 2011), and added benefits, such as increased aerobic capacity (Escalante et al., 2011). Future studies should nonetheless evaluate the effects of exercise on structural disease progression, as it is unclear whether exercise can in fact modify the long-term prognosis in osteoarthritis.

Summary

One of the most discussed and controversial management strategies for musculoskeletal conditions is exercise. 'Do I need to exercise?', and 'will exercise in fact exacerbate my condition?', are questions patients frequently ask themselves or their clinicians. In fact, conservative non-pharmacological strategies, particularly exercise, are recommended by all clinical guidelines for the management of osteoarthritis. For the majority of sufferers, a combination of aerobic and strengthening exercises is optimal to address the spectrum of impairments associated with the conditions. However, this may not necessarily be practical and the choice of one type of exercise over another will be based on an assessment of the individual patient. Therefore, over and above all else, individualisation of exercise training is key.

Study tasks

1   William is seventy-four, overweight, is finding activities of daily living increasingly hard to carry out, and has recently been diagnosed as having osteoarthritis. He looks up the condition on the internet and surmises from his own research that resistance exercise is the way to go. William has never been a typical gym user, however, and would like to maximise the benefits from his gym sessions. How should he go about his training programme?

2   Jocelyn is a healthy woman in her early forties. She is conscious that there is a history of osteoporosis in her family, and is therefore a keen runner, in order to strengthen her bones. In addition, Jocelyn looks after her diet by supplementing it with a multitude of dairy products. Nonetheless, Linda has been feeling pain in her joints and is losing weight in spite of her overtly healthy lifestyle.

Are there contraindications to the prescription of high-impact endurance exercise for Jocelyn? Is there any evidence that exercise can ameliorate the inflammation associated with her potential development of osteoarthritis?

3   Lilian is a life-long wearer of high heels in her mid-thirties. She wears them all the time, since wearing flat shoes leads to a dull continuous pain in her lower limbs that will remain for days after the event. Her physiotherapist has prescribed a twelve-week calves-stretch exercise programme. Whilst the physiotherapy is helping, the fact remains that Lilian feels as though the pain is now 'shifting' to the knee joints. What could be the issues here?

Further reading

An up-to-date review of the interlinks between exercise, inflammation, and joint diseases, written with a strong emphasis on cellular mechanisms:

Filaire, E. and Toumib, H. (2012). Reactive oxygen species and exercise on bone metabolism: Friend or enemy? *Joint Bone Spine*, 79, 341–346.

An illustration of the importance of considering joint angles during resistance exercise (open access: http://dx.doi.org/10.5772/56386):

Onambélé-Pearson, G. L., McMahon, G., Morse, C. I., Burden, A. and Winwood, K. How deep should you squat to maximise a holistic training response? Electromyographic, energetic, cardiovascular, hypertrophic and mechanical evidence. In H. Turker, (ed). (2013). *Electrodiagnosis in New Frontiers of Clinical Research*. pp 155–74.

A concise overview of the role of joint mechanics in the development, and, hence, management, of osteoarthritis:

Reeves, N. D. and Bowling, F. L. (2011). Conservative biomechancial strategies for knee osteoarthritis. *Nature Reviews: Rheumatology*, 7, 113–22.

References

American Geriatrics Society (AGS) (2001). Exercise prescription for older adults with osteoarthritis pain: consensus practice recommendations. a supplement to the AGS Clinical Practice Guidelines on the management of chronic pain in older adults. *Journal of the American Geriatrics Society*, 49(6), 808–23.

Anderson, J. J., and Felson, D. T. (1988). Factors associated with osteoarthritis of the knee in the first national Health and Nutrition Examination Survey (HANES I). Evidence for an association with overweight, race, and physical demands of work. *American Journal of Epidemiology*, 128(1), 179–89.

Arthritis Research, UK. (2008). *Arthritis in the UK – key facts*. Available at: http://www.arthritisresearchuk.org/arthritis-information/data-and-statistics.aspx.

Barrios, J. A., Higginson, J. S., Royer, T. D., and Davis, I. S. (2009). Static and dynamic correlates of the knee adduction moment in healthy knees ranging from normal to varus-aligned. *Clin Biomech (Bristol, Avon)*, 24, 850–4.

Beecher, B. R., Martin, J. A., Pedersen, D. R., Heiner, A. D., and Buckwalter, J. A. (2007). Antioxidants block cyclic loading induced chondrocyte death. *Iowa Orthop J*, 27, 1–8.

Bellucci, G., and Seedhom, B. B. (2001). Mechanical behaviour of articular cartilage under tensile cyclic load. *Rheumatology*, 40(12), 1337–45.

Bennell, K. L., and Hinman, R. S. (2011). A review of the clinical evidence for exercise in osteoarthritis of the hip and knee. *Journal of Science and Medicine in Sport/Sports Medicine Australia*, 14(1), 4–9. doi: 10.1016/j.jsams.2010.08.002.

Bennell, K. L., Hunt, M. A., Wrigley, T. V., Hunter, D. J., McManus, F. J., Hodges, P. W., Li, L., Hinman, R. S. (2010). Hip strengthening reduces symptoms but not knee load in people with medial knee osteoarthritis and varus malalignment: a randomised controlled trial. *Osteoarthritis and Cartilage/OARS, Osteoarthritis Research Society, 18*(5), 621–8. doi: 10.1016/j.joca.2010.01.010.

Block, J. A., and Shakoor, N. (2010). Lower limb osteoarthritis: biomechanical alterations and implications for therapy. *Curr Opin Rheumatol*, 22, 544–50.

Borjesson, M., Robertson, E., Wiedenhielm, L., Mattsson, E., and Olsson, E. (1996). Physiotherapy in knee osteoarthrosis: effect on pain and walking. *Physiotherapy Research International*, 1(2), 89–97. doi: 10.1002/pri.6120010205.

Brismee, J.-M., Paige, R. L., Chyu, M.-C., Boatright, J. D., Hagar, J. M., McCaleb, J. A., Quintela, M. M., Feng, D., Xu, K. T., and Shen, C. L. (2007). Group and home-based tai chi in elderly subjects with knee osteoarthritis: a randomized controlled trial. *Clin Rehabil*, 21(2), 99–111.

Brosseau, L., Wells, G. A., Tugwell, P., Egan, M., Dubouloz, C. J., Casimiro, L., Bugnariu N., Welch, V. A., De Angelis, G., Francoeur, L., Milne, S., Loew, L., McEwan, J., Messier, S. P., Doucet, E., Kenny, G. P., Prud'homme, D., Lineker, S., Bell, M., Poitras, S., Li, J. X., Finestone, H. M., Laferrière, L., Haines-Wangda, A., Russell-Doreleyers, M., Lambert, K., Marshall, A. D., Cartizzone, M., and Teav, A. (2011). Ottawa Panel evidence-based clinical practice guidelines for the management of osteoarthritis in adults who are obese or overweight. *Physical Therapy*, 91(6), 843–61. doi: 10.2522/ptj.20100104.

Chang, A., Hurwitz, D., Dunlop, D., Song, J., Cahue, S., Hayes, K., and Sharma, L. (2007). The relationship between toe-out angle during gait and progression of medial tibiofemoral osteoarthritis. *Annals of the Rheumatic Diseases*, 66(10), 1271–5. doi: 10.1136/ard.2006. 062927.

Covinsky, K. (2006). Aging, arthritis, and disability. *Arthritis and Rheumatism*, 55(2), 175–6. doi: 10.1002/art.21861.

Covinsky, K. E., Lindquist, K., Dunlop, D. D., Gill, T. M., and Yelin, E. (2008). Effect of arthritis in middle age on older-age functioning. *Journal of the American Geriatrics Society*, 56(1), 23–8. doi: 10.1111/j.1532-5415.2007.01511.x.

Dunlop, D. D., Hughes, S. L., and Manheim, L. M. (1997). Disability in activities of daily living: patterns of change and a hierarchy of disability. *American Journal of Public Health*, 87(3), 378–83.

Dunlop, D. D., Manheim, L. M., Song, J., and Chang, R. W. (2001). Arthritis prevalence and activity limitations in older adults. *Arthritis and Rheumatism*, 44(1), 212–21. doi: 10.1002/1529-0131(200101)44:1<212::AID-ANR28>3.0.CO;2-Q.

Englund, M. (2010). The role of biomechanics in the initiation and progression of OA of the knee. *Best Practice and Research. Clinical Rheumatology*, 24, 39–46.

Escalante, Y., Garcia-Hermoso, A., and Saavedra, J. M. (2011). Effects of exercise on functional aerobic capacity in lower limb osteoarthritis: a systematic review. *Journal of Science and Medicine in Sport/Sports Medicine Australia*, 14(3), 190–8. doi: 10.1016/j. jsams.2010.10.004.

Felson, D. T. (1988). Epidemiology of hip and knee osteoarthritis. *Epidemiol Rev*, 10, 1–28.

Felson, D. T., Lawrence, R. C., Dieppe, P. A., Hirsch, R., Helmick, C. G., Jordan, J. M., Kington, R. S., Lane, N. E., Nevitt, M. C., Zhang, Y., Sowers, M., McAlindon, T., Spector, T. D., Poole, A. R., Yanovski, S. Z., Ateshian, G., Sharma, L., Buckwalter, J. A., Brandt, K. D., and Fries, J. F. (2000). Osteoarthritis: new insights. Part 1: the disease and its risk factors. *Annals of Internal Medicine*, 133(8), 635–46.

Felson, D. T., and Radin, E. L. (1994). What causes knee osteoarthrosis: are different compartments susceptible to different risk factors? *The Journal of Rheumatology*, 21, 181–3.

Fransen, M., McConnell, S., and Bell, M. (2002). Therapeutic exercise for people with osteoarthritis of the hip or knee. A systematic review. *The Journal of Rheumatology*, 29(8), 1737–45.

Fransen, M., Nairn L., Winstanley J., Lam P., and Edmonds J. (2007). The Physical Activity for Osteoarthritis Management (PAFORM) study. A randomised controlled clinical trial evaluating hydro-therapy and Tai Chi classes. *Arthritis Care Res*, 57, 407–14.

Fukubayashi, T., and Kurosawa, H. (1980). The contact area and pressure distribution pattern of the knee. A study of normal and osteoarthrotic knee joints. *Acta Orthopaedica Scandinavica*, 51(6), 871–9.

Guo, M., Axe, M. J., and Manal, K. (2007). The influence of foot progression angle on the knee adduction moment during walking and stair climbing in pain free individuals with knee osteoarthritis. *Gait Posture*, 26(3), 436–41. doi: 10.1016/j.gaitpost.2006.10.008.

Hall, A. C., Urban, J. P., and Gehl, K. A. (1991). The effects of hydrostatic pressure on matrix synthesis in articular cartilage. *Journal of Orthopaedic Research*, 9(1), 1–10. doi: 10.1002/jor.1100090102.

Hamel, K. A., Okita, N., Bus, S. A., and Cavanagh, P. R. (2005). A comparison of foot/ground interaction during stair negotiation and level walking in young and older women. *Ergonomics*, 48, 1047–56.

Huang, M. H., Lin, Y. S., and Lee, C. L. (2003). A comparison of various therapeutic exercises on the functional status of patients with knee osteoarthritis. *Semin Arthritis Rheum*, 32(6), 398–406.

Hurley, M. V., Walsh, N. E., Mitchell, H. L., Pimm, T. J., Patel, A., Williamson, E., Jones, R. H., Dieppe, P. A., and Reeves, B. C. (2007). Clinical effectiveness of a rehabilitation program integrating exercise, self-management, and active coping strategies for chronic knee pain: a cluster randomized trial. *Arthritis and Rheumatism*, 57(7), 1211–19. doi: 10.1002/art.22995.

Hurwitz, D. E., Ryals, A. B., Case, J. P., Block, J. A., and Andriacchi, T. P. (2002). The knee adduction moment during gait in subjects with knee osteoarthritis is more closely correlated with static alignment than radiographic disease severity, toe out angle and pain. *Journal of Orthopaedic Research*, 20, 101–7.

Hurwitz, D. E., Sumner, D. R., Andriacchi, T. P., and Sugar, D. A. (1998). Dynamic knee loads during gait predict proximal tibial bone distribution. *J Biomech*, 31, 423–30.

Jan, M. H., Lin, J. J., Liau, J. J., Lin, Y. F., and Lin, D. H. (2008). Investigation of clinical effects of high- and low-resistance training for patients with knee osteoarthritis: a randomized controlled trial. *Physical Therapy*, 88(4), 427–36. doi: 10.2522/ptj.20060300.

Jansen, M. J., Viechtbauer, W., Lenssen, A. F., Hendriks, E. J., and de Bie, R. A. (2011). Strength training alone, exercise therapy alone, and exercise therapy with passive manual mobilisation each reduce pain and disability in people with knee osteoarthritis: a systematic review. *Journal of Physiotherapy*, 57(1), 11–20. doi: 10.1016/S1836-9553(11)70002-9.

Kakihana, W., Akai, M., Nakazawa, K., Takashima, T., Naito, K., and Torii, S. (2005). Effects of laterally wedged insoles on knee and subtalar joint moments. *Archives of Physical Medicine and Rehabilitation*, 86(7), 1465–71.

Keefe, F. J., Blumenthal, J., Baucom, D., Affleck, G., Waugh, R., Caldwell, D. S., Beaupre, P., Kashikar-Zuck, S., Wright, K., Egert, J., and Lefebvre, J. (2004). Effects of spouse-assisted coping skills training and exercise training in patients with osteoarthritic knee pain: a randomized controlled study. *Pain*. 110(3), 539–49.

Kerrigan, D. C., Lelas, J. L., and Karvosky, M. E. (2001). Women's shoes and knee osteoarthritis. *Lancet*, 357, 1097–8.

Kerrigan, D. C., Todd, M. K., and Riley, P. O. (1998). Knee osteoarthritis and high-heeled shoes. *Lancet*, 351, 1399–1401.

Kirkley, A., Webster-Bogaert, S., Litchfield, R., Amendola, A., MacDonald, S., McCalden, R., and Fowler, P. (1999). The effect of bracing on varus gonarthrosis. *The Journal of Bone and Joint Surgery. American Volume*, 81(4), 539–48.

Kristensen, J., and Franklyn-Miller, A. (2012). Resistance training in musculoskeletal rehabilitation: a systematic review. *British Journal of Sports Medicine*, 46(10), 719–26. doi: 10.1136/bjsm.2010.079376.

Lawrence, J. S., Bremner, J. M., and Bier, F. (1966). Osteo-arthrosis. Prevalence in the population and relationship between symptoms and X-ray changes. *Annals of the Rheumatic Diseases*, 25(1), 1–24.

Lim, B. W., Hinman, R. S., Wrigley, T. V., Sharma, L., and Bennell, K. L. (2008). Does knee malalignment mediate the effects of quadriceps strengthening on knee adduction moment, pain, and function in medial knee osteoarthritis? A randomized controlled trial. *Arthritis and Rheumatism*, 59(7), 943–51. doi: 10.1002/art.23823.

Lopez, H. L. (2012a). Nutritional interventions to prevent and treat osteoarthritis. Part I: focus on fatty acids and macronutrients. *PM R*, 4(5 suppl.), S145–54. doi: 10.1016/j.pmrj.2012.02.022.

Lopez, H. L. (2012b). Nutritional interventions to prevent and treat osteoarthritis. Part II: focus on micronutrients and supportive nutraceuticals. *PM R*, 4(5 suppl.), S155–68. doi: 10.1016/j.pmrj.2012.02.023.

Mallen, C. D., Peat, G., Thomas, E., Lacey, R., and Croft, P. (2007). Predicting poor functional outcome in community-dwelling older adults with knee pain: prognostic value of generic indicators. *Annals of the Rheumatic Diseases*, 66(11), 1456–61. doi: 10.1136/ard.2006.067975.

McDonough, C. M., and Jette, A. M. (2010). The contribution of osteoarthritis to functional limitations and disability. *Clinics in Geriatric Medicine*, 26(3), 387–99. doi: 10.1016/j.cger.2010.04.001.

Messier, S. P., Thompson, C. D., and Ettinger, W. H. (1997). Effects of long term aerobic or weight training regimens on gait in older, osteoarthritic population. *J Appl Biomech*, 13, 205–225.

Miyazaki, T., Wada, M., Kawahara, H., Sato, M., Baba, H., and Shimada, S. (2002). Dynamic load at baseline can predict radiographic disease progression in medial compartment knee osteoarthritis. *Annals of the Rheumatic Diseases*, 61(7), 617–22.

Nagi, S. (1965). Some conceptual issues disability and rehabiliation. In M. Sussman (ed.), *Sociology and Rehabilitation*. American Sociology Association; Washington, DC. pp. 100–13.

Nagi, S. (1979). The concept and measurement of disability. In E. D. Berkowitz (ed.), *Disability Policies and Government Programs*: New York: Praeger.

National Collaborating Centre for Chronic Conditions (UK). (2008). *Osteoarthritis: national clinical guideline for care and management in adults*. London: Royal College of Physicians.

National Institute for Health and Care Excellence (NICE) (2014). Osteoarthritis: care and management in adults. NICE guidelines [CG177], London, UK: NICE.

Nelson, M. E., Rejeski, W. J., Blair, S. N., Duncan, P. W., Judge, J. O., King, A. C., Macera, C. A., and Castaneda-Sceppa, C. (2007). Physical activity and public health in older adults: recommendation from the American College of Sports Medicine and the American Heart Association. *Medicine and Science in Sports and Exercise*, 39(8), 1435–45. doi: DOI 10.1249/mss.0b013e3180616aa2.

Peat, G., Thomas, E., Duncan, R., Wood, L., Hay, E., and Croft, P. (2006). Clinical classification criteria for knee osteoarthritis: performance in the general population and primary care. *Annals of the Rheumatic Diseases*, 65(10), 1363–7. doi: DOI 10.1136/ard.2006.051482.

Penninx, B. W., Beekman, A. T., Honig, A., Deeg, D. J., Schoevers, R. A., van Eijk, J. T., and van Tilburg, W. (2001). Depression and cardiac mortality: results from a community-based longitudinal study. *Arch Gen Psychiatry*, 58(3), 221–7.

Pollo, F. E., Otis, J. C., Backus, S. I., Warren, R. F., and Wickiewicz, T. L. (2002). Reduction of medial compartment loads with valgus bracing of the osteoarthritic knee. *Am J Sports Med*, 30(3), 414–21.

Radin, E. L., Ehrlich, M. G., Chernack, R., Abernethy, P., Paul, I. L., and Rose, R. M. (1978). Effect of repetitive impulsive loading on the knee joints of rabbits. *Clinical Orthopaedics and Related Research* (131), 288–93.

Radin, E. L., Martin, R. B., Burr, D. B., Caterson, B., Boyd, R. D., and Goodwin, C. (1984). Effects of mechanical loading on the tissues of the rabbit knee. *Journal of Orthopaedic Research*, 2(3), 221–34. doi: 10.1002/jor.1100020303.

Reeves, N. D., and Bowling, F. L. (2011). Conservative biomechancial strategies for knee osteo-arthritis. *Nature Reviews Rheumatology*, 7, 113–22.

Reeves, N. D., Spanjaard, M., Mohagheghi, A. A., Baltzopoulos, V., and Maganaris, C. N. (2009). Older adults employ alternative strategies to operate within their maximum capabilities when ascending stairs. *J Electromyogr Kinesiol*, 19, e57–68.

Roddy, E., Zhang, W., and Doherty, M. (2005). Aerobic walking or strengthening exercise for osteoarthritis of the knee? A systematic review. *Annals of the Rheumatic Diseases*, 64(4), 544–8. doi: 10.1136/ard.2004.028746.

Roos, E. M., Bremander, A. B., Englund, M., and Lohmander, L. S. (2008). Change in self-reported outcomes and objective physical function over 7 years in middle-aged subjects with or at high risk of knee osteoarthritis. *Annals of the Rheumatic Diseases*, 67(4), 505–10. doi: 10.1136/ard.2007.074088.

Roos, E. M., and Dahlberg, L. (2005). Positive effects of moderate exercise on glycosaminogly-can content in knee cartilage: a four-month, randomized, controlled trial in patients at risk of osteoarthritis. *Arthritis and Rheumatism*, 52(11), 3507–14. doi: 10.1002/art.21415.

Sasaki, T., and Yasuda, K. (1987). Clinical evaluation of the treatment of osteoarthritic knees using a newly designed wedged insole. *Clin. Orthop. Relat. Res.*, 221, 181–7.

Segal, N. A., Torner, J. C., Felson, D., Niu, J., Sharma, L., Lewis, C. E., and Nevitt, M. (2009). Effect of thigh strength on incident radiographic and symptomatic knee osteoarthritis in a longitudinal cohort. *Arthritis and Rheumatism*, 61(9), 1210–17. doi: 10.1002/art.24541.

Shakoor, N., and Moisio, K. (2004). A biomechanical approach to musculoskeletal disease. *Best Practice and Research. Clinical rheumatology*, 18, 173–86.

Shakoor, N., Sengupta, M., Foucher, K. C., Wimmer, M. A., Fogg, L. F., and Block, J. A. (2010). Effects of common footwear on joint loading in osteoarthritis of the knee. *Arthritis Care Res (Hoboken)*, 62(7), 917–23. doi: 10.1002/acr.20165.

Sharma, L., Cahue, S., Song, J., Hayes, K., Pai, Y. C., and Dunlop, D. (2003). Physical function-ing over three years in knee osteoarthritis: role of psychosocial, local mechanical, and neu-romuscular factors. *Arthritis and Rheumatism*, 48(12), 3359–70. doi: 10.1002/art.11420.

Song, R., Lee, E. O., Lam, P., and Bae, S. C. (2003). Effects of tai chi exercise on pain, balance, muscle strength, and perceived difficulties in physical functioning in older women with osteo-arthritis: a randomized clinical trial. *J Rheumatol*, 30(9), 2039–44.

Tak, E., Staats, P., Van Hespen, A., and Hopman-Rock M. (2005). The effects of an exercise program for older adults with osteoarthritis of the hip. *J Rheumatol*, 32(6), 1106–13.

Thorp, L. E., Sumner, D. R., Block, J. A., Moisio, K. C., Shott, S., and Wimmer, M. A. (2006). Knee joint loading differs in individuals with mild compared with moderate medial knee osteoarthritis. *Arthritis and Rheumatism*, 54(12), 3842–9. doi: 10.1002/art.22247.

Thorp, L. E., Wimmer, M. A., Foucher, K. C., Sumner, D. R., Shakoor, N., and Block, J. A. (2010). The biomechanical effects of focused muscle training on medial knee loads in OA of the knee: a pilot, proof of concept study. *J Musculoskelet Neuronal Interact*, 10(2), 166–73.

Tsai, P. F. (2005). Predictors of distress and depression in elders with arthritic pain. *Journal of Advanced Nursing*, 51(2), 158–65. doi: 10.1111/j.1365-2648.2005.03481.x.

van Dijk, G. M., Dekker, J., Veenhof, C., and van den Ende, C. H. (2006). Course of functional status and pain in osteoarthritis of the hip or knee: a systematic review of the literature. *Arthritis and Rheumatism*, 55(5), 779–85. doi: 10.1002/art.22244.

van Raaij, T. M., Reijman, M., Brouwer, R. W., Bierma-Zeinstra, S. M., and Verhaar, J. A. (2010). Medial knee osteoarthritis treated by insoles or braces: a randomized trial. *Clinical Orthopaedics and Related Research*, 468(7), 1926–32. doi: 10.1007/s11999-010-1274-z.

van Saase, J. L., van Romunde, L. K., Cats, A., Vandenbroucke, J. P., and Valkenburg, H. A. (1989). Epidemiology of osteoarthritis: Zoetermeer survey. Comparison of radiological osteoarthritis in a Dutch population with that in 10 other populations. *Annals of the Rheumatic Diseases*, 48(4), 271–80.

Veenhof, C., Huisman, P. A., Barten, J. A., Takken, T., and Pisters, M. F. (2012). Factors associated with physical activity in patients with osteoarthritis of the hip or knee: a systematic review. *Osteoarthritis and Cartilage/OARS, Osteoarthritis Research Society*, 20(1), 6–12. doi: 10.1016/j.joca.2011.10.006

Verbrugge, L. M., and Jette, A. M. (1994). The disablement process. *Social Science and Medicine*, 38(1), 1–14.

Verbrugge, L. M., Lepkowski, J. M., and Konkol, L. L. (1991). Levels of disability among U.S. adults with arthritis. *Journal of Gerontology*, 46(2), S71–83.

Wade, J. B., Riddle, D. L., Price, D. D., and Dumenci, L. (2011). Role of pain catastrophizing during pain processing in a cohort of patients with chronic and severe arthritic knee pain. *Pain*, 152(2), 314–19. doi: 10.1016/j.pain.2010.10.034.

Yamamoto, N., Fukuda, K., Matsushita, T., Matsukawa, M., Hara, F., and Hamanishi, C. (2005). Cyclic tensile stretch stimulates the release of reactive oxygen species from osteoblast-like cells. *Calcified Tissue International*, 76(6), 433–8. doi: DOI 10.1007/s00223-004-1188-4.

Zhang, W., Moskowitz, R. W., Nuki, G., Abramson, S., Altman, R. D., Arden, N., Bierma-Zeinstra, S., Brandt, K. D., Croft, P., Doherty, M., Dougados, M., Hochberg, M., Hunter, D. J., Kwoh, K., Lohmander, L. S., and Tugwell, P. (2007). OARSI recommendations for the management of hip and knee osteoarthritis, part I: critical appraisal of existing treatment guidelines and systematic review of current research evidence. *Osteoarthritis and Cartilage/OARS, Osteoarthritis Research Society*, 15(9), 981-1000. doi: 10.1016/j.joca.2007.06.014.

Chapter 10

Pre-operative cardiopulmonary exercise testing and prehabilitation

Lisa Loughney, Sandy Jack, and Denny Levett

Introduction

Why is there a need for a pre-operative risk stratification tool?

Recent cohort studies such as the European Surgical Outcomes Study (EuSOS) have highlighted that elective surgery is associated with significant risk. In this audit of 46,539 surgical patients, the reported hospital mortality rate of 3.6 per cent was higher than had previously been estimated (Pearse, 2012). Furthermore, there was wide variability in the mortality rate in different countries, raising the possibility that measures to improve surgical outcome could be implemented. In particular, 73 per cent of the patients who died were not admitted to critical care perioperatively, and emergency critical care admissions were associated with higher mortality than planned admissions. Such data suggest that improved patient selection for critical care may improve outcome. Post-operative morbidity (complications) is more prevalent than mortality and has an important impact on immediate post-operative recovery, as well as having long-term health implications for the patient. Prolonged post-operative morbidity, has been associated with an increased risk of death for up to three years after surgery (Moonesinghe, 2014). Thus, avoiding complications has the potential to confer significant long-term health benefits. In the United Kingdom, retrospective analyses of surgical outcome databases have identified a subgroup of 'high risk' surgical patients with increased perioperative morbidity and mortality who represent approximately 12.3 per cent of the surgical population, but account for 83.4 per cent of the post-operative mortality (Pearse, 2006). If we are to modify the outcome of this high risk group it is essential that they are reliably identified pre-operatively; cardiopulmonary exercise testing (CPET) provides a holistic means of performing this role.

What is the rationale for CPET in the pre-operative setting?

The objective of pre-operative assessment is to estimate the risk relating to surgery. In the past twenty years, a number of case cohort studies have reported an association between functional capacity measured during cardiopulmonary exercise testing and surgical outcome. As a consequence, CPET is increasingly being used preoperatively to identify patients at high risk of perioperative morbidity and mortality. This information can be used to inform operative decisions, the choice of peri- and intra-operative management, and to guide informed consent and shared decision making (Levett and Grocott, 2015a, 2015b; Older et al., 1999).

Why is CPET a good risk assessment tool?

CPET is a good pre-operative risk assessment tool because it provides an objective global assessment of the integrative responses of the pulmonary, cardiovascular, and haematological systems rather than evaluating individual organ systems' function in isolation (American Thoracic Society/American College of Chest Physicians [ATS/ACCP], 2003). This is in contrast to other objective and subjective preoperative assessments. Furthermore, as a dynamic assessment, it provides more insight into the response to physiological stress than a resting test. The perioperative period is a time of physiological stress, as the surgical stress response increases metabolic rate, and, as a consequence, tissue oxygen demand rises. By detecting abnormal exercise capacity, and, consequently, reduced physiological reserve, CPET identifies patients at increased risk of complications and mortality. Furthermore, CPET can be used to detect the cause of exercise limitation and may diagnose unsuspected cardiorespiratory disease.

Cardiopulmonary exercise testing has an established role in the evaluation of perioperative risk in a range of types of surgery. Early work focused on heart transplant and lung resection surgery (Benzo, 2007; Osada, 1998; Ong, 2000). Recently, the majority of studies have focused on major intra-abdominal surgery (Wilson, 2010; Snowden, 2010; Older et al., 1999; Hennis, 2012). Initially, CPET was primarily used to assess 'fitness for surgery', to guide the choice of location for perioperative care (intensive care or general ward), and to identify or evaluate the severity of medical co-morbidity. Recently, the focus has broadened, and CPET is used to guide collaborative decision-making between patients and clinicians (Glance et al., 2014) to evaluate the impact of neo-adjuvant therapies (including chemo- and radio-therapy) and to guide prehabilitation (prehab) programmes.

The physiology and conduct of CPET

CPET is the study of physiological events in exercising subjects, using the simultaneous measurement of respiratory gas exchange and cardiovascular variables to assess exercise capacity. During exercise, the increased demand for adenosine triphosphate (ATP) by exercising muscles requires increased tissue oxygen delivery mediated by an increase in cardiac output and ventilation. Similarly, peri-operatively, the increased ATP demand for metabolic work requires increased tissue oxygen delivery, which must be matched by increased ventilation and cardiac output, if failure of tissue perfusion and oxygenation are to be avoided. CPET assesses the capacity to increase oxygen delivery in order to meet the energy requirements of external work.

CPET integrates expired oxygen and carbon dioxide concentrations with the measurement of ventilatory flow, thus deriving oxygen uptake ($\dot{V}O_2$) and carbon dioxide production ($\dot{V}CO_2$) under conditions of varying physiological stress imposed by a range of defined external workloads. It is usually conducted on an electromagnetically-braked cycle ergometer (or in some cases an arm ergometer) with the patient breathing through a mouthpiece or facemask through which expired gas is sampled. The patient is monitored using a continuous twelve-lead ECG and oxygen saturation, with periodic measurement of blood pressure.

Despite requiring a moderate to high level of exertion, CPET is well-tolerated and safe to conduct (Weisman, 2003). It is performed by laboratory staff trained in laboratory protocols and life support. Immediate access to resuscitation equipment, oxygen and emergency drugs should be available throughout the test and recovery period with rapid access to a team with advanced life support skills (cardiac arrest team) if required.

CPET measured using an arm/cycle ergometer

Two modes of exercise, cycle ergometry and treadmill, are commonly employed in CPET, whilst arm crank ergometry is used occasionally. Cycle ergometry allows accurate determination of the external work rate, and thus evaluation of the $\dot{V}O_2$-work rate relationship, which is difficult with a treadmill (Porszasz et al., 2007). In addition, cycle ergometry requires less skill than a treadmill (performance is less affected by practice), is cheaper, and takes up less space (Porszasz et al., 2007). However, some surgical patients are unable to perform cycle ergometry because of lower limb dysfunction caused by joint arthritis, peripheral vascular disease, neurological disease, or previous amputations. CPET conducted on an arm ergometer can be used as an alternative, as it provides data on physiological responses. To date, CPET using an arm ergometer in a peri-operative setting has mainly focused on the ability to detect ECG changes in patients with coronary artery disease (Hanson et al., 1988). In healthy individuals, the maximum oxygen uptake obtained by an arm ergometer is 50–70 per cent of that measured by a leg ergometer (Davis et al., 1976). However, the same rule does not apply to the patient population. A recent study compared CPET using arm and cycle ergometers in both vascular patients and healthy individuals (Loughney et al., 2014). These data illustrated that although a relationship does exist between $\dot{V}O_2$ values for CPET as conducted by arm and cycle ergometers, this relationship was insufficient for $\dot{V}O_2$ obtained from the cycle ergometer to be accurately predicted using an arm ergometer alone. This does not prohibit the use of CPET-derived variables, ECG changes, or ventilatory limitation in the peri-operative risk stratification of patients with lower limb dysfunction using an arm ergometer. However, further evaluation of the relationship between arm ergometry CPET values and clinical outcome is required.

The CPET protocol

Although a variety of exercise protocols can be used to interrogate different elements of the exercise response, the continuous incremental exercise test (incremental ramp test) to the limit of tolerance (symptom limited) is used most widely to evaluate exercise capacity pre-operatively (Whipp et al., 1981). The incremental exercise test has a number of advantages:

- It evaluates the exercise response across the entire range of exercise capacity.
- The initial work rate is low and the duration of high intensity exercise is short.
- The entire test involves only eight to twelve minutes of exercise.
- It permits assessment of the normalcy or otherwise of the exercise response.
- It allows identification of the site of functional exercise limitation.
- It provides an appropriate frame of reference for training or rehabilitation targets.

The test protocol normally includes four phases: an initial rest phase (approximately three minutes) is employed to establish baseline values, followed by an unloaded cycling minimal workload phase. Following this, the incremental exercise phase begins, during which the set work rate increases linearly, with a corresponding increase in the intensity of the exercise. The ideal duration of the ramp is eight to twelve minutes, and a formula based on age and gender is employed to select the ramp increment to obtain this test duration (Wasserman et al., 2005):

- $\dot{V}O_{2peak}$ unloaded (ml.min^{-1}) = 150 + (6 × weight (kg)
- $\dot{V}O_{2peak}$ (ml.min^{-1}) Men = [height (cm) – age (years)] × 20
- $\dot{V}O_{2peak}$ (ml.min^{-1}) Women = [height (cm) – age (years)] × 14
- Work Rate increment (W/min) = (Peak $\dot{V}O_2$ – $\dot{V}O_2$ unloaded)/100.

The test is terminated by the patient at volitional exhaustion or by symptoms (e.g. shortness of breath, chest pain, etc.). In early perioperative CPET studies, some groups stopped tests above the anaerobic threshold but before symptom limitation because of safety concerns in this previously-unevaluated population (Older et al., 1999; Wilson et al., 2010). Subsequently, safety studies have reported very low mortality rates of approximately two to five per 100,000 in patient populations, including lung and heart transplant candidates and low significant morbidity (Myers et al., 2000; ATS/ACCP, 2003). Consequently, symptom-limited tests are now most commonly employed.

Following test completion, a recovery period of low-intensity exercise is performed to maintain venous return. Patients are observed throughout recovery until physiological variables, including heart rate, blood pressure, ventilation, and oxygen saturation have returned close to baseline levels, and any exercise-induced ECG changes have resolved (Fleisher et al., 2007; Weisman et al., 2003; Palange et al., 2007).

Pre-test assessment and baseline observations

All patients are assessed and consented prior to CPET. A medical history is taken to establish that there are no contraindications to CPET testing and whether any medications taken may interfere with the exercise response, e.g. beta-blockers. Modified test contraindications are based on the ATS and the ACCP Guidelines (Table 10.1).

CPET interpretation

The output from an incremental CPET is, by convention, represented graphically in a 9-panel plot (Figures 10.1 and 10.2 below) (ATS/ACCP, 2003; Porszasz et al., 2007). The key variables and measurements are summarised in Table 10.2. Exercise capacity can be determined, and the causes of exercise limitation are identified as patterns of abnormality in these plots. CPET can both evaluate the severity and physiological impact of known comorbidities and identify unsuspected pathology such as myocardial ischaemia (Belardinelli et al., 2003) and pulmonary hypertension (Held et al. 2014; Guazzi and Arena, 2013; Glaser et al., 2013) in the pre-operative patient.

Peak oxygen consumption ($\dot{V}O_{2peak}$) and the anaerobic threshold (AT) are indices of exercise capacity (functional capacity or physical fitness). These variables are metabolic rates expressed in mls of $\dot{V}O_2$ per minute absolute, indexed to body-weight or as percentages of predicted values. $\dot{V}O_{2peak}$ is defined as the highest oxygen uptake recorded during an incremental exercise test at the point of volitional fatigue or symptom limitation. As such, $\dot{V}O_{2peak}$ includes a volitional element (the patient

Table 10.1 Contraindications to cardiopulmonary exercise testing

Contraindications to cardiopulmonary exercise testing	
Absolute contraindications (Do not test)	Relative contraindications (Discuss with CPET doctor prior to starting test)
Acute myocardial infarction (3–5 days)	Left main coronary stenosis
Unstable angina	Moderate stenotic valvular heart disease
Uncontrolled arrhythmias causing symptoms or haemodynamic compromise	Severe untreated arterial hypertension at rest (systolic > 200mmHg, 120mm Hg diastolic)
Syncope	Tachyarrhythmia or bradyarrhythmia
Active endocarditis	High degree atrioventricular block
Acute myocarditis or pericarditis	Hypertrophic cardiomyopathy
Symptomatic severe aortic stenosis	Significant pulmonary hypertension
Uncontrolled heart failure	Advanced or complicated pregnancy
Acute pulmonary embolus or pulmonary infarction	Electrolyte abnormalities
Thrombosis of lower extremity	Orthopaedic impairment that compromises exercise performance
Suspected dissecting aneurysm	
Uncontrolled asthma	
Pulmonary oedema	
Room air desaturation at rest < 85% if no known lung pathologies	
Respiratory failure	
Acute non-cardiopulmonary disorder that may affect exercise performance	
Mental impairment leading to inability to co-operate	

American Thoracic Society/American College of Chest Physicians, 2003

may not produce a maximal effort). The anaerobic threshold (AT) (also sometimes referred to as the lactate threshold, ventilatory threshold, first gas exchange threshold, or lactic acidosis threshold) characterises the upper limit of exercise intensity that can be accomplished almost wholly aerobically (ATS/ACCP, 2003). Below the AT, exercise can be sustained indefinitely, whereas, above the AT, progressive increases in work rate result in progressive reductions in exercise tolerance (Sullivan et al., 1995). During incremental exercise, the $\dot{V}O_2$ at which there is a transition from a phase of no increase, or only a small increase in arterial [lactate], to a phase of rapidly accelerating increase in arterial [lactate] associated with a progressive metabolic acidosis is defined as the lactate threshold (LaT) (Beaver and Whipp, 1986). This point can be estimated non-invasively by breath-by-breath expired gas analysis during cardiopulmonary exercise testing, and it is then referred to as the anaerobic threshold (AT) (Beaver and Whipp, 1986). The increase in metabolic acidosis at the AT is accompanied by a rise in the pulmonary CO_2 output ($\dot{V}CO_2$) resulting from the buffering of lactate-associated protons by bicarbonate (Wasserman et al., 1990; Wasserman, 1986). This can be identified during incremental exercise testing as a change in the gradient of the $\dot{V}CO_2$-$\dot{V}O_2$ relationship (V-slope method (Beaver and Whipp, 1986) or modified V-slope method (Sue et al., 1988)), typically accompanied by a systematic rise in the

Table 10.2 Measurements and variables collected during CPET

Measurement	Variables	Symbol
External work	Work rate	WR
Exercise capacity	Peak oxygen uptake	$\dot{V}O_{2peak}$
	Anaerobic threshold	AT
Metabolic gas exchange	Oxygen uptake	$\dot{V}O_2$
	Carbon dioxide production	$\dot{V}CO_2$
	Respiratory exchange ratio	RER
Ventilatory	Minute ventilation	$\dot{V}E$
	Tidal volume	$\dot{V}T$
	Respiratory rate	RR
	Breathing reserve	BR
	Maximum voluntary ventilation	MVV
Pulmonary gas exchange	Ventilatory equivalents for	$\dot{V}E/\dot{V}CO_2$
	Ventilatory equivalents for	$\dot{V}E/\dot{V}O_2$
	End tidal oxygen	$PETO_2$
	End tidal CO_2	$PETCO_2$
	Oxygen saturations	SpO_2
Cardiovascular	Heart rate	HR
	Non-invasive blood pressure	NIBP
	Oxygen pulse	$\dot{V}O_2/HR$
	Heart Rate Reserve	HRR
Symptoms	Dyspnoea, fatigue, chest pain, leg pain	

ventilatory equivalent for oxygen ($\dot{V}E/\dot{V}O_2$) and in end-tidal PO_2 ($PETO_2$) without a concomitant decrease in end-tidal PCO_2 ($PETCO_2$) (Whipp et al., 1986). Several investigators have demonstrated that these indirect approaches provide a valid estimate of the LaT, both in healthy volunteers and in patients with cardiac disease and COPD (Simonton et al., 1988; Matsumura et al., 1983, Dickstein et al., 1990; Patessio et al., 1993). The AT is independent of patient effort. Some controversy remains surrounding the physiological basis for deriving the AT (Hopker et al., 2011); however, it can be reliably identified; the inter-observer variability for experienced clinicians is acceptable (Sinclair et al., 2009); and it has been reliably associated with surgical outcome (Levett and Grocott, 2015b, 2015a).

The ($\dot{V}E/\dot{V}O2$) and ventilatory equivalents for CO_2 ($\dot{V}E/\dot{V}CO_2$) are related to the dead space fraction (deadspace [V_D]/ tidal volume [V_T]) and increase as dead space increases (although they also increase with hyperventilation). Abnormally high ventilatory equivalents are thus evident in any pathological condition with increased dead space – for example COPD, pulmonary fibrosis, heart failure, and pulmonary embolic disease.

The AT and $\dot{V}E/\dot{V}O_{2peak}$ have been consistently associated with both post-operative morbidity and mortality in a variety of general surgical patient groups (Levett and Grocott, 2015a). The relationship between ventilatory equivalents for CO_2 and outcome is less consistent, but, in several case series, high ventilatory equivalents have been associated with a poor outcome. Consequently, these three variables are most commonly used to stratify risk for non-cardiopulmonary surgery.

A systematic approach to test interpretation is important. Firstly, test quality should be evaluated, checking for appropriate calibration (RER > 0.7 at rest) and identifying pre-test hyperventilation (RER > 1 at rest), which can interfere with interpretation of the anaerobic threshold causing a pseudothreshold (Whipp, 2007). Exercise capacity is then evaluated from the $\dot{V}O_{2peak}$ and AT. If abnormal exercise capacity is identified, patterns of abnormality in the other plots may identify possible limiting factors. Table 10.3 provides a reference for suggestive limitations that may be identified using CPET.

Other factors that have an impact on CPET interpretation include obesity, anaemia, chemotherapy, and radiotherapy for cancer and beta-blockers. In obesity, the increased body mass increases the $\dot{V}O_2$ and $\dot{V}CO_2$ for a given external work rate, increasing the metabolic work load, which increases the work of breathing. In some individuals a pattern of ventilatory limitation may be observed (Wasserman et al., 2012). Anaemia is associated with reduced arterial oxygen content and early onset of metabolic acidosis during exercise, and, consequently, a reduced anaerobic threshold (Wasserman et al., 2012). Beta-blockers are medications used extensively in cardiovascular clinical practice to treat ischaemic heart disease and left ventricular dysfunction. Their effects perioperatively have been a source of controversy, since by limiting heart rate, they may limit maximum cardiac output, and thus peak oxygen delivery, but, conversely, may avoid myocardial ischaemia. A recent study investigating the effects of acute beta blockade in vascular surgical patients (who have very high incidence of ischaemic heart disease), reported no significant change in the anaerobic threshold or $\dot{V}O_{2peak}$ after the acute introduction or withdrawal of beta-blockade, although peak work rate and oxygen pulse increased when beta-blockers were introduced. Conversely, chronic beta-blockade was associated with a lower $\dot{V}O_{2peak}$ (West et al., 2015). Finally, cancer therapies (chemotherapy and radiotherapy) are associated with a decrease in exercise capacity ($\dot{V}O_{2peak}$ and anaerobic threshold), which is greater in those receiving surgery and radiotherapy in combination with chemotherapy, compared to those who receive

Table 10.3 Suggestive limitations to exercise as identified by CPET

Suggestive Limitation	Reference
Aerobic fitness - deconditioning	• Reduced Anaerobic Threshold • Reduced $\dot{V}O_{2peak}$
Cardiovascular	• Reduced anaerobic threshold and $\dot{V}O_{2peak}$ • Flattened oxygen pulse • $\dot{V}O_2$/WR slope decreased gradient or flattened • ECG evidence of ischaemia with > 2mm flat or downsloping ST depression
Respiratory	• Reduced $\dot{V}O_{2peak}$ • Reduced or absent anaerobic threshold • Reduced breathing/ventilatory reserve at $\dot{V}O_{2peak}$ • Increased ventilatory equivalents for $\dot{V}E/\dot{V}CO_2$ and $\dot{V}E/\dot{V}CO_2$ at the anaerobic threshold • Increased heart rate reserve at $\dot{V}O_{2peak}$

Wasserman et al. 2005

radiotherapy alone or surgery alone (Moros et al., 2010). Jack and colleagues have shown that the insult of cancer therapy and surgery in patients with both lower- and upper-gastrointestinal cancers is associated with poor surgical outcome (West et al., 2014a; Jack et al., 2014). The reduction in anaerobic threshold associated with cancer therapies can potentially shift patients from a low-risk group into the high-risk category for major surgery. Thus, CPET reporting requires careful review of the patient history.

CPET case studies

Two case studies are presented below including a healthy volunteer and a patient CPET.

CPET case 1: healthy volunteer

Exercise protocol

The volunteer performed exercise on a cycle ergometer. He pedalled at sixty revolutions per minute (rpm) without added load for three minutes, after which work rate was increased by thirty watts per minute. He stopped exercise due to leg fatigue.

Results

The CPET was formally reported by a physiologist and a consultant. The anaerobic threshold was identified using the three point confirmation described above: the V-slope method, the ventilatory equivalents for oxygen, and the end tidal oxygen (illustrated in Figure 10.1).

Panel 1 illustrates the V-Slope method of anaerobic threshold determination – at the anaerobic threshold the gradient of the $\dot{V}O_2$-$\dot{V}CO_2$ relationship increases above one. The AT is confirmed by evaluation of the ventilatory response to the excess CO_2 in panel 4 –$\dot{V}E/\dot{V}CO_2$ panel 7 – end tidal oxygen, and panel 9 – ventilatory equivalents against workload. The breakpoint marked by the red vertical line is the anaerobic threshold (See Table 10.5 for variable identification).

CPET report

- Excellent $\dot{V}O_{2peak}$, greater than predicted for age and gender; peak workload achieved 309 watts.
- No evidence of cardiovascular or ventilatory limitation to exercise.

Table 10.4 Healthy individual characteristics

Patient characteristics	
Gender	Male
Age	37 years
Height	1.90 m
Weight	85 kg
BMI	23.5 kg·m²
Previous medical history	Nil of note

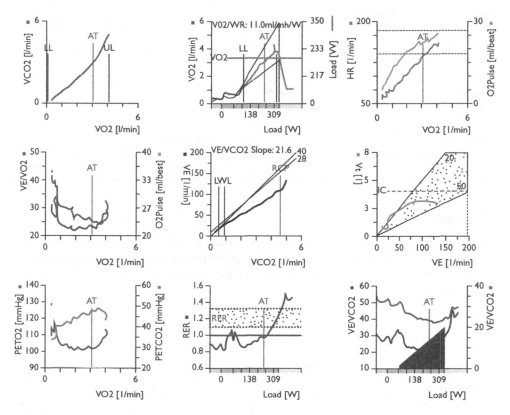

Figure 10.1 9 panel plot.

CPET case 2: pre-operative patient

Exercise protocol

The patient performed exercise on a cycle ergometer. She pedalled at sixty rpm without added load for three minutes, after which work rate was increased by 10 watts per minute. She stopped exercise because of leg fatigue.

Table 10.5 CPET variables from Test 1

CPET variables	
Anaerobic threshold (mL·kg⁻¹·min⁻¹)	36.4
Anaerobic threshold (mL·min⁻¹)	3090
$\dot{V}O_{2peak}$ (mL·min⁻¹)	48.2
$\dot{V}O_{2peak}$ (mL·min⁻¹)	4100
$\dot{V}E/\dot{V}CO_2$ (at anaerobic threshold (mL·kg⁻¹·min⁻¹)	21.6

Table 10.6 Patient characteristics

Patient characteristics	
Gender	Female
Age	77 years
Height	1.58 m
Weight	55 kg
BMI	22 kg · m^2
Reason for referral	Laparoscopic liver resection
Previous medical history	Upper lobectomy, laparoscopic right hemicolectomy
	(Recent adjuvant chemotherapy treatment × 4 cycles)

CPET results

The CPET was formally reported by a physiologist and a consultant. The anaerobic threshold was identified using the three point confirmation described above: the V-slope method, the ventilatory equivalents for oxygen, and the end tidal oxygen (illustrated in Figure 10.2).

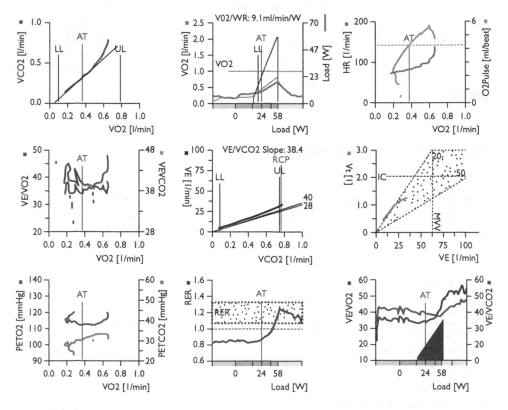

Figure 10.2 9 panel plot.

Table 10.7 CPET variables

CPET variables	
Anaerobic threshold ($mL \cdot kg^{-1} \cdot min^{-1}$)	6.7
Anaerobic threshold ($mL \cdot min^{-1}$)	370
$\dot{V}O_{2peak}$ ($mL \cdot kg^{-1} \cdot min^{-1}$)	12
$\dot{V}O_{2peak}$ ($mL \cdot min^{-1}$)	660
$\dot{V}E/\dot{V}CO_2$ at anaerobic threshold ($mL \cdot kg^{-1} \cdot min^{-1}$)	39.7

Panel 1 illustrates the V-Slope method of anaerobic threshold determination – at the anaerobic threshold the gradient of the $\dot{V}O_2$-$\dot{V}CO_2$ relationship increases above one. The AT is confirmed by evaluation of the ventilatory response to the excess CO_2 in panels 4, 7, and 9. The breakpoint marked by the vertical line is the anaerobic threshold. (See Table 10.7 for variable identification.)

CPET report

• Severely impaired exercise capacity.
• The increased $\dot{V}E/\dot{V}CO_2$ indicates increased dead space, which may reflect inefficient gas exchange, although no mechanical ventilatory limitation was identified.

The reduced anaerobic threshold and $\dot{V}O_{2peak}$, and increased ventilatory equivalents ($\dot{V}E/\dot{V}O_2$ and $\dot{V}E/\dot{V}CO_2$) put the patient at increased risk of postoperative morbidity and mortality. The overall findings may reflect the debilitating effects of chemotherapy and the deconditioning effects of two previous major surgeries this year. Risk category: very high.

Evidence supporting pre-operative CPET

CPET-derived variables must be associated with post-operative outcome if CPET is to have utility as a pre-operative risk stratification tool. Although CPET had been used for risk stratification in cardiothoracic patients, Older and colleagues in Australia were the first group to publish research that used CPET for pre-operative assessment in general surgery during the early 1990s. In a cohort study of 184 patients undergoing major elective abdominal surgery, they reported that a lower AT was associated with increased post-operative mortality (Older et al., 1993). Hospital mortality was less than 1 per cent in patients with an AT above 11 $mL \cdot kg^{-1} \cdot min^{-1}$, 18 per cent in patients with an AT below 11 $mL \cdot kg^{-1} \cdot min^{-1}$, and 50 per cent in patients with an AT below 8 $mL \cdot kg^{-1} \cdot min^{-1}$. Subsequently, more than twenty studies of preoperative CPET in patients having major intra-abdominal surgery have been reported (see Table 10.8 for detailed analysis). This data has been synthesised in several systematic reviews that demonstrate a remarkably consistent relationship between physical fitness, defined using CPET-derived variables, and postoperative outcome (Hennis et al., 2011; West et al., 2011). In the majority of studies, both AT and $\dot{V}O_{2peak}$ were associated with outcome, although this association was statistically stronger for the AT in most cases (Table 10.8). Abnormal ventilatory equivalents for carbon dioxide reflecting increased dead space were also associated with both mortality and morbidity in some case series (Carlisle and Swart, 2007, Wilson et al., 2010, Junejo et al., 2012), but not in others (Snowden et al., 2010, McCullough et al., 2006).

The AT threshold of 11 $mL \cdot kg^{-1} \cdot min^{-1}$ to identify high-risk patients initially proposed by Older to identify high risk patients was based on criteria used for the diagnosis of heart failure. Subsequently, the area under the receiver operating curve analysis has been used in a number of case series to identify predictive cut-off points for discriminating between low–risk, moderate-risk, and high-risk patient groups. As is evident from Table 10.8, more recent case series in general have reported a lower AT threshold in the region of 9–10 $mL \cdot kg^{-1} \cdot min^{-1}$. This may reflect different patient populations, changes in surgical technique with greater laparoscopic surgery (and a reduced surgical stress response), or improvements in perioperative care with more critical care provision. It may be that some types of surgery present a greater physiological challenge (for example, open Whipples procedure compared with laparoscopic colectomy) – or that the process of care is different for different sub-specialties. For example, in the United Kingdom some populations are routinely admitted to a critical

Table 10.8 Overview of preoperative CPET studies

Author, year	Patients	n	Design	AT Threshold	$\dot{V}O_2$ Peak	$\dot{V}E/ \dot{V}CO_2$	Outcome
(Older et al., 1993)	MIA	187	NR	< 11	NR	Y	CV Mortality
(Nagamatsu et al., 1994)	Upper GI	52	NR	NR	Y	NR	CP comp
(Nugent et al., 1998)	AAA	30	Pros.	NR	< 20	NR	Mortality
(Older, 1999)	MIA (> 60 years)	548	N/B Pros.	< 11	NR	NR	Mortality
(Nagamatsu, 2001)	Upper GI	91	N/B. Pros.	Y	Y	NR	CP Comps
(Epstein et al., 2004)	Hepatic transplant	59	N/B Pros	Y	Y	NR	Mortality
(McCullough, 2006)	Bariatric	109	Blinded Observ.	Y	< 15.6	NR	Composite
(Carlisle and Swart, 2007)	AAA	130	Observ.	Y	Y	> 42	Mortality
(Forshaw et al., 2008)	Upper GI	78	N/B Observ.	Y	Y	NR	CP comps
(Wilson, 2010)	MIA	847	N/B. Retrosp.	< 10.9	NR	> 34	Mortality
(Snowden, 2010)	MIA (incl. HPB)	116	Blinded Comp.	< 10.1	Y	Y	POMS (Day 7)
(Hightower et al.,2010)	MIA	32	Blinded Pilot	-	Y	Y	Morbidity

(Hennis, 2012)	Bariatric	106	N/B Prosp. (Single centre)	< 11	Y	Y		Morbidity and POMS
(Prentis et al., 2012a)	Urology radical cystectomy	82	Blinded (Single centre)	< 12	Y	NR		Morbidity and LOS
(Hartley et al., 2012)	AAA	415	N/B Prosp. Pilot (2centre)	< 10.2	< 15	Y		Mortality 30 and 90 day
(Prentis et al., 2012b)	AAA	185	Blinded Prosp. (Single centre)	< 10	Y	NR		LOS and morbidity
(Junejo, 2012)	Hepatic resection (> 65 years/ comorb.	131	N/B Prosp. (Single centre)	Y	Y	> 34.5		Mortality and morbidity
(Chandrabalan et al., 2013)	Pancreatic	100	N/B, retrosp. (Single centre)	< 10	NS	NS		LOS, post-operative adverse events
(Prentis, 2012a)	Liver transplant	165	Blinded Observ.	< 9	Y	Y		Mortality, Critical care LOS
(Ausania et al., 2012)	Pancreas	124	Blinded Prosp.	< 10.1	Y	Y		Pancreatic leak, morbidity, LOS
(Snowden, 2013)	HPB	389	Blinded Prosp.	Y	Y	Y		Mortality and LOS
(West, 2014a)	Colonic Ca	136	Blinded Observ.	< 10.1	< 16.7	Y		POMS (Day 5) and Morbidity
(Goodyear et al., 2013)	AAA	230	N/B Retrosp. Control	< 11	NR	NR		Mortality, LOS, Cost
(West, 2014b)	Rectal	105	Blinded Observ.	< 10.6	< 18.6	NR		POMS (Day 5) and Morbidity
(Dunne et al., 2014)	Liver	197	N/B Observ.	NS	NS	NS		Comps, LOS
(Brunelli et al., 2014)	Lung (NSCLC)	157	Observ.	NR	60%	NR		Survival

Abbreviations: AT: anaerobic threshold (measured in $mL \cdot kg^{-1} \cdot min^{-1}$), $\dot{V}O_{2peak}$: oxygen consumption at peak exercise (measured in $mL \cdot kg^{-1} \cdot min^{-1}$), $\dot{V}_E/\dot{V}CO_2$: ventilatory equivalents ventilation/volume of carbon dioxide, MIA: major intra-abdominal, NR: not reported, Y: yes, CV: cardiovascular, GI: gastro intestinal surgical patients, CP: Cardiopulmonary, Comp: complications, AAA: abdominal aortic aneurysm, Pros.: prospective, N/B.: not blinded, Observ: observation, Retrosp.: retrospective, POMS: post operative mortality score, HPB: hepatobiliary, LOS: length of stay, Comorb.: comorbidity, NS: not significant, NSCLC: non small cell lung cancer.

care environment post-operatively (eg. oesophagectomy, liver resection), whereas others are routinely cared for on general wards (eg. colorectal surgery). Thus, perioperative care in a critical care environment may compensate for a reduced physiological reserve. Further studies are required to explore this variability. Table 10.8 provides an overview of CPET-derived variables and thresholds associated with predicting outcome in different surgical patient groups.

The strength of the association between AT and postoperative morbidity and mortality may be underestimated in many of these case series because clinicians were not blinded to the CPET results and used them to make clinical decisions. A high-risk test would be likely to result in the institution of management to reduce risk, such as changing the choice of surgical procedure, electively admitting the patient to critical care or optimising comorbidities pre-operatively. The effect of this confounding by indication would be to dilute the strength of the association between risk and outcome (Grocott and Pearse, 2010).

CPET has also been used to guide clinicians' decision making when deciding on the appropriate choice of operative procedure and perioperative care environment. Patients defined as high-risk for adverse outcome may be scheduled for less physiologically challenging procedures or for non-surgical management. More commonly, CPET data has been used to guide the choice of postoperative care, with less-fit patients being allocated to a critical care environment post-operatively. Older and colleagues used CPET-derived variables (AT, ventilatory equivalents for oxygen, myocardial ischaemia), along with magnitude of surgery, to allocate patients to intensive care, high-dependency care, and ward care (Older et al., 1999). There was no cardiovascular mortality in the patients allocated to ward care and the mortality rates in critical care were lower than historical control data from the same institution. This study is limited by the non-randomised design and historical control data, and, consequently, does not meet the criteria for the demonstration of a causal link between the intervention (postoperative care allocated by CPET-derived variables) and outcome (mortality), but merits further investigation. Subsequently, a case-controlled study of outcome in colorectal patients with an AT of less than 11 mL·kg^{-1}·min^{-1} who were randomly assigned to either ward care or critical care, reported increased cardiac events in those allocated to the ward again, suggesting that intervening on the basis of AT may improve outcomes (Swart and Carlisle, 2012). Further studies exploring the impact of CPET-guided direction of post-operative care on outcome are needed, but the difficulty of evaluating such a complex intervention has so far limited the available data. An alternative perspective on CPET is that it can identify low-risk patients who are safe to triage to the general ward post-operatively and should have high chance of following an enhanced recovery-type pathway without deviation. CPET can thus be used to target resources to those patients whose need is greatest, which is vital in a resource constrained health care environment.

Prehabilitation

Prehabilitation is defined as 'the process of enhancing the functional capacity of the individual to enable him or her to withstand a stressful event' (Ditmyer, 2002). CPET risk stratification can also be used to identify patients who may benefit from pre-operative exercise training to increase fitness and thereby improve outcome – prehabilitation.

Preliminary data has confirmed the feasibility of this approach in colo-rectal cancer patients and has produced encouraging pilot data (West, 2014b). The advent of neoadjuvant therapies has opened up a time window to train patients prior to major cancer operations, where previously the pressure of reducing the time between diagnosis and surgery precluded such an intervention. This is a relatively new area of research, and the evidence base is currently limited. However, it is of note that there are currently more than twenty ongoing clinical trials evaluating exercise-training programmes in surgical patients registered with the clinical trials database. Improved understanding of the optimal duration, pattern, intensity, and qualities of such interventions will be needed to maximise efficacy, and should be forthcoming in the near future. Major surgery is also associated with unanticipated fear, anxiety, and psychological stresses. In addition to its effects on exercise capacity, a six-week prehabilitation exercise programme, supervised in-hospital, has been shown to promote positive changes in rectal cancer patient's behaviours and helped them view their lives in a way that was fuller, richer, and more meaningful (Burke et al., 2013). The currently-available evidence supporting prehabilitation in surgical patients is reviewed below.

Abdominal aortic aneurysm surgery

Physical fitness levels in abdominal aortic aneurysm (AAA) patients are poor as a consequence of co-morbid disease processes, sedentary lifestyle, and age. Morbidity and mortality after surgery for vascular disease are generally high (Sukhija et al.; 2004, Aronow and Ahn, 1994). The endovascular aneurysm repair (EVAR 2) and the National Quality Improvement Programme strongly advocate the optimisation of preoperative-patient fitness with the aim of improving overall outcomes. Kothmann and colleagues studied the effects of a short-term exercise programme in AAA patients awaiting surgical repair (n = 20 exercise group [EG] and n = 10 control group [CG]) (Kothmann et al., 2009). This pilot study illustrated that physical fitness increased by 10 per cent in the EG compared to the CG (p = 0.007). Myers and colleagues combined aerobic endurance and resistance training protocol in a randomised controlled trial (RCT) of AAA patients (n = 108 recruited, n = 57 follow-up data) (Myers et al., 2010). At one year the increased exercise capacity was maintained in the intervention group. More recently, Tew and colleagues demonstrated a significant increase in the anaerobic threshold in the EG following a twelve-week exercise programme in patients with small AAA disease (n = 14 EG and n = 14 CG) (Tew et al., 2012). Barakat and colleagues further support the idea that preoperative exercise training in AAA repair patients is beneficial, illustrating a significant improvement of 1.4 mL·kg^{-1}·min^{-1} following their exercise programme (Barakat et al., 2014). This group suggested more intense sessions may be beneficial, which merits further investigation. All studies agree that moderate aerobic exercise training is feasible in this patient group.

Colorectal surgery

Kim and colleagues undertook a pilot study in colorectal cancer patients awaiting surgery to assess the feasibility of a four-week progressive aerobic exercise training programme (n = 14 EG, n = 7 CG) (Kim et al., 2009). This programme was home-based and reported no change in $\dot{V}O_{2peak}$ in the EG, even with a 74 per cent adherence rate. Carli and colleagues compared the extent to which an in-hospital bike and strengthening programme (EG; n = 58) optimised recovery of functional walking capacity following surgery, compared to a home-based walking and breathing programme (CG; n = 54) (Carli et al., 2010). This study found no difference between the two programmes on functional walking capacity as measured by a 6-minute walk distance (6MWD) test. However, overall, a greater proportion of patients in the light walking and breathing exercise group had a clinical improvement in walking capacity. This group then investigated the effect of a prehabilitation programme on exercise capacity (as measured by 6MWD) (Mayo et al., 2011). They reported that, following the prehabilitation programme, 33 per cent of subjects improved their physical function, 38 per cent remained within twenty metres of their baseline score, and 29 per cent deteriorated. In the post-operative phase, the patients who had improved with training pre-operatively were also more likely to have recovered to their baseline walking capacity (77 per cent vs. 59 per cent and 32 per cent; p= 0.0007). In contrast, patients who deteriorated during prehabilitation were at greater risk of complications requiring re-operation and/or intensive care management. In 2013, Li and colleagues initiated a tri-modal prehabilitation intervention in colorectal cancer patients, which incorporated an exercise programme, nutritional counselling, protein supplementation, and anxiety reduction (n = 42 EG and n = 45 CG) (Li et al., 2013). This four-week programme improved functional walking capacity and was associated with better postoperative recovery. Recently, West and colleagues have shown that implementing a six-week in-hospital exercise intervention immediately post neoadjuvant chemoradiotherapy prior to surgery is safe and feasible in locally advanced rectal cancer patients (West et al., 2014b). This exercise programme consisted of interval training on a cycle ergometer, and exercise training intensities were responsive to each individual CPET at week zero and week three (informed and altered according to measured work rates according to variables associated with the AT and $\dot{V}O_{2peak}$). The interval-training programme consisted of alternating moderate (80 per cent of work rate at AT) and severe (50 per cent of difference between the work rate at AT and $\dot{V}O_{2peak}$) exercise intensities. They reported a clinically-significant increase in the anaerobic threshold in the exercise group, compared to the non-exercise control group, suggesting that a six-week exercise intervention can reverse the deleterious effects of neo-adjuvant chemoradiotherapy. This group are currently investigating a similar nine-week exercise programme in a prospective randomised controlled trial (ClinicalTrials, 2013).

Lung resection surgery

Complications following lung resection are significant and depend on the patient's cardiopulmonary reserves, existing comorbidities, and the extent of the surgery. Approximately two in three males and one in two females with newly-diagnosed lung cancer suffer from COPD (Loganathan et al., 2006). Previous studies have suggested that preoperative rehabilitation may reduce pulmonary complications and length of hospital stay, but this is controversial (Benzo et al., 2011). Jones and colleagues were the first to exercise non-small cell lung cancer (NSCLC) patients undergoing surgical resection (Jones et al., 2007). NSCLC patients (n = 20) exercised for five consecutive days per week for four to six weeks prior to surgery. This programme was progressive and individually tailored over the four- to six-week period, and resulted in an increase of 2.4 mL·kg^{-1}·min^{-1} in $\dot{V}O_{2peak}$ and 40m in 6MWD. Furthermore, when only considering those who adhered to the programme, > 80 per cent of such patients achieved an increase of 3.3 mL·kg^{-1}·min^{-1} in $\dot{V}O_{2peak}$ and 49m in 6MWD. Although exercise capacity decreased post-surgery, it did not fall below the pre-exercise training baseline values. Bobbio and colleagues investigated the effect of a four-week prehabilitation programme on pulmonary function and exercise performance in COPD patients undergoing lung resection for NSCLC (n = 12) (Bobbio et al., 2008). They reported a significant increase in anaerobic threshold, $\dot{V}O_{2peak}$ and O_2 pulse. Similarly, Mujovic and colleagues undertook a two- to four-week prehabilitation pulmonary rehabilitation programme in NSCLC patients with COPD (Mujovic et al., 2014). They reported that the proportional improvement in FEV_1 and 6MWD was greatest in those with the worst initial respiratory function and functional capacity, who carry the highest surgical risk. This suggests that the benefits of prehabilitation may be greatest in the patient group at most need. Another important effect of prehabilitation may be to increase the number of patients who are fit enough to tolerate chemotherapy post-operatively. Adjuvant chemotherapy is now considered standard care after surgical lung resection in lung cancer. However, previous trials have reported that 5–24 per cent of patients received no chemotherapy, and only 57–69 per cent completed planned therapy (Alam et al., 2005). Prehabilitation may thus play a crucial role in preparing patients for the 'multiple hit' of surgery and the adjuvant cancer treatment. Table 10.9 below provides a brief overview of the prehabilitation literature.

Prehabilitation summary

Overall, exercise training for surgical patients appears to be safe and feasible. However, identifying which patients will benefit most from training requires further clarification. Other areas for investigation are the optimal frequency, intensity, duration, and type of training. Furthermore, whether training at home is as effective as supervised training in hospital needs to be established. Although home programmes may be cheaper and more convenient for the patient, to date, the evidence suggests that they may not be as effective. Overall, the early data is encouraging – significant improvements in physical fitness can be achieved in a short period of time, implying that prehabilitation could be readily integrated into the surgical patient pathway without delaying surgery.

Future research

Future research studies should focus on the following:

- Randomised controlled trials using CPET-derived risk stratification to direct perioperative care and thus improve surgical outcome;
- Randomised controlled trials to establish the relationship between exercise training and improved exercise capacity and surgical outcome;
- 'Dose-response' exercise intervention studies to identify the minimum duration of training required to produce an improvement in surgical outcome;

Table 10.9 Overview of prehabilitation studies

Author, year	Surgery (n=)	Study design	Exercise programme	Location	Frequency	Intensity	Exercise mode	Duration	Adherence	Primary outcome
(Asoh and Tsuji, 1981)	Gastrointestinal (29)	Observ.	Aerobic continuous	In-hospital	2 times/day × 1-3 weeks	Individual (HR < 130bpm)	Cycle/Treadmill	20min	NR	*PPC's
(Debigaré et al., 1999)	Lung (23)	Observ.	Aerobic continuous, strength	Home-based	5/week × 10-12 weeks	≥ 50% VO_2 peak	Walking	15-45min	97%	*6MWD
(Arthur et al., 2000)	CABG (246)	RCT	Aerobic interval	In-hospital	2 times × 8 weeks	40-70% functional capacity	Cycle/arm/treadmill/stair climb	90 min	(mean 14 classes)	*LOS; (IG) V's (CG)-6 V's 7 days
(Hulzebos et al., 2006)	CABG (279)	RCT	IMT	Home-based (6day/week) In-hospital (1day/week)	Daily × 2 weeks	Prog. PImax	IMT loading device	20min	NR	*PPC's
(Jones, 2007)	Lung (25)	Pilot, single arm, prospective	Aerobic	In-hospital	5 days/week ×	Prog; 60-65% VO_2 peak	Cycle ergometer	Prog; 20-30min	72%	*VO_{2peak}
(Bobbio et al., 2008)	Lung resection (12)	Pilot, Observ.	Aerobic continuous, IMT, Stretching	Home-based	IMT; 2/day Aerobic; 5/ days/week × 4 weeks	40-65% HRR and RPE	Portable Cycle ergometer	90min	NR	*VO_{2max}
(Kothmann, 2009)	AAA (30)	Pilot, RCT	Continuous aerobic	In-hospital	2/week × 6 weeks	Moderate;RPE (6-20), BORG (12-14)	Cycle	30min	NR	*VO_2 at LT
(Kim, 2009)	Colorectal (21)	RCT, Pilot	Aerobic continuous	Home-based	5 times × 4 weeks	40-65% HRR& RPE	Cycle	20-30	74%	*Various responsive measures of CV fitness

Study	Cancer (n)	Design	Intervention	Setting	Frequency	Intensity	Mode	Duration	Adherence	Outcome
(Carli, 2010)	Colorectal (112)	RIT	Bike + strength programme/ walking + breathing programme	Home-based (1 weekly visit)	Daily × 7–8 weeks	Bike + strength; Prog; 50% HR max	Cycle/ Walking	20–45 min	16%	6MWD
(Dronkers et al, 2010)	Gastrointestinal (42)	RIT	Aerobic continuous/ strength /breathing	In-hospital (+ home) V's Home-based	2 times/day × 2–4 weeks	Aerobic varied on HR max; BORG, IMT; prog.	Cycle/ Walking/ IMT device	60min	In-hospital ~97%. Home-NR	*Feasibility/ measure of functional capacity
(Timmerman et al., 2011)	Abdominal/ thoracic (15)	Observ, Pilot	Aerobic continuous/ strength	Supervised	2/week × 5 weeks	Aerobic; 65–85% HRR Strength; 60–80% 1-RM	Cycle/ Cross-trainer/ Treadmill	120min	84%	*Feasibility *Cardio. Fitness *Muscle strength
(Rao et al., 2012)	Breast (10)	Pilot, RCT	Boot camp programme	Home-based	3/week × 4–6 months	NR	Varied (Circuit type)	60min	> 80%	*Feasibility
(Tew, 2012)	AAA (28)	Pilot, RCT	Endurance	Supervised, exercise suite	3/week × 12 weeks	Moderate; RPE (12–14)	Treadmill walking/ cycle	35–45min	94%	*Feasibility
(Coats et al., 2013)	Lung (16)	Non-R, Interv.	Aerobic, strength	Home-based	3–5/week × 4 weeks	60–80% peak workload	Walking/ Cycle	30–45min	81%	*Feasibility

(continued)

Table 10.9 (continued)

Author, year	Surgery (n=)	Study design	Exercise programme	Location	Frequency	Intensity	Exercise mode	Duration	Adherence	Primary outcome
(Barakat, 2014)	AAA repair (20)	RCT, Pilot	Aerobic	In-hospital	3/week × 6 weeks	NR	Mixed (circuit type)	60min	70–100%	*$\dot{V}O_2$ at AT, *$\dot{V}O_{2peak}$
(Mujovic, 2014)	COPD with NSCLC (83)	Prosp, Observ.	Pulmonary	In-hospital	3 daily × 5 days/week × 2–4 weeks	Prog.	Aerosol therapy/ elastic bands	45min	NR	*Lung function, *6MWD
(West, 2014)	Rectal (39)	Rand.	Aerobic Interval	In-hospital	3/week × 6 weeks	Prog. (Moderate-severe)	Cycle	40min	96%	*$\dot{V}O_2$ at LT

List of abbreviations: *: significant ($p < 0.05$), NR: not reported, IG: intervention group, CG: control group, NR: reported, Observ.: observational, Prosp.: prospective, Prog.: progressive, retrosp.: retrospective, CV: cardiovascular, HR: heart rate, BPM: beats per minute, QoL: quality of life, IMT: inspiratory muscle training, RCT: randomised control trial, Non-R: non-randomised, Rand: randomised, RIT: randomised intervention trial comparing intervention with sham intervention, LOS: length of stay, CABG: coronary artery bypass surgery, PImax: maximal inspiratory mouth pressure, PPC: pulmonary postoperative complications, HR max: maximum heart rate, RPE: rating of perceived exertion, 6MWD: 6 minute walk distance, 1RM:1 repetition maximum, HRR: heart rate reserve, cardio.: cardiorespiratory, COPD: chronic obstructive pulmonary disease, NSCLC: non small cell lung cancer, AT: anaerobic threshold, LT: lactate threshold, $\dot{V}O_{2max}$: oxygen consumption at maximal exercise, $\dot{V}O_{2peak}$: oxygen consumption at peak exercise.

- Studies to identify the characteristics of patients who respond well and poorly to exercise interventions, and thus identify which patients will benefit most from prehabilitation
- Studies of training during chemotherapy to evaluate whether this can reduce the decrease in exercise capacity.

Summary

Reduced exercise capacity, defined by a low AT or $\dot{V}O_{2peak}$, is associated with increased post-operative morbidity and mortality. CPET-derived variables can be used to risk stratify patients, and thus improve the precision of outcome prediction. CPET also helps the process of informed consent, and thus contributes to collaborative decision-making. Furthermore, CPET can be used to guide the choice of surgical procedure and to decide on the most appropriate postoperative care environment, although further clinical trial evidence is required in this area. In this way, scarce resources can be concentrated on the highest-risk patients. In the future, CPET may be used to guide prehabilitation training programmes, improving fitness and thereby reducing perioperative risk, although data confirming the efficacy of this approach is awaited.

Study tasks

1 Surgery is a large insult to the human body and poses an even greater risk to patients who are deconditioned. A very high-risk patient is adamant that they want surgery even though the clinicians know the outcome will be unsuccessful. Why might performing a CPET be useful to demonstrate the risk of surgery to the patient?

2 It is clear from this chapter that some patients would benefit from exercise training prior to surgery. You are a clinical exercise physiologist who routinely provides pre-operative CPET sessions for patients; what information would you provide to a patient to encourage their participation in six weeks of exercise before their surgery?

3 Exercise intensity above the AT is clearly related to improved outcomes in preoperative patients; how would you programme home-based exercise to facilitate this intensity, and what information might you require from any CPET to help inform this?

Further reading

Jack, S., West, M.A., Raw, D., Marwood, S., Ambler, G., Cope, T.M., Shrotri, M., Sturgess, R.P., Calverley, P.M., Ottensmeier, C.H., Grocott, M.P. (2014). The effect of neoadjuvant chemotherapy on physical fitness and survival in patients undergoing oesophagogastric cancer surgery. *Eur J Surg Oncol*, 40 (10), 1313–20.

Levett, D.Z., Grocott, M.P. (2015). Cardiopulmonary exercise testing, prehabilitation, and Enhanced Recovery After Surgery (ERAS). *Can J Anaesth*, 62 (2), 131–42.

Loughney, L., West, M., Pintus, S., Lythgoe, D., Clark, E., Jack, S., Torella, F. (2014). Comparison of oxygen uptake during arm or leg cardiopulmonary exercise testing in vascular surgery patients and control subjects. *Br J Anaesth*, 112 (1), 57–65.

Moonesinghe, S.R., Harris, S., Mythen, M.G., Rowan, K.M., Haddad, F.S., Emberton, M., Grocott, M.P. (2014). Survival after postoperative morbidity: a longitudinal observational cohort study. *Br J Anaesth*, 113 (6), 977–84.

Older, P., Courtney, P., Hone, R. (1993). Preoperative evaluation of cardiac failure and ischemia in elderly patients by cardiopulmonary exercise testing. *Chest*, 104 (3), 701–4.

Older, P., Hall, A., Hader, R. (1999). Cardiopulmonary Exercise Testing as a screening test for perioperative management of major surgery in the elderly. *Chest*, 116 (2), 355.

Wasserman, K., Hansen, J., Sue, D., Whipp, B. (2005). *Principles of exercise testing and interpretation: pathophysiology and clinical applications*. 4th ed. Baltimore, Maryland: Lippincott Williams and Wilkins.

West, M., Jack, S., Grocott, M.P. (2011). Perioperative cardiopulmonary exercise testing in the elderly. *Best Pract Res Clin Anaesthesiol*, 25 (3), 427–37.

West, M.A., Loughney, L., Barben, C.P., Sripadam, R., Kemp, G.J., Grocott, M.P., Jack, S. (2014a). The effects of neoadjuvant chemoradiotherapy on physical fitness and morbidity in rectal cancer surgery patients. *Eur J Surg Oncol*, 40 (11), 1421–8.

West, M.A., Loughney, L., Lythgoe, D., Barben, C.P., Sripadam, R., Kemp, G.J., Grocott, M.P.W., Jack, S. (2014b). Effect of prehabilitation on objectively measured physical fitness after neoadjuvant treatment in preoperative rectal cancer patients: a blinded interventional pilot study. *Br J Anaesth*, 114 (2), 244–51.

West, M.A., Lythgoe, D., Barben, C.P., Noble, L., Kemp, G.J., Jack, S., Grocott, M.P. (2014). Cardiopulmonary exercise variables are associated with postoperative morbidity after major colonic surgery: a prospective blinded observational study. *Br J Anaesth*, 112 (4), 665–71.

West, M.A., Parry, M., Asher, R., Key, A., Walker, P., Loughney, L., Pintus, S., Duffy, N., Jack, S., Torella, F. (2015). The effect of beta-blockade on objectively measured physical fitness in patients with abdominal aortic aneurysms – a blinded interventional study. *Br J Anaesth*, pii: aev026.

References

Alam N, Shepherd FA, Winton T, Graham B, Johnson D, Livingston R et al. (2005). Compliance with post-operative adjuvant chemotherapy in non-small cell lung cancer. An analysis of National Cancer Institute of Canada and intergroup trial. *Lung Cancer*, 47, 385–94.

Aronow WS, Ahn C (1994). Prevalence of coexistence of coronary artery disease, peripheral arterial disease, and atherothrombotic brain infarction in man and women > 62 years of age. *Am J Cardiol*, 74, 64, 64–5.

Arthur HM, Daniels C, McKelvie R, Hirsh J, Rush B (2000). Effect of a preoperative intervention on preoperative and postoperative outcomes in low-risk patients awaiting elective coronary artery bypass graft surgery. *Ann Intern Med*, 133(4), 253–62.

Asoh, T, Tsuji, H (1981). Preoperative physical training for cardiac patients requiring non-cardiac surgery. *Japanese Journal of Surgery*, 11(4), 251–5.

ATS/ACCP 2003. American Thoracic Society and American College of Chest Physicians Statement on cardiopulmonary exercise testing. *Am J Respir Crit Care Med*, 167, 211–77.

Ausania F, Snowden CP, Prentis JM, Holmes LR, Jaques BC, White SA, French JJ, Manas DM, Charnley RM (2012). Effects of low cardiopulmonary reserve on pancreatic leak following pancreaticoduodenectomy. *Br J Surg*, 99(9), 1290–4.

Barakat HM, Shahin Y, Barnes R, Gohil R, Souroullas P, Khan J et al. (2014). Supervised exercise program improves aerobic fitness in patients awaiting abdominal aortic aneurysm repair. *Ann Vasc Surg*, 28, 74–9.

Beaver WL, Wasserman K, Whipp BJ (1986). A new method for detecting anaerobic threshold by gas exchange. *J Appl Physiol*, 60, 2020–7.

Belardinelli R, Lacalaprice F, Carle F, Minnucci A, Cianci G, Perna G, D'eusanio G (2003). Exercise-induced myocardial ischaemia detected by cardiopulmonary exercise testing. *Eur Heart J*, 24, 1304–13.

Benzo R, Kelley GA, Recchi L, Hofman A, Sciurba F (2007). Complications of lung resection and exercise capacity: a meta-analysis. *Respir Med*, 101, 1790–7.

Benzo R, Wigle D, Novotny P, Wetzstein M, Nichols F, Shen RK et al. (2011). Preoperative pulmonary rehabilitation before lung cancer resection: results from two randomized studies. *Lung Cancer*, 74, 441–5.

Bobbio A, Chetta A, Ampollini L, Primomo GL, Internullo E, Carbognani P et al. (2008). Preoperative pulmonary rehabilitation in patients undergoing lung resection for non-small cell lung cancer. *Eur J Cardiothorac Surg*, 33, 95–8.

Brunelli A, Pompili C, Salati M, Refai M, Berardi R, Mazzanti P, Tiberi M (2014). Preoperative maximum oxygen consumption is associated with prognosis after pulmonary resection in stage I non-small cell lung cancer. *Ann Thorac Surg*, 98(1), 238–42.

Burke SM, Brunet J, Sabiston CM, Jack S, Grocott MP, West MA (2013). Patients' perceptions of quality of life during active treatment for locally advanced rectal cancer: the importance of preoperative exercise. *Support Care Cancer*, 10, 12, 3345–53.

Carli F, Charlebois P, Stein B, Feldman L, Zavorsky G, Kim DJ et al (2010). Randomized clinical trial of prehabilitation in colorectal surgery. *Br J Surg*, 97, 1187–97.

Carlise J, Swart M (2007). Mid-term survival after abdominal aortic aneurysm surgery predicted by cardiopulmonary exercise testing. *Br J Surg*, 94, 966–9.

Chandrabalan VV, McMillan DC, Carter R, Kinsella J, McKay CJ, Carter CR, Dickson EJ (2013). Pre-operative cardiopulmonary exercise testing predicts adverse post-operative events and non-progression to adjuvant therapy after major pancreatic surgery. *HPB* (Oxford), 15(11), 899–907.

Clinical Trials (2013). The effects of a 9 week exercise programme on fitness and quality of life in rectal cancer patients after chemoradiotherapy and before surgery (SRETP): https://clinicaltrials.gov/ct2/show/NCT01914068.

Coats V, Maltais F, Simard S, Fréchette E, Tremblay L, Ribeiro F, Saey D (2013). Feasibility and effectiveness of a home-based exercise training program before lung resection surgery. *Can Resp J*, 20(2), e10–16.

Davis JA, Vodak P, Wilmore JH, Vodak J, Kurtz P (1976). Anaerobic threshold and maximal aerobic power for three modes of exercise. *J Appl Physiol*, 41.

Debigaré R, Maltais F, Whittom F, Deslauriers J, LeBlanc P (1999). Feasibility and efficacy of home exercise training before lung volume reduction. *J Cardiopulm Rehabil*, 19(4), 235–41.

Dickstein K, Barvik S, Aarsland T, Snapinn S, Karlsson J (1990). A comparison of methodologies in detection of the anaerobic threshold. *Circulation*, 81, 1138–46.

Ditmyer MM, Topp R, Pifer M (2002). Prehabilitation in preparation for orthopaedic surgery. *Orthopaedic Nursing*, 21, 43–54.

Dronkers JJ, Lamberts H, Reutelingsperger IM, Naber RH, Dronkers-Landman CM, Veldman A, van Meeteren NL (2010). Preoperative therapeutic programme for elderly patients scheduled for elective abdominal oncological surgery: a randomized controlled pilot study. *Clin Rehabil*, 24(7), 614–22.

Dunne DF, Jones RP, Lythgoe DT, Pilkington FJ, Palmer DH, Malik HZ, Poston GJ, Lacasia C, Jack S, Fenwick SW. (2014). Cardiopulmonary exercise testing before liver surgery. *J Surg Oncol*, 110(4), 439–44.

Epstein, SK, Freeman, RB, Khayat, A, Unterborn, JN, Pratt, DS, Kaplan, MM (2004). Aerobic capacity is associated with 100-day outcome after hepatic transplantation. *Liver Transpl*, 10(3), 418–24.

Fleisher LA, Beckamn JA, Brown KA, Calkins H, Chaikof E, Fleischmann KE et al. (2007). ACC/AHA 2007 guidelines on perioperative cardiovascular evaluation and care for noncardiac surgery: a report of the American College of Cardiology/American Heart Association Task Force on Practice Guidelines. *Circulation*, 116, 17, 418–99.

Forshaw, MJ, Strauss, DC, Davies, AR, Wilson, D, Lams, B, Pearce, A, Botha, AJ, Mason, RC (2008). Is cardiopulmonary exercise testing a useful test before esophagectomy? *Ann Thorac Surg*, 85(1), 294–9.

Glance LG, Osler TM, Neuman MD (2014). Redesigning surgical decision making for high-risk patients. *N Engl J Med*, 370 (15), 1379–81.

Glaser S, Obst A, Koch B, Henkel B, Grieger A, Felix SB et al (2013). Pulmonary hypertension in patients with idiopathic pulmonary fibrosis – the predictive value of exercise capacity and gas exchange efficiency. *PLoS ONE*, 8, 6, e65643.

Goodyear SJ, Yow H, Saedon M, Shakespeare J, Hill CE, Watson D et al. (2013). Risk stratification by pre-operative cardiopulmonary exercise testing improves outcomes following elective abdominal aortic aneurysm surgery: a cohort study. *Perioperative Medicine*, 2(1), 10.

Grocott MP, Pearse RM (2010). Prognostic studies of perioperative risk: robust methodology is needed. *Br J Anaesth*, 105, 3, 243–5.

Guazzi M, Cahalin LP, Arena R (2013). Cardiopulmonary exercise testing as a diagnostic tool for the detection of left-sided pulmonary hypertension in heart failure. *J Card Fail*, 19, 461–7.

Hanson P, Pease M, Berkoff H, Turnipseed W, Detmer D (1988). Arm exercise testing for coronary artery disease in patients with peripheral vascular disease. *Clin Cardiol*, 11, 70–4.

Hartley RA, Pichel, AC, Grant SW, Hickey GL, Lancaster PS, Wisely NA, McCollum CN, Atkinson D (2012). Preoperative cardiopulmonary exercise testing and risk of early mortality following abdominal aortic aneurysm repair. *Br J Surg*, 99(11), 1539–46.

Held M, Grun M, Holl R, Hubner G, Kaiser R, Karl S et al (2014). Cardiopulmonary exercise testing to detect chronic thromboembolic pulmonary hypertension in patients with normal echocardiography. *Respiration*, 87, 379–87.

Hennis PJ, Meale PM, Grocott MP (2011). Cardiopulmonary exercise testing for the evaluation of perioperative risk in non-cardiopulmonary surgery. *Postgrad Med J*, 87, 1030, 550–7.

Hennis PJ, Meale PM, Hurst RA, O'Doherty AF, Otto J, Kuper M et al. (2012). Cardiopulmonary exercise testing predicts postoperative outcome in patients undergoing gastric bypass surgery. *Br J Anaesth*, 109, 4, 566–71.

Hightower CE, Riedel, BJ, Feig, BW, Morris, GS, Ensor, JE Jr, Woodruff, VD, Daley-Norman, MD, Sun, XG (2010). A pilot study evaluating predictors of postoperative outcomes after major abdominal surgery: physiological capacity compared with the ASA physical status classification system. *Br J Anaesth*, 104(4), 465–71.

Hopker JG, Jobson SA, Pandit JJ (2011). Controversies in the physiological basis of the 'anaerobic threshold' and their implications for clinical cardiopulmonary exercise testing. *Anaesthesia*, 66, 2, 111–23.

Hulzebos EHJ, Helders PJ, Favie NJ, De Bie RA, Brutel de la Riviere A, Van Meeteren NLU (2006). Preoperative intensive inspiratory muscle training to prevent postoperative pulmonary complications in high risk patients undergoing CABG surgery. *JAMA*, 296(15), 1851–7.

Jack S, West MA, Raw D, Marwood S, Ambler G, Cope TM et al. (2014). The effect of neoadjuvant chemotherapy on physical fitness and survival in patients undergoing oesophagogastric cancer surgery. *Eur J Surg Oncol*, 40, 10, 1313–20.

Jones LW, Peddle CJ, Eves ND, Haykowsky MJ, Courneya KS, Mackey JR et al. (2007). Effects of presurgical exercise training on cardiorespiratory fitness among patients undergoing thoracic surgery for malignant lung lesions. *Cancer*, 110, 3, 590–8.

Junejo MA, Mason JM, Sheen AJ, Moore J, Foster P, Atkinson D et al. (2012). Cardiopulmonary exercise testing for preoperative risk assessment before hepatic resection. *Br J Surg*, 99, 8, 1097–104.

Kim DJ, Mayo NE, Carli F, Montgomery Dl, Zavorsky GS (2009). Responsive measures of prehabilitation in patients undergoing bowel resection surgery. *Tohoku J. Exp. Med*, 217, 109–15.

Kothmann E, Batterham AM, Owen SJ, Turley AJ, Cheesman M, Parry A, Danjoux G (2009). Effect of short-term exercise training on aerobic fitness in patients with abdominal aortic aneurysms: a pilot study. *Br J Anaesth*, 103, 505–10.

Levett DZ, Grocott MP (2015a). Cardiopulmonary exercise testing for risk prediction in major abdominal surgery. *Anesthesiol Clin*, 33, 1–16.

Levett DZ, Grocott MP (2015b). Cardiopulmonary exercise testing, prehabilitation, and Enhanced Recovery After Surgery (ERAS). *Can J Anaesth*, 62, 2, 131–42.

Li C, Carlie F, Lee L, Charlebois P, Stein B, Liberman AS et al (2013). Impact of a trimodal prehabilitation program on functional recovery after colorectal cancer surgery: a pilot study. *Surg Endosc*, 27, 4, 1072–82.

Loganathan RS, Stover DE, Shi W, Venkatraman E (2006). Prevalence of COPD in women compared to men around the time of diagnosis of primary lung cancer. *Chest*, 129, 1305–12.

Loughney L, West M, Pintus S, Lythgoe D, Clark E, Jack S, Torella F (2014). Comparison of oxygen uptake during arm or leg cardiopulmonary exercise testing in vascular surgery patients and control subjects. *Br J Anaesth*, 112, 1, 57–65.

Matsumura N, Nishijima H, Kojuma S, Hashimoto F, Minami M, Yasuda H (1983). Determination of anaerobic threshold for assessment of functional state in patients with chronic heart failure. *Circulation*, 68, 360–7.

Mayo NE, Feldman L, Scott S, Zavorsky G, Kim DJ, Charlebois P et al (2011). Impact of preoperative change in physical function on postoperative recovery: argument supporting prehabilitation for colorectal surgery. *Surgery*, 150, 505–14.

Mccullough PA, Gallagher MJ, Dejong AT, Sandberg KR, Trivax JE, Alexander D et al. (2006). Cardiorespiratory fitness and short-term complications after bariatric surgery. *Chest*, 130, 2, 517–25.

Moonesinghe SR, Harris S, Mythen MG, Rowan KM, Haddad FS, Emberton M, Grocott MP (2014). Survival after postoperative morbidity: a longitudinal observational cohort study. *Br J Anaesth*, 113, 6, 977–84.

Moros MT, Ruidiaz M, Caballero A, Serrano E, Martínez V, Tres A (2010). Effects of an exercise training program on the quality of life of women with breast cancer on chemotherapy. *Rev Med Chil*, 138, 6, 715–22.

Mujovic N, Subotic D, Marinkovic M, Milovanovic A, Stojsic J et al. (2014). Preoperative pulmonary rehabilitation in patients with non-small cell lung cancer and chronic obstructive pulmonary disease. *Arch Med Sci*, 10, 1, 68–75.

Myers J, Voodi L, Umann T, Froelicher VF (2000). A survey of exercise testing: methods, utilization, interpretation, and safety in the VAHCS. *J Cardiopulm Rehabil*, 20, 251–8.

Myers JN, White JJ, Narasimhan B, Dalman RL (2010). Effects of exercise training in patients with abdominal aortic aneurysm: preliminary results from a randomized trial. *Journal of Cardiopulmonary Rehabilitation and Prevention*, 30, 374–83.

Nagamatsu Y, Shima, I, Yamana, H, Fujita, H, Shirouzu, K, Ishitake, T (2001). Preoperative evaluation of cardiopulmonary reserve with the use of expired gas analysis during exercise testing in patients with squamous cell carcinoma of the thoracic esophagus. *J Thorac Cardiovasc Surg*, 121(6), 1064–8.

Nagamatsu Y, Yamana, H, Fujita, H, Hiraki, H, Matsuo, T, Mitsuoka, M, Hayashi, A, Kakegawa, T (1994). The simultaneous evaluation of preoperative cardiopulmonary functions of esophageal cancer patients in the analysis of expired gas with exercise testing. *Nihon Kyobu Geka Gakkai Zasshi*, 42(11), 2037–40.

Nugent, AM, Riley, M, Megarry, J, O'Reilly, MJG, MacMahon J, Lowry R. (1998). Cardiopulmonary exercise testing in the pre-operative assessment of patients for repair of abdominal aortic aneurysm. *Irish Journal of Medical Science*, 167(4), 238–41.

Older P, Hall A, Hader R (1999). Cardiopulmonary exercise testing as a screening test for perioperative management of major surgery in the elderly. *Chest*, 116, 355–362.

Older P, Smith R, Courtney P, Hone R (1993). Preoperative evaluation of cardiac failure and ischemia in elderly patients by cardiopulmonary exercise testing. *Chest*, 104(3), 701–4.

Ong KC, Bendicto JP, Chan AH, Tan YS, Ong YY (2000). Cardiopulmonary exercise testing in heart transplant candidates. *Ann Acad Med Singapore*, 29, 442–6.

Osada N, Chaitman BR, Miller LW, Cishek MB, Wolford TL, Donohue TJ (1998). Cardiopulmonary exercise testing identifies low risk patients with heart failure and severely impaired exercise capacity considered for heart transplantation. *J Am Coll Cardiol*, 31, 577–82.

Palange P, Ward SA, Carlsen K-H, Casaburi R, Gallagher CG, Gosselink R et al. (2007). Recommendations on the use of exercise testing in clinical practice. *The European Respiratory Journal: Official Journal of the European Society for Clinical Respiratory Physiolog*, 29, 1, 185–209.

Patessio A, Casaburi R, Carone M, Appendini L, Donner C, Wasserman K (1993). Comparison of gas exchange, lactate, and lactic acidosis thresholds in patients with chronic obstructive pulmonary disease. *Am Rev Respir Dis*, 148, 622–6.

Pearse RM, Harrison DA, James P, Watson D, Hinds C, Rhodes A et al (2006). Identification and characterisation of the high-risk surgical population in the United Kingdom. *Critical Care*, 10, 3.

Pearse RM, Moreno RP, Bauer P, Pelosi P, Metnitz P, Spies C, Vallet B, Vincent J-L, Hoeft A, Rhodes A (2012). Mortality after surgery in Europe: a 7 day cohort study. *The Lancet*, 380, 1059–65.

Porszasz J, Stringer W, Casaburi, R (2007). Equipment, measurements and quality control. In: Ward SA, Palange, P. eds. *Clinical exercise testing: European respiratory monograph*. Sheffield: European Respiratory Society.

Prentis JM, Manas, DM, Trenell MI, Hudson M, Jones DJ, Snowden CP (2012a). Submaximal cardiopulmonary exercise testing predicts 90-day survival after liver transplantation. *Liver Transpl*, 18(2), 152–9.

Prentis JM, Trenell, MI, Jones DJ, Lees T, Clarke M, Snowden CP (2012b). Submaximal exercise testing predicts perioperative hospitalization after aortic aneurysm repair. *J Vasc Surg*, 56(6), 1564–70.

Rao R, Cruz V, Peng Y, Harker-Murray A, Haley BB, Zhao H, Xie XJ, Euhus D (2012). Bootcamp during neoadjuvant chemotherapy for breast cancer: a randomized pilot trial. *Breast Cancer*, 6, 39–46.

Simonton C, Higginbotham M, Cobb F (1988). The ventilatory threshold: quantitative analysis of reproducibility and relation to arterial lactate concentration in normal subjects and in patients with chronic congestive heart failure. *Am J Cardiol*, 62, 100–7.

Sinclair RC, Danjous GR, Goodridge V, Batterham AM (2009). Determination of the anaerobic threshold in the pre-operative assessment clinic: inter-observer measurement error. *Anaesthesia*, 64, 11, 1192–5.

Snowden CP, Prentis JM, Aderson HL, Roberts DR, Randles D, Renton M, Manas DM (2010). Submaximal cardiopulmonary exercise testing predicts complications and hospital length of stay in patients undergoing major elective surgery. *Ann Surg*, 251, 535–41.

Sue DY, Wasserman K, Moricca RB, Casaburi R (1988). Metabolic acidosis during exercise in patients with chronic obstructive pulmonary disease. Use of the V-slope method for anaerobic threshold determination. *Chest*, 94, 931–8.

Sukhija R, Aronow WS, Yalamanchili K, Sinha N, Babu S (2004). Prevalence of coronary artery disease, lower extremity peripheral arterial disease, and cerebrovascular disease in 110 men with an abdominal aortic aneurysm. *Am J Cardiol* 94, 1358.

Sullivan CS, Casaburi R, Storer TW, Wasserman K (1995). Non-invasive prediction of blood lactate response to constant power outputs from incremental exercise tests. *Eur J Appl Physiol Occup Physiol*, 71, 349–54.

Swart M, Carlisle J (2012). Case-controlled study of critical care or surgical ward care after elective open colorectal surgery. *Br J Surg*, 99, 295–9.

Tew GA, Moss J, Crank H, Mitchell PA, Nawaz S (2012). Endurance exercise training in patients with small abdominal aortic aneurysm: a randomized controlled pilot study. *Arch Phys Med Rehabil*, 93, 2148–53.

Timmerman H, de Groot, JF, Hulzebos HJ, de Knikker R, Kerkkamp HE, van Meeteren NL (2011). Feasibility and preliminary effectiveness of preoperative therapeutic exercise in patients with cancer: a pragmatic study. *Physiother Theory Pract*, 27(2), 117–24.

Wasserman K (1986). The anaerobic threshold: definition, physiological significance and identification. *Adv Cardiol*, 35, 1–23.

Wasserman K, Beaver WL, Whipp BJ (1990). Gas exchange theory and the lactic acidosis (anaerobic) threshold. *Circulation*, 81, II14–30.

Wasserman K, Hansen JA, Sue DY, Stringer WW, Sietsema KE, Sun X-G, Whipp B (2012). *Principles of exercise testing and interpretation including pathophysiology and clinical applications.* 5th ed., Baltimore, Maryland: Lippincott Williams and Wilkins.

Wasserman K, Hansen JA, Sue DY, Whipp B (2005). *Principles of exercise testing and interpretation: pathophysiology and clinical applications.* 4th ed., Baltimore, Maryland: Lippincott Williams and Wilkins.

Weisman IM, Idelle M, Martinez FJ, Sciurba F, Sue D, Myers J et al (2003). ATS/ACCP Statement on cardiopulmonary exercise testing. *American Journal of Respiratory and Critical Care Medicine.* 167, 2.

West M, Jack S, Grocott M P (2011). Perioperative cardiopulmonary exercise testing in the elderly. *Best Pract Res Clin Anaesthesiol*, 25, 427–37.

West MA, Loughney L, Barben CP, Sripadam R, Kemp GJ, Grocott MP, Jack S (2014a). The effects of neoadjuvant chemoradiotherapy on physical fitness and morbidity in rectal cancer surgery patients. *Eur J Surg Oncol*, 40, 1421–8.

West MA, Loughney L, Lythgoe D, Barben CP, Sripadam R, Kemp GJ, Grocott MPW, Jack S (2014b). Effect of prehabilitation on objectively measured physical fitness after neoadjuvant treatment in preoperative rectal cancer patients: a blinded interventional pilot study. *Br Journal Anaesth*, 114, 244–51.

West MA, Parry M, Asher R, Key A, Walker P, Loughney L, Pintus S, Duffy N, Jack S-Torella, F (2015). The Effect of beta-blockade on objectively measured physical fitness in patients with abdominal aortic aneurysms – a blinded interventional study. *Br J Anaesth*, 114,6, 878–85.

Whipp BJ (2007). Physiological mechanisms dissociating pulmonary CO2 and O2 exchange dynamics during exercise in humans. *Exp Physiol*, 92, 347–55.

Whipp BJ, Davis JA, Torres F, Wasserman K (1981). A test to determine parameters of aerobic function during exercise. *J Appl Physiol*, 50, 217–21.

Whipp BJ, Ward SA, Wasserman K (1986). Respiratory markers of the anaerobic threshold. *Adv Cardiol*, 35, 47–64.

Wilson RJ, Davies S, Yates D, Redman J, Stone M (2010). Impaired functional capacity is associated with all-cause mortality after major elective intra-abdominal surgery. *Br J Anaesth*, 105, 297–303.

Chapter 11

Influencing health behaviour

Applying theory to practice

Lynne Johnston and Andrew Hutchison

Introduction

Literature regarding the psychology of health and exercise behaviour has been strongly influenced by theoretical models developed within the wider health psychology domain (Hutchison et al., 2013). Limited attempts have also been made to explicitly state how to incorporate existing theory into day-to-day clinical practice. Arguably, one reason for this void between theory and practice is the fact that most of the published material on the psychology of health-related behaviour change has been written by academic psychologists who do not regularly work clinically with clients. Instead, their clinical experience has tended to be within the context of a research trial (e.g. Mutrie et al., 2004). The inclusion and exclusion criteria for such trials often result in a particular type of client being included (i.e. adherent people with no known comorbidities) that is very different to the typical clinical client seen within a routine clinical caseload. Consequently, we have previously argued that attempts to apply theory to practice within exercise psychology are often not sensitive enough to account for the levels of individual variation common in real-life clinical settings (Hutchison and Johnston, 2013). A further limitation with the existing health and exercise psychology literature is that intervention protocols are rarely disseminated in sufficient detail to fully understand and assess what a practitioner actually does in 'practice' (Müller-Riemenschneider et al., 2008). This can make it difficult to fully evaluate studies in terms of the specific intervention processes.

This chapter argues that the psychology of health behaviour needs to be inherently embedded within a wider case-conceptualisation process. It will focus on the pragmatic aspects of the clinical assessment and formulation[1] process within a Specialist Weight Management context. The chapter is written by two clinical psychologists who work on a daily basis with a clinical case load. We both hold previous PhDs in exercise psychology and have worked as academic psychologists publishing on the theoretical aspects of the psychology of exercise behaviour. We left our academic positions to return to clinical practice because we felt frustrated by the schism between theory and practice. To address some of the limitations within exercise psychology, we have argued for the use of clinical formulations (Johnston et al., 2011; Hutchison and Johnston, 2013). The aim of the current chapter is to further our original arguments and, using practical examples, illustrate how these clinical tools can facilitate more theoretically-informed pragmatic approaches to influencing health behaviours. Our aim is to open further debate about the way in which we study health and exercise psychology as a discipline, how we assess and formulate our clients' difficulties, and how a clinical intervention protocol can develop from a detailed clinical formulation. We also hope to open a debate about the training of future clinical health and exercise psychologists, and argue for a greater influence from clinical psychology.

Dominant trends in health and exercise psychology

Although exercise psychology represents a well-established academic field, it remains a relatively new area of interest, which has evolved from other sub-disciplines of psychology and the health sciences (Buckworth et al., 2013). Inevitably, the literature regarding the psychology of health and exercise behaviour has been influenced by theoretical models and understandings developed within a number of other pre-existing domains (e.g. health sciences, behavioural psychology, social psychology, neurophysiology). Consequently, a wealth of potentially-relevant knowledge has always been available to those interested in studying the psychology of exercise and health behaviours. With so much readily available information, it is no surprise that fields such as exercise psychology developed rapidly as scientific disciplines. However, despite an increasing emphasis on public health promotion and the role of physical activity (PA) within it, this chapter argues that any applied benefits of the theoretical advances observed remain relatively limited. Specifically, although a range of PA intervention strategies have been developed and implemented, research has demonstrated only limited support for their efficacy. While short-term changes are sometimes noted, long-term changes (i.e. maintenance) appear more difficult to achieve (Hillsdon et al., 2005; Müller-Riemenschneider et al., 2008).

One explanation for this concerns the fact that intervention practices have evolved largely from rigorous research trials devised predominantly within academic settings. While rigorous scientific approaches (e.g. RCTs) typically represent the gold standard for obtaining new levels of understanding, their ecological validity can be called into question. For example, in order to exert a high level of control over extraneous variables and maximise internal validity, studies often implement strict environmental controls and narrowly-defined inclusion and exclusion criteria. As these conditions do not mirror the complexities and individual variation that may be typical in real-life clinical settings, considerable caution should be exercised when attempting to extrapolate findings to routine clinical practice.

Arguably, the same level of caution should be exercised when applying existing theory to fields such as PA intervention development. For example, while a considerable body of literature exists that addresses the underlying psychological mechanisms associated with PA behaviour, it is important to recognise that the associated interventions being developed and tested still appear to operate at a generalisable level. Specifically, most existing theories and models represent frameworks designed to operate at a macro level, and are not formal blueprints, which are directly applicable to individual cases. To illustrate the above point, it is worth considering applications of the Transtheoretical Model (TTM), which is a commonly-adopted framework for informing the development and implementation of PA interventions (Breckon et al., 2008). Central to interventions based on the TTM is the concept of stage-matching, whereby people are classified according to a readiness continuum. As we have previously argued, whilst this provides a useful overview of the extent to which a person is motivated to engage in PA, it does not conceptualise and explain why this is the case for that particular individual (Hutchison and Johnston, 2013).

Typically, in healthcare settings, the treatment framework adopted conforms to a philosophy of classifying people according to their presenting symptoms, which, in turn, are matched to a specific treatment (Wade and Halligan, 2004). Although this 'Medical Model' approach is likely to have considerable merit when a diagnosis or classification is closely associated with a common cause or aetiology, if a common aetiology and prognosis cannot be identified, attempts to apply diagnostic labelling are likely to hinder the treatment process. For example, if a problem is deemed to be closely intertwined with a person's own history and personal experiences, then the predictability, in terms of identifying a common cause and prognosis, is likely to be lacking (Mace and Binyon, 2005). Consequently, it may be ineffective to apply an inflexible, standardised treatment. Therefore, a more individualistic process may be required to identify the underlying causes, maintaining factors, and a client-centred plan. Poor treatment outcomes when adopting a Medical Model approach could suggest that the diagnosis has failed to identify the underlying problem(s). As a result, the treatment may not address the real issue. For example, while sedentary behaviour may have resulted in someone developing physical health problems, the underlying cause of the inactivity may be complex, multifaceted, and individualistic. When an individual is labelled as sedentary and lacking in motivation, the underlying causes of this are unlikely to be generalisable. Consequently, prescribing PA to combat the symptoms of obesity is arguably akin to placing a sticking plaster on an infected wound, because the solution does not necessarily address the root of the problem. For many years, the field of clinical psychology has made an important distinction between people's overt, observable difficulties (e.g. being overweight, lack of motivation to engage in PA) and the underlying psychological mechanisms that underpin those overt difficulties (e.g. low self-esteem, depression) (See Persons, 1989). Therefore, while diagnostic labelling may help identify and diagnose people's overt difficulties, they are unlikely to consistently elicit the underlying psychological mechanisms that cause and maintain those difficulties.

In the previously-mentioned example, the TTM is arguably being used to inform a classification system, which allows for a diagnostic label to be applied and a subsequent standardised solution to be identified. To facilitate this process, there is another dimension of TTM, called the 'processes of change'. These are ten strategies that describe the techniques that individuals use to modify cognitions, emotions, and behaviours (Prochaska and Norcross, 1994). The first five processes, which are commonly classified as experiential, have been shown to be associated with the earlier stages of change (Velicer et al., 1998). The last five processes, classified as behavioural, are hypothesised to be associated with the later stage transitions (Velicer et al., 1998). Consequently, the TTM lends itself to a Medical Model philosophy, whereby individuals can be stage-matched within an intervention. Whilst these popular stage-matched interventions do represent individually-tailored approaches, at no point do they attempt to identify an individually-situated, motivational aetiology. Rather, they focus on matching generic solutions to theoretically-derived motivational symptoms, but not their underlying causes.

Existing PA intervention practices tend to acknowledge the extent to which people meet the American College of Sports Medicine's (ACSM) PA guidelines (Haskell et al., 2007) as a primary desired outcome (Gidlow and Murphy, 2009). These represent physiology-centred recommendations dictated by a dose-response relationship inherent in the evidence-based literature. Consequently, current intervention strategies (e.g. Physical Activity Referral Schemes: PARS) are primarily physiologically, and not psychologically, driven. Arguably, they need to include both components. This can be seen within existing PARS initiatives that often differentiate between physical and mental health referrals (Crone et al., 2008). Evidence suggests that mental health referrals have considerably lower adherence rates compared to physical health referrals (James et al., 2009). Consequently, existing PARS may be less well equipped to address people's needs from a psychological perspective. Arguably, it is inappropriate to differentiate between physical and mental health referrals if it is accepted that a relationship exists between individuals' observable difficulties (e.g. being overweight) and the underlying psychological mechanisms that underpin those overt difficulties and/or that maintain their difficulties (e.g. bereavement/loss issues, trauma, low self-worth, depression, avoidance associated with social anxiety, etc.). The existing theoretical literature often largely ignores historical influences, social and contextual factors, and any potentially relevant psychological comorbidities (e.g. depression, social anxiety).

Due to the explanatory level at which existing theories operate, they cannot be applied according to a 'one size fits all' philosophy. Instead, they should be used as guiding frameworks to direct the development of broad interventions, which then need to be applied at a person-centred level. Whilst health and exercise psychology practitioners may be aware of this need, a key problem is that there is no agreed framework for the implementation of individualised, holistic interventions in fields such as exercise psychology. There is arguably a need to look beyond a Medical Model philosophy of treatment and prevention. Mechanisms ultimately need to be identified that can help practitioners relate existing theory to practice in such a way that recognises the complex, individualistic nature of clients and their exercise-/health-related behaviours. As such, the remaining sections of this chapter discuss the use of a case formulation-based approach, as a means of facilitating the careful consideration of variations in the development, manifestation, and maintaining mechanisms of people's problematic health behaviours (e.g. inactivity, weight-cycling, portion control).

Case formulation

The concept of case formulation has been an increasingly prominent feature within clinical psychology and psychotherapy since the 1950s (British Psychological Society, 2011; Crellin, 1998). It was introduced within the context of psychological assessment as offering a distinctive role compared to psychiatric diagnosis. Specifically, it refers to the process of performing an individualised assessment of a clinical case, which is sensitive to variations in the development, manifestation, and maintaining mechanisms of individuals' psychological problems (Tarrier, 2006). Therefore, it accounts for the limitations associated with a Medical Model approach (i.e. treating people in the same way because they demonstrate particular symptoms, regardless of differences in underlying reasons). Although case formulation is central to the day-to-day practice of clinical psychologists and other psychotherapists, it has only recently begun to emerge in other areas of applied psychology (e.g. Gardner and Moore, 2005; Hutchison and Johnston, 2013). To explore the potential of case formulation within health and exercise behaviour change settings, the subsequent sections of this chapter provide an overview of case formulation and demonstrate how it is currently being used to enhance practice within a Specialist Weight Management Service (SWMS).

Defining case formulation

Case formulation has been interpreted and described in a variety of ways to account for different theoretical perspectives, therapeutic models, and presenting difficulties. Therefore, it can be viewed on an epistemological continuum ranging from the dominant cognitive behavioural theory/therapy (CBT) standpoint (e.g. Dudley and Kuyken, 2006) to the social constructionist (e.g. Harper and Spellman, 2006) and social inequalities perspectives (e.g. Miller and McClelland, 2006). Within these broad categories, more explicit approaches to formulation have also emerged in response to specific theoretical and therapeutic developments. Earlier case formulation definitions, rooted in the CBT approach, appeared to emphasise that formulations are theory-driven and that a hypothesis-testing approach is adopted to understand a patient's problems and inform treatment. It involves collecting and assimilating relevant information, in collaboration with a client or patient, to check, aid, and refine interpretation and meaning. Collaboration is frequently noted as a defining feature of most formulation-based approaches (Kuyken et al., 2009; Tarrier, 2006). This sentiment is central to the definition by Harper and Moss (2003), where formulation is viewed as being 'engaged in a process of collaborative sense making'(p. 8). Formulation is also typically seen as an iterative process that should be continually revisited as new information is discovered. Consequently, a case formulation appears to represent a process of developing a case-specific theory about a client's presenting issues, which can then be tested through the application of a range of treatment strategies and methods. Kuyken et al. (2009) have highlighted ten key functions of case conceptualisation (formulation) within CBT (Box 11.1).

Box 11.1 Functions of case conceptualisation in CBT (Kuyken et al., 2009, p. 6)

1 Synthesizes client experience, CBT theory, and research
2 Normalizes presenting issues and is validating
3 Promotes client engagement
4 Makes numerous complex problems more manageable
5 Guides the selection, focus and sequence of interventions
6 Identifies client strengths and suggests ways to build client resistance
7 Suggests the simplest and most cost effective interventions
8 Anticipates and addresses problems in therapy
9 Helps understand nonresponse in therapy and suggests alternative routes for change
10 Enables high quality supervision.

Recently, within the context of clinical exercise psychology, we introduced the concept of case formulation using a model commonly referred to as the 'Five Ps' framework (Hutchison and Johnston, 2013). The Five Ps has been described as an atheoretical model of case formulation, in that it is not aligned to any particular therapeutic style or psychological understanding of distress (Dudley and Kuyken, 2006). Consequently, it was deemed suitable for demonstrating the potential utility of case formulation, with reference to a hypothetical case study. The Five Ps framework describes five levels, which help structure the formulation process by encouraging the identification of the specific presenting issue(s), possible predisposing factors, potentially-relevant precipitating factors, perpetuating or maintaining factors, and protective factors (Johnstone and Dallos, 2006). See Table 11.1 for a description of the Five Ps and their potential application to PA behaviour change.

Typically, the development of a case formulation occurs as a result of information gathered during a routine consultation. Within a PA behaviour-change context, this could be a consultation with a primary healthcare worker (e.g. nurse, PARS worker, family physician, exercise psychologist). During this time, the health professional and client might work together to identify and explore the five areas identified in Table 11.1. This process should assist with the collective identification of an individualised treatment plan, which seeks to address the underlying mechanisms responsible for that person's presenting problems.

When a practitioner is working within a particular theoretical framework, such as CBT, the process of formulation is likely to be influenced by pre-existing knowledge

Table 11.1 The 'Five Ps' of formulation

The Five Ps	Potential application to health-related behaviour change
Presenting issues Statement of the client's presenting problems in terms of emotions, cognitions, and behaviours.	This goes beyond diagnosis because it attempts to define the current problems a person faces. Consequently, it does not involve categorising the person according to pre-existing criteria, but introduces specificity and individualisation.
Predisposing factors The distal external and internal factors that increase the person's vulnerability to their current problems (i.e. what led to the problems starting?).	Encourages the development of a longitudinal understanding of a person's problems. This is intended to encourage the identification of more in-depth interventions that aim to maintain change and prevent re-lapse.
Precipitating factors The proximal external and internal factors that triggered the current presenting issues.	Encourages the identification and exploration of the activating events and associated beliefs linked to a person's presenting issues.
Perpetuating factors The internal and external factors that maintain the current problems.	Helps provide a focus for the intervention by identifying the factors that need to be addressed to break the maintenance cycle.
Protective factors The person's resilience and strengths that help maintain emotional health.	Provides a path of least resistance by identifying strategies that build on existing resilience and strengths.

(Adapted from Johnstone and Dallos, 2006)

of different CBT treatment models and therapeutic manuals. However, practitioners need to be aware of the danger of merely fitting the client to a pre-existing model. The opposite problem is simply describing a client's difficulties without any level of conceptual linkage or integration (i.e. being so descriptive that the formulation is atheoretical). Kuyken, et al. (2009) discuss three guiding principles within a CBT case conceptualisation approach, which aim to avoid these dual dangers: levels of conceptualisation; collaborative empiricism; and strengths focus.

As their name would suggest, CBT-based approaches draw on both cognitive and behavioural theory to inform an understanding of people's presenting issues and subsequently highlight potential intervention strategies. Central to most CBT-based understandings of distress is the assumption that perceptions about ourselves, other people, and the world, shape our emotions and behaviours (Beck, 1976). Therefore, from this perspective, psychological distress is not a direct result of negative experiences; instead, it is the result of peoples' interpretations of those experiences. Therefore, CBT-based models typically facilitate the gathering of information about how antecedent factors, intervening beliefs, and emotional, physiological, behavioural, and cognitive consequences interact to maintain the client's difficulties (Carr and McNulty, 2006). Alongside this, they also attempt to elicit insight into developmental factors and underlying core beliefs that increase a person's vulnerability to subsequent negative cognitive appraisals (Johnston and Dallos, 2006).

Within CBT, a number of prominent disorder-specific models have been proposed to inform different understandings of psychological distress from this theoretical perspective. For example, see Shafran et al. (2013) for a review of CBT treatment models for anxiety. For the treatment of depression using a cognitive approach, see Beck et al. (1979). For a behavioural activation (BA) approach see Martell et al. (2010). Dimidjian et al (2006) point to the renewed interest in BA approaches over the last twenty years, including complex and comorbid physical health conditions. Given the high levels of comorbidity between obesity and depression (Pagoto et al., 2013), evidence for the use of BA to treat both conditions is emerging. One hypothesis is that, in depressed patients, obesity could be a consequence of the use of food to emotionally regulate, as well as behavioural avoidance (i.e. decreased physical activity and increased sedentary behavioural patterns) (Pagoto et al., 2006).

Case study

The following case study provides a sample of a typical case seen within a SWMS. The majority of clients referred into this service have comorbid physical and mental health difficulties. Each client referred receives input from a principle clinical psychologist, exercise practitioner, and senior dietician. The initial formulation (see Table 11.2), offers an insight into the way in which the interdisciplinary team made sense of the patient's presenting problems. This then enabled them to identify a treatment plan that addressed the range of maintaining difficulties (e.g. social anxiety) rather than simply focussing on the presenting (observable) symptoms (e.g. obesity). The psychological work provided for this patient involved the co-ordination of the case formulation and the delivery of a twelve-week psycho-educational group for weight management. Additional specific work using CBT for the treatment of social anxiety (SA)[2] was undertaken because it was apparent that the development/

maintenance of the patient's obesity was inextricably linked with her SA. Therefore, the Cognitive Model of Social Phobia (Clark and Wells, 1995) was used to inform a more 'disorder specific' understanding of the patient's SA related difficulties and the application of a CBT intervention.

Personal history and presenting problems

The patient, AM[3], was referred to the SWMS by her GP for 'morbid obesity', alongside a range of additional health conditions (i.e. low mood, anxiety, diabetes, sleep apnoea, hypertension, hyperlipidaemia). The referral provided demographic information and medical history only. AM was thirty four years old, unmarried, heterosexual, with no children. She lived alone, in a rented flat, in an urban area in the North East of England. She described her early childhood as 'quite normal'. Her parents divorced when she was eleven. She described her father as 'an abusive alcoholic' and viewed their relationship as 'difficult'. She left home at eighteen to live in the south of England and moved back to the North East at the age of twenty five (catalyst: breakdown of a romantic relationship). Her weight increased from the age of eighteen and was associated with poor dietary/alcohol choices (e.g. skipping breakfast, long gaps between meals, excessive use of convenience foods, increased levels of daily alcohol use, weekend binge-drinking), lack of a good quality sleep routine, and a lack of PA. At the point of referral she weighed 160 kg (BMI=55 kgm^{-2}) and was employed in a call centre. She described a close, positive, relationship with her maternal family. However, she also reported showing a lack of emotional reaction to losses and used food to regulate her emotions.

Case formulation

To make sense of AM's difficulties, the Five Ps framework was utilised to guide an initial formulation (see Table 11.2). This process involved gathering potentially-relevant information to obtain not only a detailed description of AM's difficulties, (1) but also insight into the factors which may increase her susceptibility to them, (2) trigger their onset (3), and contribute to their maintenance (4). In addition, the Five Ps also encouraged the identification of AM's strengths and sources of support (5). By gathering this depth of information, it was possible to construct an initial intervention plan based on a hypothesised understanding of her difficulties (Table 11.2).

Having identified SA and its symptoms as being central to AM's on-going difficulties, it was then possible to adopt a more theoretically-derived approach to understanding and supporting AM. The following section provides a further description of the specific CBT work for SA. This was viewed as an integral part of AM's treatment, as it was judged unlikely that she would be able to become independently active without addressing her SA.

Problem map for social anxiety

The links between AM's weight and her SA are shown in Figure 11.1. AM described a gradual process of social avoidance over the previous nine years. At referral, AM was leaving her house to go to work (usually by taxi), visit family members ('in safe

Table 11.2 5 Ps Framework for AM

| 1 | Presenting Issues: obesity, low mood, social anxiety |

Emotional impact of poor quality of life due to deteriorating mental (anxiety/depression) and physical health [EMOTIONS]

Overestimation of perceived risks of engagement in social/PA outside of family 'safe zones' [THOUGHTS]

Maladaptive behavioural coping responses: Inactivity, social withdrawal, comfort eating, distraction via films/TV, staying indoors/avoidance of social interaction [BEHAVIOURS]

2 Predisposing	3 Precipitating	4 Perpetuating	5 Protective
Mother and father divorce (age 11)	Weight gain increasingly (from age 18)	Avoidance of unnecessary activity outside home (e.g. refusal of social invitations)	Strong maternal family support
Poor relationship with father (from age 11)	Drank heavily (from age 18–27)	'Netflix'; excessive time alone immersing self in films (emotional avoidance)	Employed Work colleagues
Poor emotional repertoire; tendency to internalise negative affect (age 11 or earlier)	Moved away from family/ social support network (from age 18) Sport injury (age 23) ('shattered knee') ended playing career. Reduced PA patterns and increasing lack of physical fitness/social isolation (age 24)	Minimises travel to work via public transport Sedentary job (call centre) Over-estimates threat of negative comments from others regarding size; adoption of various 'safety behaviours'	Changed problematic behaviours previously (e.g. alcohol misuse) Motivation to change Sister source of support
High standards of self in social performance situations (e.g. school/ teenage 'banter'; sport club 'banter'; early work life 'banter')	Critical incident: Alton Towers 'too big to fit on ride' (age 24). Negative verbal comments regarding physical size from strangers age 24 +)	Perceived inability to cope with negative comments from others/concern regarding over-reaction /loss of control over anger	
Avoidant coping strategies	Relationship break-up (age 25); moved back to North East (age 25) Diagnosed with obesity, hypertension, hyperlypidemia (age 26) Increasing levels of social avoidance (from age 27) Sedentary job (call centre from age 27/28) Verbal abuse (bus stop, age 27/28) Grandfather's death (age 32) Increasing levels of social isolation outside work environment (age 27+)	Use of taxis to travel small distances Avoidance of emotional expression (e.g. anger at father; feelings regarding physical size) Avoidance of busy locations – over- estimation of risk of catastrophic humiliation Weight gain/maintenance (food used as emotional comfort; sedentary behaviour at home and work) Lack of intimate relationship	

Plan
12-week psycho-educational work for biological, social, and psychological factors in weight
    management
Individual psycho-educational work with a dietician trained in Motivational Interviewing
Individual Work with a PA Specialist trained in Motivational Interviewing
CBT work for social anxiety-psycho-education, formulation, specific interventions
Graded exposure work for increasing activity outside the home/ work environments (including PA)
    and increasing social contact (Easyline, Tier 2 exercise referral; psych-educational group).

zones'), attend medical appointments, and (occasionally) visit local shops. She had not
been to the city centre for five years. She ordered food online and was not attending
social events. Consequently, AM had essentially confined herself to her home. She was
predominantly sedentary; her level of social contact was minimal; and her comfort
eating increased.

Assessment of social anxiety

Social anxiety is defined as a 'marked fear or anxiety about one or more social situations in which the individual is exposed to possible scrutiny by others' (American
Psychiatric Association, 2013: p.202). AM described this across a range of situations.
Anxiety symptoms must almost always occur when the person is exposed to a social
situation (e.g. speaking, eating, or travelling in public) (Wells, 1997). AM described
experiencing anxiety whenever she was in a public space (i.e. upon leaving her home).
She described considerable distress due to increasing avoidance of social contact. This
was impacting negatively upon her quality of life and was identified as a key barrier to
activity (Johnston et al. 2009).

Whilst most people experience some anxiety in novel situations, the distress caused
in those with diagnosed SA is disproportionate to the level of threat posed. If another
medical condition, such as obesity, exists, 'the fear, anxiety, or avoidance' experienced needs to be either unrelated or excessive. The Social Phobia Inventory (SPIN)

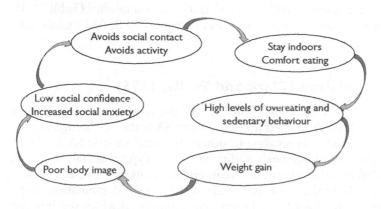

Figure 11.1 Initial problem map for AM.

(Connor, et al., 2000) was administered (after three sessions of weight management assessment) to establish whether AM was experiencing a clinically significant level of SA and if this was excessive. AM's initial score of forty three confirmed that she was experiencing severe levels of SA; above the clinical cut-off of nineteen. An examination of her subscale scores (16 – fear, 18 – avoidance, and 9 – physiological) identified that they were all in line with clinical norms (Connor et al., 2000). An examination and clinical discussion of her individual responses confirmed that her experience of SA was excessive, but clearly related to her obesity.

Treatment plan

The agreed treatment plan was to provide individual CBT based on Clark and Wells (1995). The NICE clinical guidelines (2013) state that the treatment of SA with CBT should consist of up to fourteen sessions of ninety minutes' duration over approximately four months, and include the following:

- Education about social anxiety
- Experiential exercises to demonstrate the adverse effects of self-focused attention and safety-seeking behaviours
- Video feedback to correct distorted negative self-imagery
- Systematic training in externally-focused attention
- Within-session behavioural experiments to test negative beliefs with linked home-work assignments
- Discrimination training or re-scripting to deal with problematic memories of social trauma
- Examination and modification of core beliefs
- Modification of problematic pre- and post-event processing
- Relapse prevention.

(NICE, 2013: p.195)

Treatment goals

At the outset of treatment, collaboratively agreed SA goals were established (Table 11.3). In line with the principles of goal-setting (Locke and Latham, 2002), AM's goals were continually refined and revised.

Social anxiety formulation (Clark and Wells, 1995)

As explained previously, the CBT model utilised with the current case was that of Clark and Wells (1995). They argue that a key aspect of SA is the heightened importance of presenting a favourable impression to others (in social situations), whilst at the same time being insecure about one's ability to do so. Typical social situations (triggers) may be divided into those that 'involve interaction, observation, and performance' (NICE, 2013: p.14). In the Clark and Wells model it is the combination of the trigger situation and the activation of core beliefs and assumptions which result in the individual perceiving the situation as threatening. An individual with SA can worry

Table 11.3 Initial agreed treatment goals

Type of goal	Goal statement
Engagement	To contact the SWMS in the event of cancellations.
	To complete agreed homework before each session.
	To engage collaboratively within sessions.
	To highlight difficulties in a timely manner.
Psycho-educational and conceptual	To demonstrate a working understanding of the CBT approach generally.
	To undertake regular 'homework' tasks and be honest in any difficulties encountered.
	To demonstrate a working understanding of Clark and Wells (1995).
	To complete schematic representations of SA using Figure 9.2 from Butler and McManus (2013, p. 263).
Behavioural	To identify and work through an agreed hierarchy of exposure tasks to reverse the process of social avoidance. To reduce reliance on safety behaviours alongside this.
	To be truthful about difficulties in any exposure tasks, behavioural experiments, or surveys.
	To attend an eight-week exercise class.
	To attend a twelve-week psycho-educational weight management group and engage with others in this group via informal discussion tasks.
Cognitive	To be open and honest about internal thoughts, images and emotions, and to be prepared to discuss and scrutinise them.
	To complete negative automatic thought (NAT) records to highlight evidence for and against NATs.
	To describe internal images attached to NATs.
	To work on challenging NATs when evidence against exists.

excessively in advance of a 'feared social situation'. Typical worries relate to doing or saying something that will result in catastrophic social consequences (i.e. perceived negative evaluation by others), which results in a loss of status or rejection alongside excruciating embarrassment and humiliation. Negative automatic thoughts (NATs) are thought to activate three responses which create a maintenance cycle: safety behaviours; self-consciousness; and somatic and cognitive symptoms of anxiety.

Safety behaviours

Someone with SA may avoid certain situations or employ safety behaviours to help cope with anticipated threats. Salkovskis et al. (1999) suggest that safety behaviours 'are intended to avoid disaster, and these responses have the secondary effect of preventing disconfirmation that would otherwise take place' (p.573). Thus, whilst safety behaviours can offer a short-term coping response, in the longer term they have the effect of maintaining a person's anxiety.

Processing self as a social object

Self-consciousness in SA refers to the phenomenon of shifting the focus of attention to the processing of the self. This is often done from the observer perspective (Wells, 1997). However, because this is based on what the person perceives themselves to look like, and is strongly influenced by interoceptive (i.e. bodily or physical sensations) feedback, this results in an exaggerated, inaccurate internal image (i.e. what the person thinks others see).

Somatic and cognitive symptoms

Somatic symptoms of anxiety, which occur in response to the perceived threat, (e.g. increased heart rate, sweating, temperature) maintain the cycle by providing physiological signs of a threat response. This offers feedback to the threat appraisal via NATs and internal images. As well as 'anticipatory threat appraisals', Wells (1997) suggests that socially-anxious individuals engage in 'post-event rumination' (a 'cognitive post-mortem'). This tends to be biased towards an internal focus with an overemphasis on negative aspects. This perpetuates the NATs, feelings, and images, and reinforces the individual's underlying beliefs and assumptions.

Formulation applied to Clark and Wells (1995)

Figure 11.2 conceptualises one example (cross-sectional) formulation (using Clark and Wells, 1995) of a weekly avoidance situation for AM. This often resulted in AM extending her journey home (by an hour). AM felt it was easier to stay on the bus (safety behaviour), and wait until everyone else had left the bus, than risk attempting to exit under the humiliating scrutiny (feared consequence) of others. She viewed this as a functional coping behaviour rather than a safety behaviour. Further, she engaged in considerable pre- and post- event rumination and imagined a wide range of catastrophic outcomes (e.g. getting stuck/squashing others; everyone on the bus pointing and laughing at her), if she did not 'cope' (avoid) by staying on the bus. She visualised herself as 'Eleroo' (elephant TV character) and estimated her size as similar to an 'elephant on two legs'. She felt her use of a 'cartoon character' made it easier to cope with her tragic sense of reality.

AM reported engaging in pre- and post-rumination of various feared situations/consequences on a daily basis (i.e. especially whenever she left her home). She discussed a number of examples where she had felt frozen to the spot and unable to move. This occurred regularly whenever she was in a public space (e.g. waiting for buses, travelling on buses, walking to and from a bus stop, etc.).

Safety behaviours

AM described various behaviours which had become stronger and more prevalent. At the extreme, this involved complete avoidance. Examples of safety behaviours included: refusing to attend job interviews; using back alleyways/lanes when walking; leaving and returning home during school hours (to avoid children). She moved from attending supermarkets at quieter times to ordering all her shopping online. She

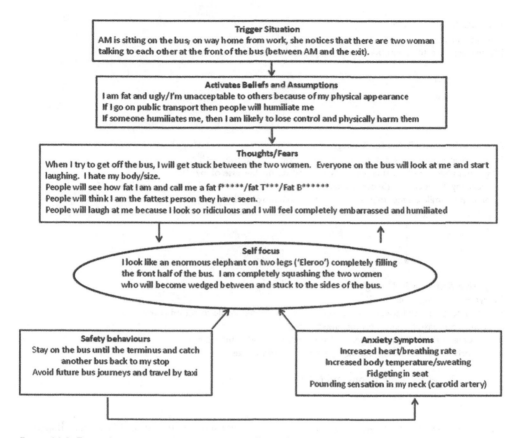

Figure 11.2 Formulation based on Clark and Wells (1995).

rebuffed social engagements with her immediate family ('safe zones'). AM described wearing several T-shirts to 'hide' her sweat and layers of fat. Further, she had worn a hooded top as a 'security blanket' for seven years to hide her 'rolls of fat'.

Somatic and cognitive symptoms

AM's anxiety symptoms included increases in heart/breathing rates; body temperature, and sweating. She described these as worst when anticipating an event rather than during post-event processing. Her typical NATs pertained to over-estimation of threats of humiliation and inability to cope (See Figure 11.2).

Processing self as a social object

AM's visual self-images were both distorted and exaggerated. Her perception of her size was completely out of proportion: viewing herself as an elephant character (Eleroo) with an enormous stomach. Further, she exaggerated the level and visibility of her sweating, especially under her arms. The longitudinal aspects relating to

Core Beliefs:
I am fat and ugly
I'm unacceptable to others because of my physical appearance

Assumptions and Rules for Living:
If I go out in a busy public space, then everyone will stare at me
If I go on public transport then people will humiliate me because of my size
If I wear my 'hooded top' (Security Blanket) then people will be less likely to see my layers of fat
If someone humiliates me, then I am likely to lose control and physically harm them

Negative Automatic Thoughts
Everyone is staring at me
I'm going to get stuck between two people on a bus and be unable to get off at my stop
I'm going to squash the person sitting next to me
The people at the bus stop are going to verbally abuse and humiliate me
People driving passed me are staring at me because of my size

Figure 11.3 Beliefs, assumptions and NATs.

her underlying beliefs and assumptions are represented in Table 11.2 (pre-disposing and precipitating). Figure 11.3 shows examples of how AM's beliefs and assumptions linked to her NATs. The aforementioned formulations were conceptualised in collaboration with AM.

Process of therapy

Having developed a shared understanding of AM's difficulties, the next phase of the formulation-informed intervention involved engaging AM in some psycho-education and graded exposure work. In addition, CBT work incorporated experiential exercises to demonstrate the adverse effects of self-focused attention, and the modification of problematic pre and post-event processing using behavioural experiments with linked thought records. This was followed by a discussion of interpersonal processes and relapse prevention.

Psycho-education and graded exposure

Self-help materials (Butler and McManus, 2013) were provided as a psycho-educational resource. Initially, AM found it difficult to understand the subtle differences between adaptive avoidant coping responses and safety behaviours (Thwaites and Freeston, 2005). She viewed her (avoidant) coping as entirely functional. For example, when initially challenging her avoidance of public space/scrutiny, AM employed various 'safety behaviours' (e.g. using headphones to walk to the local shops). The use of Socratic Dialogue (Padesky, 1993) helped AM to understand the rationale for dropping safety behaviours, and she subsequently reduced their use.

Exercises to demonstrate adverse effects of self-focused attention and safety seeking

AM systematically worked through her graded exposure tasks (Table 11.4) alongside work to shift her attentional focus. Initially, in-session experiments, practicing switching from an internal to external focus of attention (e.g. hearing the air conditioning system; music from the gym), helped AM to understand the adverse effect of self-focussed attention. Next, imagery was used to help AM experience socially-anxious situations (e.g. walking to the shops; travelling by bus), and to rate her levels of anxiety (0–10 scale) when internally or externally focused. AM discovered that when she was self-focussed (thinking everyone was looking, pointing, sniggering), her anxiety ratings were higher. When she switched to an external focus, her anxiety ratings decreased. We built on this work via *in-vivo* exposure (e.g. in the gym/studio/reception), at increasingly busier times. She was able to see others were not looking at her. Next, she practiced outside therapy. Over time, AM worked through her exposure hierarchy and reduced her safety behaviours (Table 11.4).

Use of behavioural experiments and linked thought records.

As AM worked through her graded exposure tasks, she kept Thought Record Sheets (www.getselfhelp.co.uk) to help her to identify her NATs, linked emotions (e.g. fear) and behaviours. AM identified her unhelpful images (e.g. getting 'stuck' or 'squashing others' in a cinema/bus/theatre; 'everyone looking'; 'pointing and laughing') and formulated various examples (e.g. Figure 11.2). This strengthened her conceptualisation of her SA and helped her understand the importance of challenging her NATs with balanced thoughts. As she dropped the safety behaviours/avoidance, she was able to progress through her exposure hierarchy.

Relapse prevention work

Arguably, as with therapeutic endings (Malan, 2001), relapse prevention work begins early in the therapeutic journey. Viewing lapses as normal, expected, and something to learn from was encouraged from the start (Collins, 2005). An early lapse, reframed as 'an opportunity', involved size-related negative comments from teenagers. Padesky (1997; 2008) argues that encouraging SA clients to practice the 'Assertive Defence of Self' can be useful, when the threat of negative evaluation is probable, and that this may be used alongside Clark and Wells (1995). Given AM's task of engaging in exposure tasks within a lower socio-economic area of the North East of England, it was deemed likely she may be exposed to negative comments. Consequently, we were able to develop useful internal phrases for AM to utilise alongside her exposure work (e.g. Yes I am overweight, but I'm doing something about it; I've lost three stone in the last year; I'm now making effective changes to my food intake and activity

Table 11.4 AM's graded exposure tasks

Process goal	Previous safety behaviour or avoidance	Target days	Done
Walk to the local shops via main public route	Travel via back alley	7–14	✓
Purchase meat from a local butcher	Online shopping	14–28	✓
Purchase fresh fruit/vegetables via local shop	Online shopping	14–28	✓
Attend weekly Psych-educational group on weight management	Avoidance	60	✓
Attend local cinema with sister	'Netflix'	60	✓
Attend local cinema alone	'Netflix'	90	✓
Travel to work via bus (weekly to daily)	Taxi or lift	14–90	✓
Attend 'Easyline (exercise) Classes'	Avoid	90–180	✓
Attend work social event (daytime)	Avoid	90–180	✓
Attend a work social event (evening)	Avoid	120–180	✓
Attend large social event	Avoid	180	✓
Purchase bike and build up the length of cycle trips	Avoid	210	✓
Shopping in the city centre (weekday)	Avoid	180–240	✓
Bowling with family members	Avoid	240	✓
Attend 15 week-Exercise Referral Scheme	Avoid	240	✓
Day out (beach)	Avoid	270	✓
Shopping in the city centre (weekend)	Avoid	270	✓
Attend gym minimum of twice per week	Avoid	365	✓
Cinema in the city centre (daytime)	Avoid	365	
Travel by train to London to see the show 'Wicked'	Avoid	365	
Cinema in city centre (evening)	Avoid	365	
Shopping in city centre	Avoid	365	
To start driving lessons	Avoid (seat belt size limitations)	365+	
To cycle to work	Avoid	365+	
To go on a plane to Paris	Avoid	365+	

levels). Another significant lapse occurred, after eight months, when AM fell from her bicycle. We discussed this, with appropriate humour, and identified pragmatic coping strategies to minimise reoccurrences. AM got her bike repaired and started riding again.

Clinical outcomes

At the point of writing this case study, AM was still receiving treatment from SWMS and had lost three stone. Her weight loss continued to reinforce treatment gains from the SA work. Whilst the discreet treatment intervention for SA was complete, the exposure work continued within the SWMS context. The discussion that follows focuses on the CBT SA work only.

Quantitative data

AM's scores on the Hospital Anxiety and Depression Scale (HADS) (Zigmond and Snaith, 1983) reduced for both anxiety (11 to 4) and depression (15 to 5), indicating a movement from moderate to mild levels. This supports clinical observations that AM was experiencing less anxiety and improved mood. AM's SPIN score reduced to 25 (9 – fear, 11 – avoidance, 5 – physiological), indicating a reduction (i.e. severe to moderate). While she continued to report elevated scores on some items, ongoing graded exposure tasks and the continued use of the Assertive Defence of Self helped to address her fears regarding critical comments from others. While these results are encouraging, it is arguably the qualitative data that provides the compelling human story regarding AM's treatment outcomes.

Qualitative data

AM reports that she now socialises with colleagues on a regular basis and that this has improved her interactions at work (i.e. expanded conversational repertoire). She has started applying for jobs and feels ready to attend interviews. She volunteers for the Royal National Institute of Blind People (RNIB) and recently met a regional representative in a city centre café. AM is engaging in more social activities generally. She now walks via main streets, and is attending an exercise class and the gym. She is also now planning more extensive social activities (e.g. overnight theatre trips), and her longer term goal is to travel abroad. She would also like to get to a point of cycling to work. AM's personal functioning has significantly improved. She decided to give her father 'another chance' and describes this relationship as 'improving'. She purchased a bicycle and is now cycling longer distances. She is using public transport on a regular basis and, consequently, spends less money on taxis, less time in her house, and her 'emotional eating' has reduced. AM is wearing clothes that have not fitted for over five years. Towards the end of her SA treatment, AM arrived without her blue hooded 'security blanket'. The aforementioned improvements are based on self-reports and therapist observations. However, her detailed narrative suggests a high level of authenticity. In one of her last SA appointments, AM voluntarily recalled a conversation she had earlier that day:

> The weight management service has saved my life . . . if it was not for that service, I would have become one of those people that get so fat they need a crane to get them out [the house] . . . I think I would have given up my job and totally lost my independence.
>
> AM (August 2013)

Chapter summary

This chapter has focussed on the process of applying psychological theory to practice within the context of health and exercise-related behaviour change. By presenting a detailed clinical case example, we have argued that there is a considerable need for the psychology of health behaviour to be routinely and inherently embedded within a wider case-formulation process. It is hoped that the information presented has demonstrated that the routine implementation of formulation-informed assessment and intervention work, within clinical settings, is likely to facilitate the application of relevant theory to practice and enhance clinical outcomes. However, while this chapter seeks to encourage a move toward more intensive ways of facilitating heath behaviour change, in practice, this may be difficult to achieve without some structural or organisational reforms. Specifically, although the case study presented is an accurate reflection of the clinical practices currently adopted within a SWMS, many existing health behaviour change settings and intervention practices (described in other chapters of this book) reflect the fact that limited resources and expertise are available to implement such approaches. Therefore, it may also be necessary for health service providers and authorities to consider the need for additional, clinically-trained roles within existing heath promotional structures. This may involve the provision of training for existing healthcare workers in a range of skills more commonly adopted in clinical psychology settings.

Future research

As the concept of case formulation has only recently begun to emerge within the exercise sciences literature (Gardner and Moore, 2005; Hutchison and Johnston, 2013), there remains considerable potential for future research in this area. Specifically, although compelling arguments have been presented, which appear to highlight a need for case formulation to be routinely incorporated into the psychology of exercise-related behaviour change, no attempts have yet been made to empirically examine the efficacy of such approaches. Therefore, future research is needed to examine the effectiveness and cost-effectiveness of formulation-based interventions for addressing exercise and health-related behaviour change. Additionally, most existing approaches to case formulation are informed by theory derived from the clinical psychology and psychotherapy literature. Therefore, there is a clear need for future research to explore ways of better facilitating the inclusion of existing exercise and health psychology-related theory into the formulation process. This may also necessitate further integration of existing physical and mental health-related theory, alongside further exploration of reciprocal links between physical conditions (e.g. obesity) and mental health-related difficulties (e.g. anxiety and depression).

Study tasks

1   Making reference to relevant literature, compare and contrast the collaborative case formulation-based approach described in this chapter, with other prominent intervention approaches used in exercise psychology or PARS.
2   Write a short summary, which describes what is meant by the Medical Model and discusses the pros and cons of its application to difficulties commonly encountered within applied health and exercise behaviour change settings.
3   Read and summarise the British Psychological Society's (2011) *Good practice guidelines on the use of psychological formulation* (freely available at: http:// shop.bps.org.uk/), and consider its relevance to the field of applied exercise psychology.
4   Using the 5 Ps model of formulation (see Tables 11.1 and 11.2) formulate a case from your own practice or applied experience.

Further reading

For a more detailed introduction to the theory and practice of formulation from a range of theoretical perspectives, readers are encouraged to refer to the following text:

Johnstone, L. and Dallos, R. (2006). *Formulation in psychology and psychotherapy*. London: Routledge.

For a more detailed account of how formulation has been applied to understand a range of challenging and complex presentations, to improve therapeutic/treatment outcomes, see:

Tarrier, N. (2006). *Case formulation in cognitive behaviour therapy*. London: Routledge.

For detailed guidance on how to collaboratively develop case formulations within the context of cognitive behavioural therapy work, see:

Kuyken, W., Padesky, C.A. and Dudley, R. (2009). *Collaborative case conceptualization: Working effectively with clients in cognitive-behavioral therapy*. New York: Guilford Press.

For more specific reading on the application of clinical formulation to health and exercise related clinical settings, see:

Gardner, F.L. and Moore, Z.E. (2005).Using a case formulation approach in sport psychology consulting. *The Sport Psychologist*, 19, 430–45.
Hutchison, A.J. and Johnston, L.H. (2013). Exploring the potential of case formulation within exercise psychology. *Journal of Clinical Sports Psychology*, 7, 60–76.
Johnston, L.H., Hutchison, A. and Ingham, B. (2011). The utility of biopsychosocial models of clinical formulation within stress and coping theory and applied practice. In T.J. Davenport (Ed). *Managing stress: from theory to application* (pp. 261–91). New York: Nova.

Notes

1 The terms 'case formulation' and 'case conceptualisation' are used interchangeably throughout this chapter.
2 The terms 'social phobia' and 'social anxiety' are used interchangeably within the literature. NICE (2013) guidance on social anxiety uses the term 'social anxiety' and states that it was formerly termed 'social phobia' (p.14).
3 To protect the anonymity of this case, some demographic information has been changed.

References

American Psychiatric Association (2013). *Diagnostic and statistical manual of mental disorders*. 5th ed. Arlington, VA: American Psychiatric Publishing.
Beck, A.T. (1976). *Cognitive therapy and the emotional disorders*. New York: International Universities Press.
Beck, A.T., Rush, A.J., Shaw, B.F. and Emery, G. (1979). *Cognitive therapy of depression*. New York: Guildford Press.
Breckon, J., Johnston, L. and Hutchison, A. (2008). Physical activity counseling content and competency: a systematic review. *Journal of Physical Activity and Health*, 5, 398–417.
British Psychological Society (BPS), (2011). *Good practice guidelines on the use of psychological formulation*. Leicester: BPS.

Buckworth, J., Dishman, R., O'Connor, P. and Tomporowski, P. (2013). *Exercise psychology.* 2nd ed. Champaign, Illinois: Human Kinetics.

Butler, G. and McManus, F. (2013). Social phobia. In R. Shafran, L. Brosan, and P. Cooper. *The complete CBT guide for anxiety* (pp. 243–87). London: Robinson.

Carr, A. and McNulty, M. (2006). The handbook of adult clinical psychology. An evidence based practice approach. London: Routledge.

Clark, D.M. and Wells, A. (1995). A cognitive model of social phobia. In R.G. Heimberg, M. R. Liebowitz, D.A. Hope and F.R. Schneier (Eds). *Social phobia. Diagnosis, assessment and treatment* (pp. 69–93). London: Guilford.

Collins, R.L. (2005). Relapse prevention for eating disorders and obesity. In G.A. Marlatt and D.M. Donovan, (Eds). *Relapse prevention: maintenance strategies in the treatment of addictive behaviours* (pp. 248–75). London: Guilford.

Connor, K.M., Davidson, J.R.T., Churchill, L.E., Sherwood, A., Foa, E. and Wesler, R.H. (2000). Psychometric properties of the Social Phobia Inventory (SPIN). *British Journal of Psychiatry*, 176, 379–86.

Crellin, C. (1998). Origins and social contexts of the term 'formulation' in psychological case-reports. *Clinical Psychology Forum*, 112, 18–28.

Crone, D., Johnston, L., Gidlow, C. Henley, C. and James, D. (2008). Uptake and participation in physical activity referral schemes in the UK: an investigation of patients referred with mental health problems. *Issues in Mental Health Nursing*, 29, 1088–97.

Dimidjian, S., Hollon, S.D., Dobson, K.S., Schmaling, K.B., Kohlenberg, R., Addis, M. and Jacobson, N.S. (2006). Randomized trial of behavioral activation, cognitive therapy, and antidepressant medication in the acute treatment of adults with major depression. *Journal of Consulting and Clinical Psychology*, 74, 658–70.

Dudley, R. and Kuyken, W. (2006). Formulation in cognitive behavioural therapy: 'There is nothing either good or bad, but thinking makes it so.' In L. Johnstone, and R. Dallos (Eds.), *Formulation in psychology and psychotherapy* (pp. 17–46). London: Routledge.

Gardner, F.L. and Moore, Z.E. (2005). Using a case formulation approach in sport psychology consulting. *The Sport Psychologist*, 19, 430–45.

Gidlow, C. and Murphy, R. (2009). Physical activity promotion in primary health care. In L. Dugdill, D. Crone, and R. Graham (Eds.), *Physical activity and health promotion* (pp. 21–38). Oxford: Blackwell.

Harper, D. and Moss, D. (2003). A different kind of chemistry? Reformulating 'formulation.' *Clinical Psychology*, 17, 8–11.

Harper, D. and Spellman, D. (2006). Social constructionist formulation: telling a different story. In L. Johnstone, and R. Dallos (Eds.), *Formulation in psychology and psychotherapy* (pp. 98–125). London: Routledge.

Haskell, W.L., Lee, I., Pate, R.R., Powell, K.E., Blair, S.N., Franklin, B.A., Macera, C.A., Heath, G.W., Thompson, P.D. and Bauman, A. (2007). Physical activity and public health: updated recommendation for adults from the American College of Sports Medicine and the American Heart Association. *Circulation*, 116, 1081–93.

Hillsdon, M., Foster, C., Cavill, N., Combie, H. and Naidoo, B. (2005). *The effectiveness of public health interventions for increasing physical activity among adults: a review of reviews* (2nd ed.). London: Health Development Agency.

Hutchison, A.J. and Johnston, L.H. (2013). Exploring the potential of case formulation within exercise psychology. *Journal of Clinical Sports Psychology*, 7, 60–76.

Hutchison, A.J., Johnston, L.H. and Breckon, J.D. (2013). A grounded theory of successful physical activity behavior change. *Qualitative Research in Sport, Exercise and Health*, 5(1), 109–26.

James, D.V.B., Mills, H., Crone, D., Johnston, L.H., Morris, C. and Gidlow, C.J. (2009). Factors associated with physical activity referral completion and health outcomes. *Journal of Sports Sciences*, 27, 1007–17.

Johnston, L.H., Breckon, J.D. and Hutchison, A. (2009). Influencing health behaviour: applying theory to practice. In L. Dugdill, D. Crone and R. Graham (Eds). *Physical activity and health promotion* (pp. 21–38). Oxford: Blackwell.

Johnston, L.H., Hutchison, A. and Ingham, B. (2011). The utility of biopsychosocial models of clinical formulation within Stress and Coping Theory and applied practice. In T.J. Davenport (Ed). *Managing stress: from theory to application* (pp. 261–91). New York: Nova.

Johnstone, L. and Dallos, R. (2006). Introduction to formulation. In L. Johnstone, and R. Dallos, (Eds), *Formulation in psychology and psychotherapy* (pp. 1–16). London: Routledge.

Kuyken, W., Padesky, C.A. and Dudley, R. (2009). *Collaborative case conceptualization: working effectively with clients in cognitive-behavioral therapy.* New York: Guilford Press.

Locke, L.A. and Latham, G.P. (2002). Building a practically useful theory of goal setting and task motivation: a 35 year odyssey. *American Psychologist, 57,* 705–17.

Mace, C. and Binyon, S. (2005). Teaching psychodynamic formulation to psychiatric trainees. Part 1: basics of formulation. *Advances in Psychiatric Treatment, 11,* 416–23.

Malan, D.H. (2001). *Individual psychotherapy and the science of psychodynamics.* London: Arnold.

Martell, C.R., Dimidjian, S. and Herman-Dunn, R. (2010). *Behavioural activation for depression.* London: Guilford Press.

Miller, J. and McClelland, L. (2006). Social inequalities formulation: mad, bad, and dangerous to know. In L. Johnstone, and R. Dallos (Eds), *Formulation in psychology and psychotherapy* (pp. 126–53). London: Routledge.

Muller-Riemenschneider, F., Reinhold, T., Nocon, M. and Willich, S.N. (2008). Long-term effectiveness of interventions promoting physical activity: a systematic review. *Preventive Medicine, 47*(4), 354–68.

Mutrie, A., MacIntyre, N., Kirk, P. and Fisher, M. (2004). Effects of a 12-month physical activity counselling intervention on glycaemic control and on the status of cardiovascular risk factors in people with type II diabetes. *Diabetologia, 47,* 821–32.

NICE (2013). Social anxiety disorder: recognition, assessment and treatment. London: NICE.

Padesky, C.A. (1993). Socratic questioning: changing minds or guiding discovery. Keynote address at the European Congress of Behavioural and Cognitive Therapies. London, September 24th.

Padesky, C.A. (1997). A more effective treatment focus for social phobia. *International Cognitive Therapy Newsletter, 11,* 1–3.

Padesky, C.A. (2008). CBT for social anxiety. DVD available at: http://store.padesky.com/dvd_social_anxiety.htm.

Pagoto, S.L., Spring, B., Cook, J.W., McChargue, D. and Schneider, K. (2006). High BMI and reduced frequency and enjoyment of pleasant events. *Personality and Individual Differences, 40*(7), 1421–31.

Pagoto, S., Schneider, K.L., Whited, M.C., Oleski, J.L., Merriam, P., Appelhans, B., Ma, Y., Olendzki, B., Waring, M.E., Busch, A.M., Lemon, S., Ockene, I. and Crawford, S. (2013). Randomized controlled trial of behavioural treatment for co-morbid obesity and depression in women: the Be Active Trial International. *Journal of Obesity, 37*(11), 1427–34.

Persons, J.B. (1989) Cognitive therapy in practice: a case formulation approach. London: Norton.

Prochaska, J.O. and Norcross, J.C. (1994). *Systems of psychotherapy: a transtheoretical analysis.* 4th ed. Pacific Grove, CA: Brooks Cole.

Salkovskis, P.M., Clark, D.M., Hackmann, A., Wells, A. and Gelder, M.G. (1999). An experimental investigation of the role of safety-seeking behaviours in the maintenance of panic disorder with agoraphobia. *Behaviour Research and Therapy, 37,* 559–74.

Shafran, R., Brosan, L. and Cooper, P. (2013). *The complete CBT guide for anxiety.* London: Robinson.

Tarrier, N. (2006). An introduction to case formulation and its challenges. In N. Tarrier (Ed). *Case formulation in cognitive behaviour therapy* (pp. 1–11). London: Routledge.

Thwaites, R. and Freeston, M. (2005). Safety-seeking behaviours: fact or function? How can we clinically differentiate between safety behaviours and adaptive coping strategies across anxiety disorders? *Behavioural and Cognitive Psychotherapy*, 33, 177–88.

Velicer, W.F., Prochaska, J.O., Fava, J.L., Norman, G.J. and Redding, C.A. (1998). Smoking cessation and stress management: applications of the Transtheoretical Model of behaviour change. *Homeostasis*, 38, 216–33.

Wade, D.T. and Halligan, P.W. (2004). Do biomedical models of illness make for good health-care systems? *British Medical Journal*, 329, 1398–1401.

Wells, A. (1997). Cognitive therapy of anxiety disorders. Chichester: Wiley.

Zigmond, A.S. and Snaith, R.P. (1983). The hospital anxiety and depression scale. *Acta Psychiatrica Scandinavica*, 67, 361–70.

Chapter 12

Evidence-based practice in physical activity promotion

Diane Crone and David James

Evidence-based practice in physical activity promotion: a review

The use of physical activity to promote health, and as an adjunct treatment for a range of physical and mental conditions, has been evident in the community and in health-care since the early 1990s (this is discussed in more detail in Chapter 13). The rationale for the development of such interventions was based on evidence of the role of physical activity for health improvement, treatment of some conditions, and in health maintenance (Pate et al., 1995). Programmes were initially developed in relation to the prevention of coronary heart disease, but, more latterly, for the treatment and prevention of a range of conditions including diabetes, depression, and osteoporosis. The evidence for the benefits of physical activity was developed in the latter part of the 20th Century, with much of the modern-day research starting after the Second World War. During the same period, the focus in public health was shifting from purely health education about key topics associated with poor health outcomes (e.g. sanitation) to health promotion. Today, the emphasis has shifted further to a specific focus on the modification of individual behaviours, such as smoking cessation, healthy eating, and physical activity, as evidence regarding the relationship between lifestyle behaviours and non-communicable chronic disease has become better understood. The focus on lifestyle behaviours, and specifically exercise, started to develop following confirmation of the cause and effect relationship between cardiovascular disease and exercise, and specifically the work of Morris and colleagues in the 1960s (Morris et al., 1966). Their seminal paper identified differences between activity levels and the health status of bus conductors (walking, collecting fares) versus bus drivers (sitting, driving the bus). Research continued, and the relationships between dose (i.e. how much – frequency × duration × intensity), and specific health outcomes, were becoming much better understood (Sattelmair et al., 2011), along with the impact on life expectancy and mortality (Lee et al., 2012). Policy has also developed in line with research, with published national recommendations for physical activity (Department of Health, 2011), in addition to public health promotion campaigns such as the UK government's £75 million Change4Life campaign (http://www.nhs.uk/change4life).

These advances in evidence have informed practice and led to the development of programmes, such as exercise referral schemes, that continue to be developed across both primary and secondary care (Crone et al., 2009; Gidlow and Murphy, 2009), and in the community (Crone and Baker, 2009). There is a range of interventions available for a range of population groups and medical conditions, including pro- grammes for weight management, people with cardiac or respiratory conditions, musculo-skeletal conditions (e.g. back pain, knee care programmes), mental health conditions (e.g. depression, anxiety, schizophrenia, and bi-polar), and a range of population-specific programmes, such as those targeting men (generally overweight, middle-aged, and at risk of coronary health disease), women-only exercise groups, and overweight/obese children and their families. Furthermore, since the publication of the Department of Health's *Let's get moving* document (Department of Health, 2009), there has been a surge of interest and corresponding research output integrat- ing behavioural interventions such as motivational interviewing and brief negotia- tion into existing physical activity programmes. These programmes have focused on a range of population groups and medical conditions, for example, coronary heart disease (Eman et al., 2012), diabetes (White et al., 2012), arthritis (Feinglass et al., 2012), multiple sclerosis (Dlugonski et al., 2012), obese children (Wong and Cheng, 2013), and disadvantaged groups (Hardcastle, 2012). As a consequence of this surge in behavioural intervention within a physical activity context, and some evidence, recommendations to help people to become more active (NICE, 2013) embrace these interventions. This has been despite concerns regarding efficacy, and fidelity or con- formity issues (Breckon et al., 2008; Hutchison et al., 2013). This area of evidence- based practice is discussed further in Chapter 13.

Evidence for the efficacy of many of these programmes is varied. Numerous ran- domised controlled trials (RCTs) explored the efficacy of the exercise referral scheme model with mixed findings. For example, an RCT based in Wales (Murphy et al., 2012) concluded that the exercise referral scheme was only effective in increasing physical activity among those referred for CHD risk, and that, for people referred with a mental health condition, there was no influence of physical activity, despite there being an association with reduced anxiety and depression.

Systematic reviews of this research provide further evidence. Of the most recent systematic reviews (Pavey et al., 2012, 2011; Williams et al., 2007), two of the three (Pavey et al., 2012; Williams et al., 2007) incorporated a holistic approach to the inclu- sion criteria by including both observational and population cohort studies. However, Pavey et al. (2011) adopted a stricter inclusion criterion of only including randomised controlled trials. For some years, the RCT approach has been questioned as the most appropriate method of assessing effectiveness in the area of physical activity promo- tion (Dugdill et al., 2005; Gidlow et al., 2008), given the exclusion of evidence from studies that do not meet strict inclusion criteria.

The most recent systematic review (Pavey et al., 2012) was more inclusive, with resulting conclusions more in line with the range of other published studies. They concluded that exercise referral schemes appear more suited to some population groups, and were more effective in terms of uptake and adherence for some medi- cal conditions. It was also suggested that there should be some agreement regard- ing terms such as 'uptake' and 'adherence' to enable a more consistent approach to developing robust evidence, and to better understand programme effectiveness as a health intervention.

Furthermore, some researchers in this area have either used, or called for, a range of evaluation approaches to understand more about the factors associated with outcomes (Clarke et al., 2013; Dugdill and Stratton, 2007; Gidlow and Murphy, 2009; Hanson et al., 2013; Victora et al., 2004). Pavey and colleagues (2012) echoed these calls, and have also concluded that there is a need for alternative methods of evaluation, including both qualitative and quantitative methods. Alternative approaches to evaluation provide evidence that is essential for the development of evidence-based practice. What is important is that the totality of evidence available should be used to determine and shape evidence-based practice. The range of methods and approaches, and their combination in mixed-methods evaluation design, provide evidence of effectiveness for a range of community-based interventions, including, for example, exercise referral schemes (Crone et al., 2008; Gidlow et al., 2007; Hanson et al., 2013; James et al., 2008, 2009; Mills et al., 2012; Vinson and Parker, 2012), walking programmes for people with mental health problems or cognitive impairment (Crone, 2007; van Uffelen et al., 2009), and exercise as an adjunct to therapy for specific population groups (Crone and Guy, 2008; Sharma et al., 2012). These approaches, their application in applied practice, and the evidence they have collectively (and independently) produced, provide the intelligence that should inform practice. Researchers should be mindful and appreciative that evaluating the impact of large-scale community interventions is complex, because they are multi-dimensional, for example, in terms of processes (i.e. pathways, sites for interventions, professionals involved) and the range of outcomes (i.e. physical, mental, social, economic). Therefore, a variety of evidence should be used to make recommendations for practice (Victora et al., 2004). Some of these methods will be explored in more depth later in this chapter, where examples are presented from different methodologies and methods, including quantitative, qualitative, and mixed-methods.

Current national guidance on evaluation for physical activity interventions

A number of problems have been identified in the generation and synthesis of evidence for physical activity interventions, including inconsistency in terms used by researchers, measurement of physical activity, and study duration. Such inconsistencies and differences have led to problems when trying to synthesise the available evidence. In an attempt to support practitioners and evaluators, some guidance has been produced to help inform them about areas to consider in the design, implementation, and evaluation of programmes. Key documents that can be referred to for guidance include:

- National Institute for Health and Care Excellence (NICE) 2006 guidelines for practice in physical activity interventions (NICE, 2006)
- University of Salford's guidelines document focusing specifically on the evaluation of sport and physical activity programmes, including advice on measurement, duration of interventions and evaluation methods (Dugdill and Stratton, 2007)
- The British Heart Foundation's specific guide to the evaluation of exercise referral schemes (BHF, 2010)
- NICE 2013 recommendations document on the use of behavioural interventions for physical activity programmes (NICE, 2013).

Presenting a case: a pragmatic approach to evidence-based practice in physical activity promotion

Approaches for generating evidence include quantitative, qualitative, and mixed-methods evaluation design. The value of these differing approaches is discussed by drawing on published examples from physical activity intervention evaluation in health care and the community.

Generating quantitative evidence

Quantitative approaches are varied, and traditional 'experimental' approaches (e.g. randomised controlled trials) are only a sub-set of those possible. Although the experimental approach is well established in many research areas, where variables are identified and 'controlled', the external validity of the approach and resulting findings are questionable when investigating physical activity promotion initiatives. The potential problems include participant selection, attrition rates, group matching, control of independent variables, and bias. Also, the most important questions for complex public health interventions are simply not suitably addressed through adopting a solely experimental approach (Victora et al., 2004). For example, the type of research question that often needs to be answered relates to which factors are important in uptake, attendance, and completion of the programme because the most pressing issue is increasing physical activity levels. Questions about health benefits as a result of increasing physical activity levels have largely been answered already. Therefore, research approaches that focus on process evaluation, rather than health outcomes, are arguably more useful. Observational approaches are a complementary alternative to experimental approaches, and allow the researcher to observe a number of variables without 'controlling' any of them. The researcher may then conduct analyses to explore outcomes of interest, and the factors that are associated with those outcomes. These are often process-specific (e.g. attendance at the programme), but can also include other (e.g. health) outcomes. Essentially, observational approaches trade off internal validity typical in experimental work in order to increase external (or ecological) validity (Victora et al., 2004).

Conducting observational studies may be no less demanding than experimental approaches, and requires considerable understanding of the physical activity programme (e.g. programme duration and stages), the data captured about the individual participant (e.g. area of residence, age, body mass index), or the range of process variables (e.g. categories of referring health professional, categories of medical condition). Use of data that are gathered routinely as part of the process is recommended (Hanson et al., 2013), as this not only increases study feasibility, but also relates more to actual practice (Gidlow et al., 2008). For routinely collected data to be useful and appropriate to answer important questions requires input from the evaluation team at the beginning of the intervention design process. This can ensure that data collection processes are optimised and embedded in the intervention design, and requires strong partnership between programme commissioners/deliverers and researchers. One disadvantage of routinely-collected data is the reduced possibility for data quality assurance, especially where multiple people are responsible for its collection at points along the pathway. Also, the statistical analyses are complex, and depend on large numbers of participants (usually more than 1000), to allow a range of variables to be considered. Common variables of interest fall into the category of 'explaining variables', i.e. socio-demographic characteristics (age, gender, socio-economic status), referral reason (e.g. medical condition), referring professional (general practitioner, nurse). Explaining variables can then be explored in relation to 'outcome variables', i.e. level of attendance, completion, levels of physical activity, or health outcomes such as change in mental wellbeing, blood pressure, or body mass index.

The following case study provides an example of a quantitative observational investigation of a physical activity intervention within primary care and the community.

Box 12.1 Case study 1

Factors associated with physical activity referral uptake and participation (James et al., 2008).

What was the aim of the study? To examine scheme and individual participant characteristics associated with access (i.e. from the point of initial referral), uptake, and participation in a physical activity referral scheme using a population-based longitudinal design.

What were the research questions? What factors are associated with access, uptake, and participation?

Who were the participants? Patients (n = 2958) referred from primary care into a county-wide physical activity referral scheme over a three-year period.

What was the intervention? Patients, from primary care were referred to an eight to twelve week physical activity referral scheme which involved bi-weekly, supervised exercise sessions at local leisure facilities (leisure centres). Patients' programmes of physical activity were typically gym-based, but also included swimming, circuit, and/or exercise-to-music classes.

Method - what data were collected and how? Data were collected routinely as part of the process of the referral scheme. A coordinator received the referral form from primary care, which included patient demographic information such as age, gender, postcode (for the purposes of assigning them a socio-economic position), reason for referral (e.g. overweight, cardiovascular, respiratory), referring health professional (i.e. general practitioner, practice nurse, physiotherapist) at baseline, and then recorded data for patient progress in terms of access, uptake, and participation in the scheme.

How was this analysed? A well-established technique used in epidemiological research was adopted, known as binary logistic regression. A model was developed for each of the outcomes of interest (e.g., access). Selected explaining variables were entered into each regression model (e.g., referral reason).

What were the findings? Primary referral reason was associated with the coordinator making contact with the participants. In addition to the influence of

(continued)

(continued)

referral reason, females were also more likely to agree to be assigned to a leisure provider. Referral reason and referring health professional were associated with taking up a referral opportunity and older participants and males were more likely to complete the referral.

What were the conclusions and implications for practice? The study concluded that physical activity referral schemes may be less appropriate for those more constrained by time (women, young adults) and those with certain referral reasons (overweight/obesity, mental health conditions). In terms of implications for practice, the findings suggest that more appropriate targeting at the point of referral could improve participation rates, and certain groups appear to experience barriers to participation.

Generating qualitative evidence

There is a range of possible qualitative approaches that can be used to generate evidence for physical activity promotion, including the more commonly used approaches such as ethnography, narrative, case study, grounded theory, and phenomenology (Creswell, 2012). The phenomenon under investigation, or the specific aim of the evaluation or research, determines which approach is appropriate. Explanations of the more common approaches can be found in Creswell (2012). Qualitative approaches used in the development of evidence in physical activity promotion are adopted to explore and understand a range of phenomena or 'interest areas'.

These phenomena or interest areas include, for example, understanding the experiences of the people taking part in interventions, from the point of referral or entry into the programme, and as they progress through (or not) to completion. Understanding what people experience can provide valuable evidence that can influence practice in terms of modifying a protocol for recruitment and referral, adding social support at key stages of referral and uptake, or simply being able to understand whether processes are efficient from the end user perspective. Qualitative research is also used to explore the participants' perceptions, attitudes, and opinions of the intervention, which can help to understand why some people decide to take part in interventions (or not), and about successful completion. Exploring perception and opinions can provide information regarding the social, physical, and cultural aspects associated with the experience of the interventions, and of the interactions experienced between, for example, the other 'actors'. These other actors can include the referring health professionals, the deliverers of the programmes, other people on the intervention, and also the physical environment that it takes place within. These dynamics and interactions can be explored in interviews and focus groups with those who experience them. Qualitative research can also provide further self-reported evidence and support for the outcomes from participation that might be observed in quantitative data. Perceived outcomes from involvement can be health improvements, such as feeling fitter, improved mood, feeling thinner, or behaving differently (e.g. eating more healthily, taking more physical activity, taking less medication). Many of these reported changes and outcomes are often not measurable, or are too onerous or difficult to measure using quantitative methods. There are also occasions when these outcomes are not predicted, and, thus, qualitative findings may provide insight into what can be achieved from participation in interventions that those commissioning them or delivering them had not anticipated and, therefore, what other indicators should be measured in quantitative evaluation.

Qualitative evidence can often help to explain what is actually happening in schemes and assist in understanding more about the processes, both formal and informal, that exist for all the actors within interventions. Data are typically captured through interviews and focus groups, and require in-depth interpretation rather than statistical analysis. Qualitative data are particularly suited to answering questions such as

- What is happening here and why it is happening?
- What are the experiences of the patients going through the programme?
- What are the dynamics between the different 'actors' and the impact of the processes upon experiences?
- What can we learn about interventions from the people that experience them first hand?

These interpretive questions are designed to provide evaluators with a deeper understanding of all of the dynamics associated with an intervention that is designed to promote physical activity, and also to understand more about the reasons why some people do, and some people don't become more active, or achieve the intended health outcomes.

Commonly, evaluations using qualitative methods collect and interpret data from a range of participants involved in health interventions, including participants (those that take part) (Crone, 2007; Crone et al., 2005; Hardcastle and Taylor, 2001; Little and Lewis, 2006), health professionals (those who refer patients) (Graham et al., 2005), and the providers of the actual intervention (the activity leader) (Moore et al., 2011). Some also include one or more of these participant groups and compare and contrast the findings from each group (Crone et al., 2012; Mills et al., 2012; Owens et al., 2010).

In contrast to quantitative methods, the sample size for qualitative studies is much smaller and does not always require a 'representative' sample. Sample sizes vary depending on the group and the phenomenon under investigation. For example, in Mills et al., (2012), a total of twenty-eight participants were interviewed using focus groups and individual interviews, including seventeen patients, four exercise providers, and seven referring health professionals, whereas Crone (2007) included a sample size of just four. However, the latter investigation focussed on people with severe mental illness where a larger sample size is not always possible, and might not also be necessary for the specific research question and method of analysis (e.g. Grounded Theory vs. Interpretative Phenomenology). Furthermore, a representative sample is not necessarily required for qualitative research studies. Many researchers use purposive sampling (Strauss and Corbin, 1998) where a particular population group is identified and sought to understand the specific views of that population; e.g. people that complete a programme, or people with a particular medical condition.

The following case study provides an example of a qualitative investigation of a physical activity intervention within secondary care, in a mental health care setting.

Box 12.2 Case study 2

A qualitative approach to understanding mental health service users' experiences of a sport/exercise intervention in the treatment of their mental health problem (Crone and Guy, 2008).

What was the aim of the study? To investigate the experiences and perceived role of sports therapy for service users (patients) in a mental health trust in England.

What were the research questions? Topics under investigation included service users' motivations for participation, their experiences of the intervention, their perceptions of the role of the intervention, and their perceived benefits from participation.

Who were the participants? Service users (n=11) of a mental health trust. Participants were: between eighteen and sixty five years old, a service user of the trust, involved in the physical activity intervention during 2005, and consenting to be interviewed about their experiences of the intervention.

What was the intervention? The intervention consisted of physical activity sessions twice weekly: both outpatient (away from the mental health unit) and inpatient (situated at the unit) sessions. Sessions included badminton, fitness gym, water aerobics, and occasional 10-pin bowling. Patients had to pay for the sessions that were held at local leisure facilities, such as water aerobics. Generally, sessions were for five to six people, and participants in this study had been taking part from between two months and four years.

Method - what data were collected and how? Focus groups were undertaken, and participants attended one of two groups available. Discussions were facilitated through a semi-structured interview schedule designed to elicit relevant discussions. Focus groups were recorded and transcribed verbatim, and any information that could lead to the identification of participants, physical activity staff, or specific sports groups was removed, anonymised, or replaced with pseudonyms to ensure the confidentiality of participants, sports group, and staff.

How was this analysed? The process of analysis initially involved transcripts being scrutinised through close reading, to ensure the researchers were fully immersed in the data and understood participants' perspectives. Inductive analysis, through a series of coding (a thorough sorting of text units i.e. quotations that includes refining and comparing the content of the codes to refine their final content) produced a series of themes. These themes were then analysed further using a conceptual framework (a diagrammatic representation of the findings) that supports the written text in the themes, and further helps to explain the subjective experiences of the intervention from the perspectives of these participants.

What were the findings? Central to participants' subjective experiences was the 'taking part', i.e., participating in the intervention, and factors shaping that included the theme 'factors affecting participation' that had to be overcome for participation to occur, with 'previous experience', 'attitudes and opinions', and 'perceived role of sports therapy' potentially helping people to shape a response to these factors, and to overcome them. Ultimately, the 'reasons for participation' theme was a causal condition as it impacted directly on the core category. Participation itself, or 'taking part', as a category, was a conduit, because once sports therapy had been participated in, participants had a subjective experience of it, and the consequences of perceived benefits could be enjoyed, and consequential improvements suggested.

What were the conclusions and implications for practice? A number of conclusions and recommendations were made from this study. These included:

- Mental health professionals (e.g. activity leaders, physiotherapists, psychiatrists, mental health nurses) have an important role in facilitating service user's access into physical activity programmes.
- Professionals can act as gatekeepers and have a pivotal role encouraging participation and explaining its role and evidence base.
- Health care professionals have a role in assisting patients in accessing these services, and enabling them to understand and appreciate the role of exercise, as therapy, in their treatment.
- The research added further support to the use of physical activity in mental health services, identifying its important role in the lives of the people that take part and become a more integral part of a client-centred, contemporary, evidence-based mental health service.

Generating mixed-methods evidence

The two examples presented in this chapter demonstrate that both qualitative and quantitative methods of generating evidence provide insightful and informative perspectives, and allow different research questions to be addressed (O'Cathain et al., 2008). These two approaches can also be used together (mixed or combined) to develop evidence about a combined phenomenon such as the concept of success in exercise referral schemes (Mills et al., 2012), and have been promoted as useful research responses to increasing complexity in social problems (Greene and Caracelli, 1997). In terms of being a combined approach and a method in its own right, mixed-methods research provides an interesting paradox for the traditional researcher, given the traditional discordance between the paradigms they both reside within (Onwuegbuzie and Collins, 2007).

Generating evidence in primary care-based physical activity using a mixed-methods design provides an opportunity to ask different questions. The approach captures the potential of both components by using data to develop a combined response to the research questions (Sandelowski et al., 2006). Principally, mixed-methods combines or mixes both types of evidence-generation method. There are many mixed-methods research designs (Onwuegbuzie et al., 2009; Teddlie and Tashakkori, 2009). A simple explanation of the approach would be to consider the timings of the two components and the relationship to each other in terms of data generation. For example, if the quantitative and qualitative components are undertaken at the same time, it is classed as a concurrent design; or when the two components occur one after the other, it is described as a sequential design (Onwuegbuzie and Collins, 2007; Onwuegbuzie et al., 2009). In mixed-methods research, there are many considerations regarding the placing and relationship of the two components and of the philosophical underpinnings, not just of the mixed-methods approach *per se*, but also of the design and relationship between the two components adopted, which will be different for each study (Onwuegbuzie et al., 2009). The sampling design for each component is more complicated than in quantitative or qualitative research alone, and the subsequent analysis of the data and its presentation requires careful consideration to ensure that the study utilises mixed-methods to its full extent (Onwuegbuzie and Collins, 2007). Useful texts to fully understand the nuances of mixed methods are Teddlie and Tashakkori (2009) and Creswell and Clark (2007).

The implications for practice from this pragmatic and alternative approach to evaluation potentially provide the most complete and useful results (Johnson et al., 2007). In doing so, it offers practitioners and policy makers a much richer understanding of what is happening in physical activity promotion interventions, especially in terms of the processes and outcomes of such programmes.

Box 12.3 Case study 3

Exploring the perceptions of success in an exercise referral scheme: a mixed method investigation (Mills et al., 2012)

What was the aim of the study? To understand the concept of success in an exercise referral scheme by combining a qualitative component which included exploring experiences and perceptions of the three groups of participants (the patients, exercise providers, and referring health professionals) and the analysis of quantitative measures routinely collected through the scheme. The aim was to explain the concept of 'success' and how it was perceived and understood from the perspective of all parties involved in the scheme.

What were the research questions? To explore the concept and complexity of success within the exercise referral scheme context. To explore and identify the components of 'success' through the comparison, contradiction, and integration of both the qualitative and quantitative components of the research design.

Who were the participants? For the quantitative aspect, participants were patients referred onto an exercise referral scheme (n = 1315). For the qualitative aspect, there were three groups of participants (n = 28), patients (n = 17), exercisers providers (n=4), and referring health professionals (n = 7).

What was the intervention? Patients from primary care were referred to a twenty-six-week exercise referral scheme. A physical activity programme was agreed between each patient and the exercise provider [fitness professional/exercise scientist] which included goal setting and the patients preferred type of exercise. The activity programme was reviewed every six weeks where changes were made to the goals or exercise plan, if required. Patients could take part in either/both group and individual exercise sessions, which included the gym, exercise studio, and the swimming pool, at one of five local leisure centres.

Method – what data were collected and how? Quantitative data included an observational, population-based cohort design which used routinely collected data from the exercise referral scheme. Data included patient sociodemographic characteristics (age, gender, ethnicity, occupation [which enabled a classification for socio-economic position], and primary referral reason, i.e. obesity). These explaining variables were associated with three outcome variables: completion of the referral scheme, weight loss (body mass index change), and mean arterial pressure reduction.

Qualitative data included interview transcripts from focus groups with patients ($n = 4$ focus groups) and individual interviews with exercise providers ($n = 4$) and health professionals ($n = 7$).

How was this analysed? Quantitative data were analysed using a three-stage binary logistic regression to identify patient sociodemographic characteristics with the outcome variables of completion, weight loss, and mean arterial pressure reduction. Qualitative analysis was informed by grounded theory methodology, which involves a series of sequential coding processes and an eventual development of a theoretical framework to explain the phenomena under investigation, in this case the concept of success.

The results from the two components were given equal weight and were mixed by converging the two components and then comparing and contrasting the findings of both during interpretation.

What were the findings? The qualitative findings produced a conceptual construction of success which was presented in a diagrammatic form. The diagram identified a wide range of concepts within success which included empowerment, inclusion, and confidence, and explained the interrelationships between them for participants. The quantitative data provided showed that 57% completed their exercise programme, 33.3% achieved a weight loss, and 49.2% reduced blood pressure, and demonstrated a number of relationships including completion and increased age, and a reduction in body mass index for those who completed. In mixing the methods, the findings highlighted the multidimensional and complexity of the concept of success in an exercise referral scheme and highlighted that the more traditional and accepted concepts of success such as attendance, weight loss, and blood pressure reduction featured within a more holistic view of success which incorporated the psychological and social aspects as both influences of success and outcomes associated with it for all parties.

What were the conclusions and implications for practice? The findings highlight the holistic concept of success for those that are involved in an exercise referral scheme. In highlighting these, it stresses the need for schemes in practice to ensure outcomes reflect this range of success measures and outcomes, for both the participants taking part, and for the professionals involved in their design, delivery, and evaluation.

Chapter summary

This chapter provides a critical view of what evidence-based practice can be, within the context of physical activity interventions for health. It has adopted a holistic concept of evidence and presented quantitative, qualitative, and mixed-methods approaches to evidence generation in this area of applied interventions. The three approaches presented in this chapter each have their own merits and value, and should be applied dependent on the research/evaluation questions for each phenomenon or intervention under investigation. They complement the existing epidemiological evidence regarding the role of physical activity for health improvement, and add to the controlled trial evidence that exists for specific interventions, such as exercise referral schemes. Researchers, policy makers, and practitioners should be aware of the range of approaches to generate evidence that can be used to fully understand the processes and outcomes of interventions, including highly context-specific factors that exist within interventions.

Future research

Physical activity promotion has, for many years, been informed by evidence associating physical activity levels with health outcomes. Furthermore, traditional 'experimental' approaches to evidence generation were initially applied to physical activity interventions. Whilst these approaches reveal important findings within 'controlled' environments for some research questions, most of the current questions are not addressed by this approach. Physical activity takes place within the context of a physical, economic, cultural, and social environment more generally, and there is a specific intervention environment for many initiatives. A range of alternative approaches for evidence generation are required, often necessitating a multi-disciplinary approach reflecting the complexity of the context and intervention (Crone and Baker, 2012). Future research in the area of physical activity promotion should embrace the range of available research approaches to answer the most pressing questions, taking account of the context in which the interventions are taking place. A better understanding of the factors associated with successful outcomes is required, given the persistent levels of physical inactivity in the population and the associated health and wellbeing consequences.

Study tasks

The tasks below will encourage you to consider what you have read about in this chapter in relation to evidence and practice.

1   Using a recently-published mixed-methods evaluation of a sport or physical activity programme, explain how the findings benefited from the multi-method approach.
2   Find an example of a controlled trial and an observational study and consider the limitations of each research approach.
3   For a physical activity initiative that you are familiar with, design an evaluation demonstrating that you have considered the following:

a   Identified the evaluation questions to be addressed
b   Areas of interest that the evaluation could focus on, i.e. physical, social, mental outcomes, or a holistic approach that involves all three areas
c   What data would be used in the evaluation, i.e. what data are to be collected, when and from whom?
d   The range of possible approaches, i.e. quantitative, qualitative, or mixed-methods, that could be used to undertake the evaluation.

Further reading and resources

The following articles and text books are recommended for this chapter:

British Heart Foundation (BHF) (2010). A toolkit for the design, implementation and evaluation of exercise referral schemes: a guide to evaluating exercise referral schemes. Loughborough: BHF National Centre for Physical Activity and Health.
Cresswell, J. W., and Clark, V. L. P. (2007). *Designing and conducting mixed methods research*. California: Sage.
Dugdill, L., and Stratton, G. (2007). *Evaluating sport and physical activity interventions: a guide for practitioners*. Salford: University of Salford.
NICE (2006). Four commonly used methods to increase physical activity: brief interventions in primary care, exercise referral schemes, pedometers and community-based exercise programmes for walking and cycling. *Public health intervention guidance 2*. London: National Institute for Health and Clinical Excellence.
NICE (2013). Physical activity: brief advice for adults in primary care. *NICE public health guidance 44*. London: National Institute for Health and Clinical Excellence.

References

BHF. (2010). A toolkit for the design, implmentation and evaluation of exercise referral schemes: a guide to evaluating exercise referral schemes. Loughborough: BHF National Centre for Physical Activity and Health.
Breckon, J. D., Johnston, L. H., and Hutchison, A. (2008). Physical activity counseling content and competency: a systematic review. *Journal of Physical Activity and Health*, 5(3), 398–417.
Clarke, B., Gillies, D., Illari, P., Russo, F., and Williamson, J. (2013). The evidence that evidence-based medicine omits. *Preventive Medicine*, 57(6), 745–7. doi: http://dx.doi.org/10.1016/j.ypmed.2012.10.020.
Creswell, J. W. (2012). *Qualitative inquiry and research design: choosing among five approaches*. London: Sage.
Creswell, J. W., and Clark, V. L. P. (2007). Designing and conducting mixed methods research.
Crone, D. (2007). Walking back to health: a qualitative investigation into service users' experiences of a walking project. *Issues in Mental Health Nursing*, 28(2), 167–83.
Crone, D., and Baker, C. (2009). Physical activity interventions in the community. In L. Dugdill, D. Crone and R. Murphy (Eds.), *Physical activity and health promotion: evidence-based approaches to practice* (1st ed., pp. 110–27). UK: Wiley-Blackwell.
Crone, D., and Baker, C. (2012). Promoting health in 2012: embracing alternative evaluation designs, working practices and service delivery modes. *Journal of Public Health*, 20(5), 477–8. doi: 10.1007/s10389-012-0525-8.
Crone, D., and Guy, H. (2008). 'I know it is only exercise, but to me it is something that keeps me going': a qualitative approach to understanding mental health service users' experiences of sports therapy. *International Journal of Mental Health Nursing*, 17(3), 197–207.

Crone, D., Heaney, L., and Owens, C. S. (2009). Physical activity and mental health. In L. Dugdill, D. Crone and R. Murphy (Eds.), *Physical activity and health promotion: evidence-based approaches to practice* (1st ed., pp. 198–212). UK: Wiley-Blackwell.

Crone, D., Johnston, L. H., Gidlow, C., Henley, C., and James, D. V. B. (2008). Uptake and participation in physical activity referral schemes in the UK: an investigation of patients referred with mental health problems. *Issues in Mental Health Nursing*, 29(10), 1088–97.

Crone, D. M., O'Connell, E. E., Tyson, P., Clark-Stone, F., Opher, S., and James, D. V. B. (2012). 'It helps me make sense of the world': the role of an art intervention for promoting health and wellbeing in primary care – perspectives of patients, health professionals and artists. *Journal of Public Health*, 1–6.

Crone, D., Smith, A., and Gough, B. (2005). 'I feel totally at one, totally alive and totally happy': a psycho-social explanation of the physical activity and mental health relationship. *Health Education Research*, 20(5), 600–11.

Department of Health. (2009). *Let's get moving London*: Department of Health.

Department of Health. (2011). *Start active, stay active: a report on physical activity for health from the four home countries' Chief Medical Officers*. London: HMSO.

Dlugonski, D., Motl, R. W., Mohr, D. C., and Sandroff, B. M. (2012). Internet-delivered behavioral intervention to increase physical activity in persons with multiple sclerosis: sustainability and secondary outcomes. *Psychology, Health and Medicine*, 17(6), 636–51.

Dugdill, L., Graham, R. C., and McNair, F. (2005). Exercise referral: the public health panacea for physical activity promotion? A critical perspective of exercise referral schemes; their development and evaluation. *Ergonomics*, 48(11–14), 1390–1410.

Dugdill, L., and Stratton, G. (2007). *Evaluating sport and physical activity interventions: a guide for practitioners* Retrieved from: http://usir.salford.ac.uk/3148/1/Dugdill_and_Stratton_2007.pdf.

Eman, A., Holly, B., and Richard, W. (2012). Behavioural intervention to increase physical activity among patients with coronary heart disease: protocol for a randomised controlled trial. *International Journal of Nursing Studies*, 49, 1489–93. doi: 10.1016/j.ijnurstu.2012.07.004.

Feinglass, J., Song, J., Semanik, P., Lee, J., Manheim, L., Dunlop, D., and Chang, R. W. (2012). Association of functional status with changes in physical activity: insights from a behavioral intervention for participants with arthritis. *Archives of Physical Medicine and Rehabilitation*, 93(1), 172–5.

Gidlow, C., Johnston, L. H., Crone, D., and James, D. V. B. (2008). Methods of evaluation: issues and implications for physical activity referral schemes. *American Journal of Lifestyle Management*, 2(1), 46–50.

Gidlow, C., Johnston, L. H., Crone, D., Morris, C., Smith, A., Foster, C., and James, D. V. B. (2007). Socio-demographic patterning of referral, uptake and attendance in physical activity referral schemes. *Journal of Public Health*, 29(2), 107–13.

Gidlow, C., and Murphy, R. (2009). Physical activity promotion in primary health care. In L. Dugdill, D. Crone and R. Murphy (Eds.), *Physical activity and health promotion: evidence-based approaches to practice* (1st ed., pp. 87–102). UK: Wiley-Blackwell.

Graham, R. C., Dugdill, L., and Cable, N. T. (2005). Health professionals' perspectives in exercise referral: implications for the referral process. *Ergonomics*, 48(11–14), 1411–22.

Greene, J. C., and Caracelli, V. J. (1997). Defining and describing the paradigm issue in mixed-method evaluation. *New Directions for Evaluation*, 1997(74), 5–17. doi: 10.1002/ev.1068

Hanson, C. L., Allin, L. J., Ellis, J. G., and Dodd-Reynolds, C. J. (2013). An evaluation of the efficacy of the exercise on referral scheme in Northumberland, UK: association with physical activity and predictors of engagement. A naturalistic observation study. *BMJ Open*, 3(8). doi: 10.1136/bmjopen-2013-002849.

Hardcastle, S. N. M. (2012). The effectiveness of a motivational interviewing primary-care based intervention on physical activity and predictors of change in a disadvantaged community. *Journal of Behavioral Medicine*, 35(3), 318–33. doi: 10.1007/s10865-012-9417-1.

Hardcastle, S., and Taylor, A. H. (2001). Looking for more than weight loss and fitness gain: psychosocial dimensions among older women in a primary-care exercise-referral program. *Journal of Aging and Physical Activity*, 9(3), 313–28.

Haynes, B., and Haines, A. (1998). Education and debate. Getting research findings into practice: barriers and bridges to evidence based clinical practice . . . fourth in a series of eight articles. *BMJ: British Medical Journal (International Edition)*, 317(7153), 273–6. doi: 10.1136/bmj.317.7153.273.

Hutchison, A. J., Johnston, L. H., and Breckon, J. D. (2013). A grounded theory of successful long-term physical activity behaviour change. *Qualitative Research in Sport, Exercise and Health*, 5(1), 109–26.

James, D. V. B., Johnston, L. H., Crone, D., Sidford, A. H., Gidlow, C., Morris, C., and Foster, C. (2008). Factors associated with physical activity referral uptake and participation. *Journal of Sports Sciences*, 26(2), 217–24.

James, D. V. B., Mills, H., Crone, D., Johnston, L. H., Morris, C., and Gidlow, C. J. (2009). Factors associated with physical activity referral completion and health outcomes. *Journal of Sports Sciences*, 27(10), 1007–17.

Johnson, R. B., Onwuegbuzie, A. J., and Turner, L. A. (2007). Toward a definition of mixed methods research. *Journal of Mixed Methods Research*, 1(2), 112–33.

Lee, I. M., Shiroma, E. J., Lobelo, F., Puska, P., Blair, S. N., and Katzmarzyk, P. T. (2012). Effect of physical inactivity on major non-communicable diseases worldwide: an analysis of burden of disease and life expectancy. *Lancet*, 380(9838), 219–29.

Little, A., and Lewis, K. (2006). Influences on long-term exercise adherence in older patients with cardiac disease. *International Journal of Therapy and Rehabilitation*, 13(12), 543–50.

Mills, H., Crone, D., James, D. V. B., and Johnston, L. H. (2012). Exploring the perceptions of success in an exercise referral scheme: a mixed method investigation. *Evaluation Review*, 36(6), 407–29.

Moore, G., Moore, L., and Murphy, S. (2011). Facilitating adherence to physical activity: exercise professionals' experiences of the National Exercise Referral Scheme in Wales. A qualitative study. *BMC Public Health 2011*, 935(11), 935.

Morris, J. N., Kagan, A., Pattison, D. C., and Gardner, M. J. (1966). Incidence and prediction of ischaemic heart-disease in London busmen. *Lancet*, 2(7463), 553–9.

Murphy, S. M., Edwards, R. T., Williams, N., Raisanen, L., Moore, G., Linck, P., Hounsome, N., Din, N. U., and Moore, L. (2012). An evaluation of the effectiveness and cost effectiveness of the National Exercise Referral Scheme in Wales, UK: a randomised controlled trial of a public health policy initiative. *Journal of Epidemiology and Community Health*, 66(8), 745–53. doi: 10.1136/jech-2011-200689.

NICE. (2006). Four commonly used methods to increase physical activity: brief interventions in primary care, exercise referral schemes, pedometers and community-based exercise programmes for walking and cycling. *Public health intervention guidance 2*. London: National Institute for Health and Clinical Excellence.

NICE. (2013). Physical activity: brief advice for adults in primary care *NICE public health guidance 44*. London: National Institute for Health and Care Clinical Excellence.

O'Cathain, A., Murphy, E., and Nicholl, J. (2008). The quality of mixed methods studies in health services research. *Journal of Health Services Research and Policy*, 13(2), 92–8.

Onwuegbuzie, A. J., and Collins, K. M. (2007). A typology of mixed methods sampling designs in social science research. *Qualitative Report*, 12(2), 281–316.

Onwuegbuzie, A. J., Johnson, R. B., and Collins, K. M. T. (2009). Call for mixed analysis: a philosophical framework for combining qualitative and quantitative approaches. *International Journal of Multiple Research Approaches*, 3(2), 114–39.

Owens, C., Crone, D., Kilgour, L., and El Ansari, W. (2010). The place and promotion of wellbeing in mental health services: a qualitative investigation. *Journal of Psychiatric and Mental Health Nursing*, 17(1), 1–8. doi: 10.1111/j.1365-2850.2009.01480.x.

Pate, R. R., Pratt, M., Blair, S. N., Haskell, W. L., Macera, C. A., Bouchard, C., Buchner, D., Ettinger, W., Heath, G. W., King, A. C., Kriska, A., Leon, A. S. Marcus, B. H., Morris, J., Paffenbarger Jr, R. S., Patrick, K., Pollock, M. L., Rippe, J. M., Sallis, J., and Wilmore, J. H. (1995). Physical activity and public health: a recommendation from the Centers for Disease Control and Prevention and the American College of Sports Medicine, *JAMA.*, 273(5), 402–7.

Pavey, T. G., Taylor, A. H., Fox, K. R., Hillsdon, M., Anokye, N., Campbell, J. L., Foster, C., Green, C., Moxham, T., Mutrie, N., Searle, J., Trueman, P., and Taylor, R. S. (2011). Effect of exercise referral schemes in primary care on physical activity and improving health outcomes: systematic review and meta-analysis. *British Medical Journal*, 343. doi: 10.1136/bmj.d6462.

Pavey, T., Taylor, A., Hillsdon, M., Fox, K., Campbell, J., Foster, C., Moxham, T., Mutrie, N., Searle, J., and Taylor, R. (2012). Levels and predictors of exercise referral scheme uptake and adherence: a systematic review. *Journal of Epidemiology and Community Health*, 66(8), 737–44. doi: 10.1136/jech-2011-200354.

Sandelowski, M., Voils, C. I., and Barroso, J. (2006). Defining and designing mixed research synthesis studies. *Research in the schools: a nationally refereed journal sponsored by the Mid-South Educational Research Association and the University of Alabama*, 13(1), 29.

Sattelmair, J., Pertman, J., Ding, E. L., Kohl 3rd, H. W., Haskell, W., and Lee, I. M. (2011). Dose response between physical activity and risk of coronary heart disease: a meta-analysis. *Circulation*, 124(7), 789–95. doi: 10.1161/circulationaha.110.010710.

Sharma, H., Bulley, C., and van Wijck, F. M. J. (2012). Experiences of an exercise referral scheme from the perspective of people with chronic stroke: a qualitative study. *Physiotherapy*, 98(4), 344–50. doi: 10.1016/j.physio.2011.05.004.

Strauss, A., and Corbin, J. (1998). *Basics of qualitative research: techniques and procedures for developing grounded theory*. London: Sage.

Teddlie, C., and Tashakkori, A. (2009). *Foundations of mixed methods research: integrating quantitative and qualitative approaches in the social and behavioral sciences*. London: Sage.

van Uffelen, J. G. Z., Chinapaw, M. J. M., Hopman-Rock, M., and van Mechelen, W. (2009). Feasibility and effectiveness of a walking program for community-dwelling older adults with mild cognitive impairment. *Journal of Aging and Physical Activity*, 17(4), 398–415.

Victora, C. G., Habicht, J.-P., and Bryce, J. (2004). Evidence-based public health: moving beyond randomized trials. *American Journal of Public Health*, 94(3), 400–5.

Vinson, D., and Parker, A. (2012). Exercise, service and support: client experiences of physical activity referral schemes (PARS). *Qualitative Research in Sport, Exercise and Health*, 4(1), 15–31.

White, K. M., Terry, D. J., Troup, C., Rempel, L. A., Norman, P., Mummery, K., Riley, M., Posner, N., and Kenardy, J. (2012). An extended theory of planned behavior intervention for older adults With type 2 diabetes and cardiovascular disease. *Journal of Aging and Physical Activity*, 20(3), 281–99.

Williams, N. H., Hendry, M., France, B., Lewis, R., and Wilkinson, C. (2007). Effectiveness of exercise-referral schemes to promote physical activity in adults: systematic review. *The British Journal Of General Practice: The Journal Of The Royal College Of General Practitioners*, 57(545), 979–86.

Wong, E. M. Y., and Cheng, M. M. H. (2013). Effects of motivational interviewing to promote weight loss in obese children. *Journal of Clinical Nursing*, 22(17/18), 2519–30. doi: 10.1111/jocn.12098.

Chapter 13

Physical activity promotion in primary health care and the community

Christopher Gidlow, Diane Crone, and Michelle Huws-Thomas

Physical activity in primary care

Rationale for the primary care setting

In the early 1990s there were growing concerns regarding cardiovascular disease (CVD) and a developing epidemiological evidence base regarding the role of exercise in the treatment and prevention of CVD (Pate et al., 1996). As a result, primary care was identified as a viable setting for physical activity promotion. To date, two main types of physical activity pathway exist within primary care; clinically delivered advice, usually termed as behaviour change counselling (brief negotiation) or motivational interviewing (Bull and Milton, 2011; Department of Health, 2009), or the more traditional exercise referral scheme (ERS)[1] or physical activity referral scheme (PARS) model (Williams, 2011).

These two types of schemes have a mix of evidence underpinning their effectiveness, which will be discussed later in this chapter. Briefly, for brief negotiation, and its role in signposting people to a physical activity pathway, there is some evidence of effectiveness (Bull and Milton, 2010, 2011; Curry et al., 2011; Orrow et al., 2012). For ERS, while many papers allude to their role for specific populations groups (Crone et al., 2008; Gidlow et al., 2007; Harrison et al., 2005; James et al., 2009; James et al., 2008; Murphy et al., 2012; Williams et al., 2007), evidence from controlled research is equivocal (Pavey et al., 2011a). In some cases the two types of pathway have been merged and some recent evidence suggests that this combination can be most effective (Hardcastle et al., 2012; Hardcastle and Hagger, 2011).

Current national guidance on physical activity in primary care

Physical activity recommendations for the general population have recently been modified, and current national guidance includes recommendations for older adults, adults aged between eighteen to sixty five years, young people, and children. For the first time they have also included guidance regarding sedentary behaviour (Department of Health, 2011).

In terms of the guidance for the promotion of health generally in primary care the National Institute for Health and Care Excellence (NICE), a non-departmental public body accountable to the Department of Health, provides national guidance and advice to improve health and social care in England. NICE guidance determines the standards for health care and focuses on healthy living. The topics for its guidance documents are determined by the Department of Health and selected on the basis of their relationship to the burden of disease, socio-economic impact, and where there is a range of practice taking place across England (www.nice.org.uk).

NICE has produced a number of documents related to the promotion of physical activity, including guidance regarding the use of the environment (NICE, 2008b), the workplace (NICE, 2008c), children and young people (NICE, 2009), and older people (NICE, 2008a). In terms of guidance within primary care, they produced two key documents, recommending four commonly-used methods to increase physical activity used in primary care in 2006 and 2013, and one specific to exercise referral (NICE, 2014).

The 2006 guidance (NICE, 2006) included brief intervention, exercise referral schemes, pedometers, and walking and cycling programmes. The guidance provided recommendations on the use of these different types of physical activity interventions in primary care. The choice of the four reflected the emerging evidence and the advances in practice, i.e. the use of pedometers as an intervention to motivate patients to meet the 10,000 steps recommendations for health, and the increasing rise of nationally-supported walking and cycling programmes within the community. They also included the original exercise referral scheme model and the less-established 'brief interventions', which refers to clinically-delivered advice, such as brief negotiation, motivational interviewing, and exercise counselling.

The 2013 guidance reflects the more contemporary developments in physical activity promotion in primary care. They provide a range of recommendations on the use and implementation of behavioural interventions for physical activity promotion and advice on embedding this into the commissioning process and on commissioning training of delivery staff (NICE, 2013). In addressing these issues, the guidance goes some way to allay the concerns raised in the literature regarding the differing practices and fidelity or conformity issues in this area of practice (Breckon et al., 2008; Hutchison et al., 2008; Johnston et al., 2009). These issues are discussed later in the chapter.

The 2014 guidance was a response to uncertainty regarding the effectiveness of exercise referral following publication of numerous reviews in the area (NICE, 2014).

Clinician-delivered approaches

A common challenge faced by health professionals in primary care is that of encouraging and supporting people to change their behaviour to become more physically active. Research has shown that advice alone is often ineffective, and that ambivalence, lack of motivation, and low confidence are common motivational struggles rooted in social, economic, and cultural circumstances (Miller and Rollnick, 2012). Understanding and appreciating the complexity of difficulties such as overcoming low motivation and dealing with ambivalence, as well as developing skills and strategies to support people through the change process, are necessary to address physical activity levels within the community. The two commonly-used behaviour change interventions used in primary care include Motivational Interviewing (MI) and Behaviour Change Counselling (BCC).

There is considerable evidence for the effectiveness of MI in a range of health behaviours, including the treatment of substance abuse (VanBuskirk and Wetherell,

2013), adherence to medication (Possidente et al., 2005), eating disorders (Macdonald et al., 2012), type I and II diabetes (Martins and McNeil, 2009), oral health (Martins and McNeil, 2009), and exercise (Hardcastle et al., 2012). The success of this method is based on practice techniques and an empathic communication style (Miller and Rollnick, 2012). Behaviour Change Counselling is a briefer version of MI, which has showed promise in short consultations, such as those between a person and a health professional in, for example, a GP consultation (Rollnick et al., 1999). There is also evidence that these interventions are most effective when they are educational, focused on helping the person build skills and confidence, and correspond with person and health care professional's values (Miller and Rollnick, 2012).

Motivational interviewing and BCC are explained below in more detail, with a brief summary of the supporting evidence from physical activity promotion and the challenges for evidence-based practice.

Motivational Interviewing

Motivational Interviewing is described as 'client-centred, directive methods for enhancing intrinsic motivation to change by exploring and resolving ambivalence person centred form of guiding to elicit and strengthen motivation for change' (Miller and Rollnick, 2012, p.25). The dialogue between person and practitioner is based on eliciting and strengthening motivation for change. The core principle of the method is that the person's motivation to change is improved if there is a gentle process of negotiation in which the person, not the professional, is encouraged to discuss the benefits and costs involved in changing behaviour that personally relate to them. A conversation where the healthcare professional engages the person in a collaborative dialogue, which is person-centred and explores the discrepancy between deeply-held values and problematic current behaviour, is more likely to be successful than when the professional argues or instructs for change to occur. Motivational Interviewing includes four guiding key principles: 1) Resist the righting reflex; 2) Understand the person's own motivations; 3) Listen with empathy; and 4) Empower the person. Three core styles of communication (directing, guiding, and following) collectively provide the structure of the method to engage effectively with a person and evoke desired change (Miller and Rollnick, 2012; Rollnick et al., 2010).

In terms of the evidence from both quantitative and qualitative research, MI in physical activity promotion appears to be an effective method to support people to become more active (Hardcastle et al., 2012; Hardcastle and Hagger, 2011), especially when combined with an exercise referral scheme (Sjöling et al., 2011). This has been embraced in mainstream services through the national health trainer programme.

Behaviour change counselling

Behaviour change counselling is a brief counselling style that focuses on the same principles of MI, but in shorter consultations. The differences in techniques depend on the client, setting, and the length of consultation, although, principally, BCC includes the stages presented in Figure 13.1, and applies the elements of the five 'A's ('assess', 'advise', 'agree', 'assist', and 'arrange') (Goldstein et al., 2004).

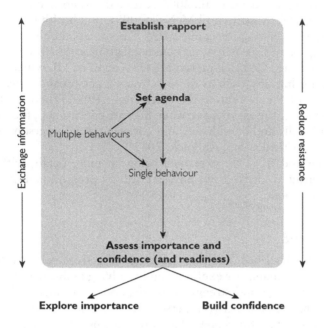

Figure 13.1 Key techniques in consultations about behaviour change (Rollnick et al., 1999; p12).

In terms of the evidence base for the shorter consultations used in BCC, there is evidence that they can be as effective and, therefore, perhaps more cost-effective than lengthier MI techniques (Spanou et al., 2010), and have been tested in a range of areas, including smoking cessation (Butler et al., 2013; Lai et al., 2010) and accident and emergency alcohol-related accidents (Monti et al., 1999). Research has demonstrated that it has been particularly useful in consultations around behaviours such as smoking (Aveyard et al., 2012), unsafe alcohol consumption (Dauer et al., 2006), and unhealthy diet and lack of exercise (Ackerman et al., 2011). However, within a cluster randomised controlled trial (RCT), it was concluded that to establish longer-term behaviour change, it was important to increase the number of client-health professional contacts (i.e. more than one) (Butler et al., 2013).

Challenges for evidence-based practice

Despite the growing evidence regarding the use of both of these techniques for a range of lifestyle behaviours in primary care, this is a developing area of evidence-based practice, and, as such, this emerging evidence has had some criticisms. These are predominantly associated with the lack of fidelity regarding the content and the delivery of the interventions, and the difficulties trying to develop a robust evidence base. A group of researchers have been reviewing the evidence since the development of these techniques in the physical activity promotion area. In the first paper, the authors undertook a systematic review of physical activity counselling and concluded that whilst interventions were predominantly based on appropriate theory, little information was reported on the specifics of the intervention in terms of duration, frequency, and the competence level of the provider (Breckon et al., 2008). They also observed that, due to the range of professionals delivering these counselling sessions and a lack of intervention control and treatment fidelity in these studies, it was difficult to draw comparisons and conclusions regarding the efficacy (Johnston et al., 2009).

Summary

There has been significant change in physical activity promotion practice over the twenty years since the original exercise on the prescription model was introduced. This change has been informed by a developing evidence base, initially from epidemiology, but more recently from the contemporary research and practice from psychology in MI and BCC. There are concerns about new models of practice, especially as the evidence base of what works for which situation and client groups is still emerging. However, the simple model of referring someone to an exercise setting has been proved to be too simplistic to address the complex adoption processes involved in being more physically active. The next section discusses in more detail models of intervention and the associated evidence in this area of physical activity promotion in primary care and the community.

Exercise referral schemes

The exercise referral model

As noted earlier in this chapter, the ERS model emerged in the early 1990s, with rapid proliferation and continued use across the UK (Gidlow and Murphy, 2009) and elsewhere (Sørensen et al., 2011). These schemes operate through the referral of a patient by a health professional to a physical activity or exercise intervention, either in the community (e.g. local leisure centre, walks programme) or a practice-based scheme where exercise takes place in-house (Crone, Johnston, and Grant, 2004). This model recognised the limited capacity and exercise-specific expertise of health professionals for intervention delivery, and made links with local exercise and physical activity providers. These programmes were initially developed for CVD prevention, but have since broadened to the treatment and prevention of a range of conditions, including diabetes, depression, osteoporosis, anxiety, hypertension, obesity, and respiratory conditions.

Originally, only general practitioners (GPs) were able to refer patients on to such schemes, hence the name 'GP referral'. However, it became clear that other members of the primary healthcare team, such as practice nurses and physiotherapists, were identifying patients who would benefit. Coupled with the name change to exercise (ERS) or physical activity referral schemes (PARS), was a broadening of 'referrers' to include the whole primary health care team. In 2001, national guidance was produced to promote greater standardisation of practice and evaluation (Department of Health, 2001), but local differences in population characteristics, needs, and resources, inevitably create variation across localities in the delivery model and the robustness of any evaluation.

Typically, ERSs include independent and group-based activity including walking, fitness activities such as the gym, swimming, exercise classes, or a combination of activities (Gidlow and Murphy, 2009). Traditionally, most activities tend to be facility-based, but there are examples of alternatives, for example: walking groups (Lamb et al., 2002) and independent home-based exercise (Stevens et al., 1998).

Within primary care settings today, a whole range of physical activity opportunities are available in health centres and general practices within the community. The popularity of physical activity referral schemes, and the simplicity in practice of a health professional referring a patient for a programme of physical activity, has developed into a plethora of opportunities for different community groups in most geographic areas in England. For example, many health centres are venues for walking groups and programmes, including led/guided walks and the publication of walk maps centred around a health centre. There may also be a physical activity element included in weight management programmes delivered at the practice or at a local community venue such as the leisure centre. Furthermore, with the emergence of health trainers, employed health-improvement professionals, and the development of brief intervention, Motivational Interviewing, and counselling techniques in primary care, physical activity referral pathways have developed significantly from the simple 'GP referral of a patient to a leisure centre model' of the 1990s.

For more detail on the background, implementation, and evaluation of exercise referral, you can refer to various sources (e.g. British Heart Foundation, 2010; Crone et al., 2004; Department of Health, 2001; Dugdill et al., 2005). The remainder of this section provides an overview of the associated evidence base.

Evidence from quantitative research

There have been numerous reviews of the exercise referral literature (Gidlow et al., 2005; Morgan, 2005; NICE, 2006; Pavey et al., 2012; Pavey et al., 2011a; Pavey, et al., 2011b; Williams et al., 2007). Despite differences in their specific focus and the types of study included, some common themes emerge, in addition to ongoing debate. Rather than replicate these reviews, the following offers a brief overview of review-level evidence and consistent themes in terms of programme reach (who gets referred to ERS), uptake and adherence (who engages and adheres), effectiveness and cost-effectiveness (do ERS promote beneficial changes in behaviour or health, and do these warrant investment in ERS?). Both quantitative and qualitative evidence is presented.

Reach

To summarise current knowledge about who gets referred to ERS (i.e. reach), it is possible to examine the characteristics of participants from programme evaluations and some RCTs. This tends to be the earliest point in ERS for which participant data are available; we are not aware of data on who is offered the referral by their health professional but refuses it. These basic data on ERS participant characteristics can indicate possible bias in referrals. As noted in an earlier review, RCT recruitment methods can limit how much we can learn about who, in practice, is referred to ERS (Gidlow et al., 2005). Depending on the trial, it might not always be valid to suggest that the sample of individuals who are subject to RCT recruitment and exclusion criteria are representative of a sample referred through the usual means.

The most commonly-reported participant characteristics are age, gender, and health indicators. Women generally account for a higher proportion of exercise referrals, with men accounting for between 16 and 43 per cent (Hanson et al., 2013; Murphy et al., 2012; Pavey et al., 2011a; Williams et al., 2007). This over-representation of women is not specific to ERS, and is commonly observed in physical activity interventions and related research (Müller-Riemenschneider et al., 2008; Orrow et al., 2012). The age of ERS participants tends to be between forty and seventy four years. In some cases, this reflects the specific programme referral criteria, which sometimes target older adults (e.g. Damush et al., 2001; Dinan et al., 2006; Munro et al., 2004). Commonly-targeted health characteristics include CVD risk factors (e.g. hypertension and overweight/obesity) and mild mental health problems, in addition to sedentariness. In practice, the latter is likely to be based on the health practitioner-patient consultant prior to referral rather than measurement of activity levels. There is some evidence that those referred to ERS are more likely to be from lower socio-economic groups (Gidlow et al., 2007). In the context of generally poorer uptake of preventive health opportunities by more deprived groups, this appears encouraging. However, it might simply reflect worse health and more frequent primary care visits in lower socio-economic groups (Goddard and Smith, 2001), and does not necessarily convert into better uptake and adherence.

Overall, and often as a result of programme referral criteria that focus on specific conditions or age groups in which such conditions tend to manifest, ERSs typically reach adults around mid-life who have one or more lifestyle-related condition, with more female than male participants.

The next step in the referral pathway that can be studied is whether or not those who are referred engage with the programme and subsequently adhere.

Uptake and adherence

Uptake of referral tends to be defined as attendance at the first appointment with the exercise professional, or attendance at one or more exercise sessions. Although less studied than adherence and effectiveness, several systematic reviews have summarised evidence on levels and predictors of uptake.

Pooled estimates of uptake of 66 per cent (95 per cent CI = 57–75 per cent) from observational studies in one review suggest that approximately one-third of those referred will drop out of ERS before starting the programme (Pavey et al., 2012; 2011b). This wide-ranging, but, generally, high level of attrition was comparable with earlier reviews (Gidlow et al., 2005; Williams et al., 2007) and raises questions about whether health professionals are referring appropriately (Johnston et al., 2005). To explore this, researchers have tried to identify if certain groups are less likely to take up referral and, therefore, should not be referred for ERS. So far, data are relatively inconclusive. Some researchers have linked higher uptake with factors such as higher age, female gender, lower deprivation, and rural residence. Differences by medical condition are difficult to discern given the various disease groups reported and how they have been compared (Pavey et al., 2012). However, there is some evidence to suggest that patients with some medical conditions such as mental health problems like anxiety and depression may require more social support than is routinely offered to help with uptake and adherence to physical activity programmes (Crone et al., 2008). The complexities around assumptions of treating people with similar conditions as homogeneous groups are well described in Chapter 11.

Adherence to ERS has been also been defined in a number of ways, from attendance at the final assessment to attendance of at least 75 or 80 per cent of exercise sessions. Similar to uptake, levels of adherence are variable, but relatively low overall, with less than half of ERS participants completing: Pavey et al. (2012; 2011a) reported 49 per cent (95 per cent CI = 40–59 per cent) in observational studies and 37 per cent (95 per cent CI = 20–54 per cent) in RCTs; Williams et al. (2007) reported 12 to 42 per cent; Gidlow et al. (2005) reported 12 to 56 per cent. Studies published after these reviews have reported adherence at the higher end of these ranges, and in relation to longer intervention periods: 44 per cent at sixteen weeks (Murphy et al., 2012); 43 per cent at twenty four weeks (Hanson et al., 2013); and 45 per cent at twenty six weeks (Tobi et al., 2012).

When predictors of adherence have been explored, older age and being male appear to increase the likelihood of completing programmes (Pavey et al., 2012). Other factors are less consistently reported, but some have found lower adherence levels in residents of more deprived and rural areas (Gidlow et al., 2007) and referrals have been from health professionals other than GPs (Dugdill et al., 2005; James et al., 2008). Once again, the process of the actual referral is bought into question, as is the suitability of the programme on offer for certain groups.

Effectiveness and cost-effectiveness

Reviews of effectiveness have summarised the extent to which ERS can increase physical activity or improve lifestyle-related health outcomes. Where meta-analyses have been used to derive pooled estimates for physical activity or health change, inclusion criteria have often delimited to controlled (or uncontrolled) trials to allow sufficient homogeneity for statistical synthesis of data (Pavey et al., 2011a; Williams et al., 2007). Other systematic reviews have been somewhat more inclusive, and provided narrative syntheses. Collectively, the evidence base suggests that ERS may increase physical activity levels in the short term. In the longer term, such as six or twelve months after referral, such increases often disappear. However, two meta-analyses and a subsequent pragmatic RCT of ERS in Wales have reported higher levels of participation in physical activity in ERS participants at follow-up ranging from 16–20 per cent (Murphy et al., 2012; Pavey et al., 2011b; Williams et al., 2007). It should be acknowledged that physical activity is almost exclusively measured through self-report, which has well-documented limitations (Prince et al., 2008; Shephard and Vuillemin, 2003). Researchers should consider more objective methods in future, such as accelerometry.

Economic evaluation of ERS is relatively limited. A common measure of cost-effectiveness is the cost of the intervention per Quality Adjusted Life Year (QALY): a measure of the incremental price of achieving a one unit improvement in health that allows different types of intervention to be compared (Gold et al., 2002; NICE, 2010). Estimates of the cost-effectiveness from reviews of ERS are close to, or within, the recommended limits for cost-effectiveness for public health interventions recommended by NICE (£20,000 to £30,000 per QALY) (Pavey et al., 2011b), and well within the limit of cost-effectiveness in the case of the subsequent Welsh RCT (£12,111 per QALY) (Murphy et al., 2012). Moreover, ERSs appear far more cost-effectiveness in sedentary individuals who have a diagnosed medical condition (Pavey et al., 2011b), as reflected in the NICE guidance (NICE, 2014).

Evidence from qualitative research

Quantitative research confirms that those who complete schemes have associated physical health benefits. Therefore, qualitative research is important to help in understanding what supports patients to engage and complete ERS. The ERS ability to successfully engage individuals (reach and uptake) includes participant acknowledgments that taking part requires an ability to cope (Crone et al., 2005) and that perceived poor health can present a barrier to participating in higher levels of activity (Little and Lewis, 2006). Interviews with health professionals have identified that people with mental health problems report having higher levels of anxiety about the exercise environment, and the important supportive role of the health professional at the point of referral to mitigate this barrier (Moore et al., 2011).

Regarding programme adherence once people have engaged with ERS, qualitative published research points to a number of key aspects. These can be considered as the social and cultural (e.g. social support of group exercise), and physical environment of the exercise setting (e.g. a non-intimidating gym environment), which appear to be associated with positive experiences and, therefore, adherence (Crone et al., 2005; Little and Lewis, 2006; Vinson and Parker, 2012). This can be promoted through staff and their professionalism in creating a support network (Vinson and Parker, 2012). Indeed, interviews with exercise professionals delivering on a national ERS identified process factors as important for adherence and effectiveness, including social support mechanisms and a post-scheme maintenance programme (Moore et al., 2011). The latter relates to quantitative evidence that short-term physical activity increases are often not maintained beyond the life of the programme.

Qualitative data also provide insight regarding the physical, mental, social, and behavioural (physical activity) effects of ERS. Participants have reported physical health changes as a consequence of participation (Crone et al., 2005; Mills et al., 2012). A range of perceived psychological benefits include a sense of achievement and control (Hardcastle and Taylor, 2001; Sharma et al., 2012), self-acceptance and a sense of purpose (Crone et al., 2005), improved self-confidence (Mills et al., 2012; Vinson and Parker, 2012; Wormald and Ingle, 2004), and empowerment and inclusion (Mills et al., 2012; Vinson and Parker, 2012). Developing a sense of belonging and an exercise identity during their engagement with programmes adds to the argument for creating conducive social and cultural environments in ERS (Crone et al., 2005; Hardcastle and Taylor, 2001).

Summary

From a national perspective, on the basis of NICE and Health Technology Assessment reviews, the use of ERS as an effective means of promoting population physical activity remains under question. The most recent NICE recommendation was that commissioners should not fund ERS unless targeting people who are 'sedentary or inactive and have existing health conditions or other factors' (NICE, 2014, p.8). However, it has long been noted that ERS can play a role for some people, and qualitative evidence highlights the potential benefits for social and psychological health. Uptake, adherence, and physical activity change apparently vary with age, gender, and disease group. Qualitative research points to important factors to create exercise environments that lead to positive experiences, which, in turn, foster the necessary engagement and adherence (e.g. social support networks). Such evidence should be considered to maximise the effectiveness and cost-effectiveness of ERS through improving not only patient targeting, but retention of inactive individuals with existing morbidities (e.g. obesity, hypertension, and depression).

Uncertainty around ERS effectiveness (NICE, 2014) and evidence supporting the use of brief interventions created the rationale for the next iteration of national physical activity programmes in the UK, the health trainer programme.

Moving physical activity promotion out of primary care

Looking beyond the primary care setting

The advantages of primary care as a setting for physical activity promotion were described earlier in the chapter. To overcome possible limitations of health professional capacity and area-specific expertise, the ERS model moved delivery outside of primary care to exercise professionals. However, two issues remain, which could account for ERS apparently working for some groups more than others, and the modest overall effects on behaviour and health. First, the type of the exercise interventions will depend on the local physical activity facilities and resources that are available. Second, the ERS approach tends to be relatively prescriptive (e.g. eight to twelve weeks of structured exercise at a local facility). This is not an issue if the referral and screening processes are effective and the delivery model suits the participant. However, in many cases, such factors can mean that programmes lack the flexibility to accommodate differences in individuals' preferences, needs, and circumstances, i.e. the individual and their environment.

Rather than taking a narrow and prescriptive approach to physical activity intervention, it is increasingly recognised that, for sustainable behaviour change, interventions need to take into account both individual and broader social ecological influences on behaviour (Stokols, 1992). We described earlier how techniques such as MI can be used to tailor support to individuals' readiness to change their behaviour, engage them in identifying their own goals (rather than prescribing), and help individuals to manage their behaviour in the context of competing social and physical environmental influences. If such interventions and follow-up support could be delivered by people with an understanding and knowledge of the local area and community, this could, theoretically, allow for behavioural support that is responsive to the individual and their local environment. It is on this basis that the health trainer model was developed: a national initiative to improve health and reduce health inequalities using community-based delivery by trained lay people.

Health trainer programme development and policy context

The 2004 government white paper, introduced the idea of accredited health trainers (Department of Health, 2004), where patients are referred from primary care to receive lifestyle support from trained lay people who are drawn from the communities that the services are trying to engage with. This is similar to the lay health worker model, which has been used mostly outside the UK to address a range of health issues (Lewin et al., 2005). The underpinning rationale is that people are more likely to respond to those they see as similar to themselves. In turn, this might allow the service to reach 'those who want to adopt healthier lifestyles, but who have little contact with services' (Michie et al., 2006; p.3). The introduction of health trainers denoted a shift from 'top-down' prescriptive intervention to 'support from next door', such that the deliverers understand the experiences of those they support (Department of Health, 2004). Key to the health trainer remit is reaching lower socio-economic groups who are often more difficult to engage in mainstream health promotion services.

The service is based on behaviour change approaches discussed earlier in the chapter. It is intended to be client-centred, in that participants attend an initial assessment meeting, and to set their own behavioural goals, with subsequent support to manage their behaviour, and the events and circumstances in their lives that they would like to change (Michie et al., 2006). Health trainers are, therefore, trained in specific competencies, including MI techniques (to help people identify what behaviour they would like to change), goal setting (plan the behaviour change), confidence building, and how to promote self-monitoring and encourage participants to build in social support. Where appropriate, signposting/referrals to local services or groups are used (e.g. weight loss groups, exercise groups), requiring links with other public and third-sector organisations, links that should have improved since the move of public health into local authority in the UK. The duration and frequency of health trainer-participant contact can vary between programmes, but typically lasts three to six months.

The Health Trainer model was introduced selectively in 2005, with national rollout from 2007. However, similar to exercise referral, this proliferation has taken place in the absence of a robust evidence base.

Evidence for health trainers

Attree et al. (2011) reviewed the health trainer evidence-base after several years of national implementation. At the time, the published evidence was mostly limited to local evaluations and audits of the national data repository used by a large number of programmes (Data Collection and Reporting System, DCRS). Few of the reviewed evaluations included robust, primary quantitative data that could demonstrate beneficial changes in participants' behaviour or health. Rather, evaluations typically recorded DCRS data, in some cases supplemented by qualitative data from participant or stakeholder interviews on process and feasibility. The review authors reported positive findings in terms of process and implementation, the type of support provided, client and health trainer experiences, and their perceived role in reaching disadvantaged communities.

Research and evaluation has since progressed, but without providing definitive evidence of effectiveness. Analysis of national data from 4418 participants showed beneficial twelve-month changes in predominantly self-reported outcomes (e.g. physical activity, fruit/vegetable consumption, intentions, and motivation), and a moderate reduction in mean Body Mass Index (BMI) (34.0 to 32.3 kgm^{-2}) (Gardner et al., 2012). However, most of these data were self-reported, including some of the BMI measures. Twelve-month clinical and health-related quality of life improvements have been observed in a sample of 994 health trainer programme participants from a city-wide programme (Gidlow et al., 2013; see Box 1). Data indicated that the programme cohort had considerable health risk at baseline (33.6 per cent with ≥ 20 per cent ten-year CVD risk; 95.7 per cent were overweight or obese), and that most lived in deprived areas (53 per cent from areas in the most deprived quintile of national rankings). Moreover, statistically significant changes in CVD risk, CVD risk factors, and self-reported health were evident, but most marked in those with high CVD risk at baseline (≥ 20 per cent ten-year CVD risk).

Although the inclusion of clinical outcomes was an important addition (Gidlow et al., 2013), the absence of a control group in both of the above studies was a limitation, and one that is often difficult to address in applied research and evaluation. There have been two UK RCTs (at the time of writing). Barton et al. (2012) completed a small trial of patients with one or more CVD risk factors who received health promotion literature and either three months of health trainer support (n = 72) or no further support (n = 38). Greater six-month improvements in health-related quality of life in the health trainer group were used to estimate a cost per QALY of £14,480, which falls within the aforementioned cost-effectiveness threshold set by NICE (£20,000–£30,000). A larger RCT reported randomised NHS Health Check patients identified as 'high risk' (≥ 20 per cent ten-year CVD risk) to either a health trainer service (n = 236) or usual care (n = 365) (Cochrane et al., 2012; Davey et al., 2010). CVD risk reduced in all participants, but with no significant additional benefit in those receiving health trainer support (31.9 per cent to 29.2 per cent) versus usual care (32.9 per cent to 29.4 per cent) (Cochrane et al., 2012).

Evidence from controlled research on similar approaches outside the UK is similarly equivocal, showing a lack of clinically or statistically significant health improvement (Carr et al., 2011; van Limpt et al., 2011). Indeed, many of the concerns about the supporting evidence for health trainer programmes noted in the earlier review still apply (Attree et al., 2011):

1   Insufficient evidence of benefit for behaviour, health, and programme cost-effectiveness.
2   Too much emphasis on nationally-available data on outputs (e.g. number of clients engaged) and process (Ball and Nasr, 2011; Shircore, 2013; South et al., 2007), rather than outcomes of health and behaviour change, which are largely self-reported (not clinical).
3   Available data suggest a degree of success in reaching lower socio-economic groups (Shircore, 2013), but more sophisticated measures of impact on health inequalities are warranted.
4   Local service evaluations are important for service development, but robust research and evaluation is warranted (e.g. use of robust, objective health data; comparison or controls tend not to be used).

Summary

The health trainer programme was born out of evidence supporting the use of brief interventions and motivational interviewing, and the need to consider local environmental influences on the sustainability of behaviour change. So far, it appears that these programmes have wide acceptability, and are viewed positively by participants and stakeholders (Ball and Nasr, 2011). Participant profiles suggest relative success in reaching lower socio-economic groups who have an established heath need (Gidlow et al., 2013; Shircore, 2013). Yet, the accompanying evidence of effectiveness and cost-effectiveness, and more specific demonstration of how programmes can help to address health inequalities, is not yet manifest. Where beneficial effects have been shown, they have been modest and/or limited to those with worse health profiles at recruitment (Gardner et al., 2012; Gidlow et al., 2013). Similar to exercise referral, the recruitment and screening process is likely to be an important contributor to effectiveness: to ensure recruitment of those with a genuine health need and who are 'ready' to change. Only the former has been demonstrated with consistency so far.

It is encouraging that the health trainer model developed around tried and tested behaviour-change techniques. Therefore, programme effectiveness is dependent on the effective delivery of complex behaviour-change techniques by individuals from a range of professional backgrounds who have received varying levels of training. It is too early to know if interventions are being delivered as effectively as expected, so further research is warranted.

Box 13.1 Case study of health trainer evaluation

One-year cardiovascular risk and quality of life changes in participants of a health trainer service (Gidlow et al., 2013)

What was the aim of the study? To estimate changes in CVD risk and self-reported health-related quality of life (HRQoL) in a sample of Health Trainer programme participants.

What were the research questions? Is engagement with a health trainer programme associated with beneficial changes in clinical or self-reported health?

Who were the participants? Patients (n = 994) were from those referred to a city-wide programme from forty-one general practices in Stoke-on-Trent, UK, between May 2009 and January 2010.

What was the intervention? Participants were assigned to one of twenty two health trainers with core competency training (based on national health trainer curriculum) and additional training (City & Guilds). Lifestyle support lasted six to twelve months. An initial consultation involved techniques such as motivational counselling and goal setting, to agree lifestyle goals and the level of support, with signposting/referral to services as appropriate (e.g. physical activity, smoking cessation). Follow-up support was provided by face-to-face meetings and telephone/text message (depending on patient preference).

Method – what data were collected and how? Quantitative data from a range of sources were linked through unique numeric identifiers: clinical data from general practice databases, data routinely gathered by health trainers, health trainer logs of signposting, additional self-reported health. Framingham 10-year CVD risk (%) was determined using clinical data (British Cardiac Society et al.,

(continued)

(continued)

2005) and HRQoL derived from the a validated self-reported measure (Quality Metric, 2006).

How was this analysed? Intention to treat (ITT) analysis was used. Main analyses were paired samples t-tests to estimate twelve-month change in CVD risk (transformed), CVD risk factors, and HRQoL.

What were the findings? At twelve months there were significant improvements in modifiable CVD risk factors (BMI, serum cholesterol, total: HDL cholesterol), but not overall CVD risk (–.25 ± 6.50 per cent). Within the subsample of participants with high CVD risk at baseline (n = 320), however, significant overall CVD risk reductions were evident (–2.34 ± 8.13 per cent). Small, significant twelve-month HRQoL improvements were also observed, but were not associated with clinical improvements.

What were the conclusions and implications for practice? Given the greater health benefit for those with high CVD risk (and lack of significant change in the total population), this study indicated that the programme should target those with CVD risk ≥ 20 per cent.

Chapter summary

This chapter has focused on primary health care as the setting or the means of accessing physical activity interventions, and the relatively recent move to more community settings. There is a clear need to strengthen the evidence base around primary care-based physical activity promotion. Even where the behaviour change techniques are evidence-based, their application within programmes warrants further robust research and evaluation. Despite the advantages of using primary care, there are limitations (e.g. the under-representation of certain groups). Where programmes are delivered outside the primary care setting, health professionals often remain the gate-keepers to them, so their role in appropriate identification and signposting should not be ignored. Overall, evidence for ERS and health trainer programmes indicates that, at best, they can have more marked health benefits for those with the worst health profiles, with modest, short-term benefits overall; at worst, they may have no effect for some people. While we work to address the gaps in the evidence, it is arguable that continued action is preferable, if the alternative is to cease funding for physical activity programmes and risk a general worsening in population physical activity levels while we wait for evidence to guide investment in specific interventions.

Further research

Across the programmes discussed in this chapter, some important considerations for future research are suggested. First, there is a need for better measurement of health and behaviour outcomes, either in routine practice or associated research/ evaluation. Physical activity measurement is problematic and rarely involves objective measures (e.g. accelerometry) given the costs and logistical challenges. Those implementing physical activity programmes should ensure that validated and reliable physical activity questionnaires are used routinely (National Obesity Observatory, 2012), and researchers should include objective physical activity assessment where possible. In terms of health, where possible, objective measures, such as clinical (e.g. blood pressure, cholesterol) and anthropometric outcomes (e.g. measured BMI, waist circumference, body fat percentage) should be included. Where self-report is necessary or preferred, validated and reliable tools are recommended. Second, the lack of long-term outcomes is a perennial issue, as tracking of participants through and beyond programmes to allow robust measurement of longer-term changes has been relatively poor to date. The growing interest in Mobile Health (mHealth) holds great potential in this regard (World Health Organization, 2011); e.g. the use mobile phones to maintain contact with, and collect basic follow-up data from participants, even with those who drop out of programmes. Third, we recognise the need for controlled research of effectiveness and cost-effectiveness, and advocate the use of pragmatic RCTs where usual processes are not manipulated at the expense of external validity. Strong academic-practice partnerships can improve the quality of routine monitoring and evaluation where controlled research is not feasible, and the breath of published evidence should be used to inform practice. Fourth, qualitative research is important to help explain the reasons for the patterns and phenomena observed in quantitative research and evaluation, to understand the processes involved, and to identify appropriate changes to practice. Finally, and specific to the health trainer model, there is a need for research to verify the fidelity of behaviour change technique delivery in health trainer programmes. At present, there is an assumption that the training provided confers the necessary expertise to foster behaviour changes. As discussed in Chapter 11, this is an assumption that we should not be afraid to challenge and test.

Study tasks

1 *Research*

Find and read the most recent systematic review of a physical activity programme of your choice, using terms like 'exercise', 'physical activity', 'intervention', and 'primary care'. Write your own critique based on the inclusion/exclusion criteria, types of evidence considered, quality of this evidence and the types of question that the review was able to answer.

2 *Applied*

Make a list of physical activity promotion programmes in your local area, and try to locate evidence of local evaluation, or evidence from the published literature that supports these approaches.

3 *Policy*

Visit the NICE website (http://www.nice.org.uk) and find guidance that relates to physical activity. Select either 'Physical activity: brief advice for adults in primary care' (2013), 'Exercise referral' (2014), or 'Four commonly used methods to increase physical activity' (2006). Consider delivery in your local area in relation to this guidance.

Further reading

The following resources are recommended for this chapter:

Attree, P., Clayton, S., Karunanithi, S., Nayak, S., Popay, J., and Read, D. (2011). NHS health trainers: a review of emerging evaluation evidence. *Critical Public Health*, 22(1), 1–14.

NICE (2006). Four commonly used methods to increase physical activity: brief interventions in primary care, exercise referral schemes, pedometers and community-based exercise programmes for walking and cycling. *Public health intervention guidance 2.* London: National Institute for Health and Clinical Excellence.

NICE (2013). Physical activity: brief advice for adults in primary care. *NICE public health guidance 44.* London: National Institute for Health and Clinical Excellence.

Michie, S., Rumsey, N., Fussell, S., Hardeman, W., Johnston, M., Newman, S., and Yardley, L. (2006). *Improving health: changing behaviour – NHS health trainer handbook.* London: Department of Health and British Psychological Society.

Miller, W. R., and Rollnick, S. (2012). *Motivational interviewing: preparing people for change.* 3rd ed. New York: Guildford.

Note

1 Exercise Referral Schemes (ERS) will be used in this chapter, as it remains the most commonly-used term. Other terms for this model include (but are not limited to) Physical Activity Referral Schemes (PARS), GP referral schemes, and Exercise on Prescription.

References

Ackerman, E., Falsetti, S. E., Lewis, P., Hawkins, A. O., and Heinschel, J. A. (2011). Motivational interviewing: a behavioral counseling intervention for the family medicine provider. *Family Medicine*, 43(8), 582–5.

Attree, P., Clayton, S., Karunanithi, S., Nayak, S., Popay, J., and Read, D. (2011). NHS health trainers: a review of emerging evaluation evidence. *Critical Public Health*, 1–14. doi: 10.1080/09581596.2010.549207.

Aveyard, P., Begh, R., Parsons, A., and West, R. (2012). Brief opportunistic smoking cessation interventions: a systematic review and meta-analysis to compare advice to quit and offer of assistance. *Addiction*, 107(6), 1066–73.

Ball, L., and Nasr, N. (2011). A qualitative exploration of a health trainer programme in two UK primary care trusts. *Perspectives in Public Health*, 131(1), 24–31. doi: 10.1177/1757913910369089.

Barton, G. R., Goodall, M., Bower, P., Woolf, S., Capewell, S., and Gabbay, M. B. (2012). Increasing heart-health lifestyles in deprived communities: economic evaluation of lay health trainers. *Journal of Evaluation in Clinical Practice*, 18(4), 835–40.

Breckon, J. D., Johnston, L. H., and Hutchison, A. (2008). Physical activity counseling content and competency: a systematic review. *Journal of Physical Activity and Health*, 5(3), 398–417.

British Heart Foundation. (2010). *A toolkit for the design, implmention and evaluation of exercise referral schemes: a guide to evaluating exercise referral schemes.* Loughborough: BHF National Centre for Physical Activity and Health.

Bull, F., and Milton, K. (2010). A process evaluation of a 'physical activity pathway' in the primary care setting. *BMC Public Health*, 10, 463–70.

Bull, F., and Milton, K. (2011). Let's Get Moving: a systematic pathway for the promotion of physical activity in a primary care setting. *Global Health Promotion*, 18(1), 59–61.

Butler, C. C., Simpson, S. A., Hood, K., Cohen, D., Pickles, T., Spanou, C., McCambridge, J., Moore, L. A. R., Randell, E., Alam, M. F., Kinnersley, P. R., Edwards, A. G., Smith, C., and Rollnick, S. (2013). Training practitioners to deliver opportunistic multiple behaviour change counselling in primary care: a cluster randomised trial. *BMJ*, 346 f1191. doi: http://dx.doi.org/10.1136/bmj.f1191.

Carr, S. M., Lhussier, M., Forster, N., Geddes, L., Deane, K., Pennington, M., Visram, S., White, M., Michie, S., Donaldson, C., and Hildreth, A. (2011). An evidence synthesis of qualitative and quantitative research on component intervention techniques, effectiveness, costeffectiveness, equity and acceptability of different versions of health-related lifestyle advisor role in improving health. *Health Technology Assessment*, 15(9), iii–iv, 1–284. doi: 10.3310/hta15090.

Cochrane, T., Davey, R., Iqbal, Z., Gidlow, C., Kumar, J., Chambers, R., and Mawby, Y. (2012). NHS health checks through general practice: randomised trial of population cardiovascular risk reduction. *BMC Public Health*, 12(1), 944.

Crone, D., Johnston, L., and Grant, T. (2004). Maintaining quality in exercise referral schemes: a case study of professional practice. *Primary Health Care Research and Development*, 5(5), 96–103.

Crone, D., Johnston, L. H., Gidlow, C., Henley, C., and James, D. V. B. (2008). Uptake and participation in physical activity referral schemes in the UK: an investigation of patients referred with mental health problems. *Issues in Mental Health Nursing*, 29(10), 1088–97.

Crone, D., Smith, A., and Gough, B. (2005). 'I feel totally at one, totally alive and totally happy': a psycho-social explanation of the physical activity and mental health relationship. *Health Education Research*, 20, 600–11.

Curry, N. R., Crone, D., James, D., and Gidlow, C. (2011). Factors influencing participation in outdoor physical activity promotion schemes: the case of South Staffordshire, England. *Leisure Studies*, 31 (4), 447–63.

Damush, T. M., Stump, T. E., Saporito, A., and Clark, D. O. (2001). Predictors of older primary care patients' participation in a submaximal exercise test and a supervised, low-impact exercise class. *Preventive Medicine*, 33(5), 485–94. doi: http://dx.doi.org/10.1006/pmed.2001.0919.

Dauer, A. R.-M., Rubio, E. S., Coris, M. E., and Valls, J. M. (2006). Brief intervention in alcohol-positive traffic casualties: is it worth the effort? *Alcohol and Alcoholism*, 41(1), 76–83.

Davey, R., Cochrane, T., Iqbal, Z., Rajaratnam, G., Chambers, R., Mawby, Y., Picariello, L., Leese, C., and Ryder, N. (2010). Randomised controlled trial of additional lifestyle support for the reduction of cardiovascular disease risk through primary care in Stoke-on-Trent, UK. *Contemporary Clinical Trials*, 31(4), 345–54. doi: 10.1016/j.cct.2010.04.002.

Department of Health. (2001). *Exercise referral systems: a national quality assurance framework*. London: HMSO.

Department of Health. (2004). Choosing health. Making healthy choices easier. White Paper (p. 207). London: Department of Health.

Department of Health. (2009). *Let's get moving – a new physical activity care pathway for the NHS. Commissioning Guidance*. London: HMSO.

Department of Health. (2011). *Start active, stay active: a report on physical activity for health from the four home countries' Chief Medical Officers*. London: HMSO.

Dinan, S., Lenihan, P., Tenn, T., and Iliffe, S. (2006). Is the promotion of physical activity in vulnerable older people feasible and effective in general practice? *British Journal of General Practice*, 56(531), 791–3.

Dugdill, L., Graham, R. C., and McNair, F. (2005). Exercise referral: the public health panacea for physical activity promotion? A critical perspective of exercise referral schemes; their development and evaluation. *Ergonomics*, 48(11), 1390–410.

Gardner, B., Cane, J., Rumsey, N., and Michie, S. (2012). Behaviour change among overweight and socially disadvantaged adults: a longitudinal study of the NHS health trainer service. *Psychology and Health*, 27(10), 1178–93. doi: 10.1080/08870446.2011.652112.

Gidlow, C. J., Cochrane, T., Davey, R., Beloe, M., Chambers, R., Kumar, J., Mawby, Y., and Iqbal, Z. (2013). One-year cardiovascular risk and quality of life changes in participants of a health trainer service. *Perspectives in Public Health*, 134(3), 135–44. doi: 10.1177/1757913913484419.

Gidlow, C., Johnston, L. H., Crone, D., and James, D. (2005). Attendance of exercise referral schemes in the UK: a systematic review. *Health Education Journal*, 64(2), 168–86. doi: 10.1177/001789690506400208.

Gidlow, C., Johnston, L. H., Crone, D., Morris, C., Smith, A., Foster, C., and James, D. V. B. (2007). Socio-demographic patterning of referral, uptake and attendance in physical activity referral schemes. *Journal of Public Health*, 29, 107–13.

Gidlow, C., and Murphy, R. (2009). Physical activity promotion in primary health care. In L. Dugdill, D. Crone and R. Murphy (Eds.), *Physical activity and health promotion: evidence-based approaches to practice* (1st ed., pp. 87–102). UK: Wiley-Blackwell.

Goddard, M., and Smith, P. (2001). Equity of access to health care services: theory and evidence from the UK. *Social Science and Medicine*, 53(9), 1149–62. doi: 10.1016/s0277-9536(00)00415-9.

Gold, M., Stevenson, D., and Fryback, D. (2002). HALYS and QALYS and DALYS, oh my: similarities and differences in summary measures of population health. *Annual Review of Public Health*, 23, 115–34.

Goldstein, M. G., Whitlock, E. P., and DePue, J. (2004). Multiple behavioral risk factor interventions in primary care: summary of research evidence. *American Journal of Preventive Medicine*, 27(2), 61–79.

Hanson, C. L., Allin, L. J., Ellis, J. G., and Dodd-Reynolds, C. J. (2013). An evaluation of the efficacy of the exercise on referral scheme in Northumberland, UK: association with physical activity and predictors of engagement. A naturalistic observation study. *BMJ Open*, 3(8). doi: 10.1136/bmjopen-2013-002849.

Hardcastle, S., Blake, N., and Hagger, M. S. (2012). The effectiveness of a motivational interviewing primary-care based intervention on physical activity and predictors of change in a disadvantaged community. *Journal of behavioral medicine*, 35(3), 318–33.

Hardcastle, S., and Hagger, M. S. (2011). 'You Can't Do It on Your Own': experiences of a motivational interviewing intervention on physical activity and dietary behaviour. *Psychology of Sport and Exercise*, 12(3), 314–23.

Hardcastle, S., and Taylor, A. H. (2001). Looking for more than weight loss and fitness gain: psychosocial dimensions among older women in a primary-care exercise-referral program. *Journal of Aging and Physical Activity*, 9(3), 313–28.

Harrison, R. A., McNair, F., and Dugdill, L. (2005). Access to exercise referral schemes – a population based analysis. *Journal of Public Health*, 27(4), 326–30.

Hutchison, A. J., Breckon, J. D., and Johnston, L. H. (2008). Physical activity behavior change interventions based on the transtheoretical model: a systematic review. *Health Education and Behavior*. 36(5), 829–45. doi: 10.1177/1090198108318491.

James, D., Mills, H., Crone, D., Johnston, L. H., Morris, C., and Gidlow, C. J. (2009). Factors associated with physical activity referral completion and health outcomes. *Journal of Sports Sciences*, 27(10), 1007–17.

James, D. V. B., Johnston, L. H., Crone, D., Sidford, A. H., Gidlow, C., Morris, C., and Foster, C. (2008). Factors associated with physical activity referral uptake and participation. *Journal of Sports Sciences*, 26(2), 217–24.

Johnston, L., Breckon, J. D., and Hutchison, A. (2009). Influencing health behaviour: applying theory to practice. In L. Dugdill, D. Crone and R. Murphy (Eds.), *Physical activity and health promotion: evidence-based approaches to practice* (1st ed., pp. 87–102). UK: Wiley-Blackwell.

Johnston, L. H., Warwick, J., De Ste Croix, M., Crone, D., and Sidford, A. (2005). The nature of all 'inappropriate referrals' made to a countywide physical activity referral scheme: implications for practice. *Health Education Journal*, 64(1), 58–69. doi: 10.1177/0017896905064 00107.

Lai, D., Cahill, K., Qin, Y., and Tang, J. L. (2010). Motivational interviewing for smoking cessation. *Cochrane Database Syst Rev*, (1), CD006936. doi: 10.1002/14651858.

Lamb, S., Bartlett, H., Ashley, A., and Bird, W. (2002). Can lay-led walking programmes increase physical activity in middle-aged adults? *Journal of Epidemiology and Community Health*, 56, 246–52.

Lewin, S. A., Babigumira, S. M., Bosch-Capblanch, X., Aja, G., van Wyk, B., Glenton, C., Scheel, I., Zwarenstein, M., and Daniels, K. (2005). Lay health workers in primary and community health care: A systematic review of trials. *Cochrane database of systematic reviews*, CD004015. Epub: 2005 Jan 25.

Little, A., and Lewis, K. (2006). Influences on long-term exercise adherence in older patients with cardiac disease. *International Journal of Therapy and Rehabilitation*, 13(12), 543–50.

Macdonald, P., Hibbs, R., Corfield, F., and Treasure, J. (2012). The use of motivational interviewing in eating disorders: a systematic review. *Psychiatry Research*, 200(1), 1–11.

Martins, R. K., and McNeil, D. W. (2009). Review of motivational interviewing in promoting health behaviors. *Clinical Psychology Review*, 29(4), 283–93.

Michie, S., Rumsey, N., Fussell, S., Hardeman, W., Johnston, M., Newman, S., and Yardley, L. (2006). *Improving health: changing behaviour – NHS health trainer handbook*. London: Department of Health and British Psychological Society.

Miller, W. R., and Rollnick, S. (2012). *Motivational interviewing: preparing people for change*. 3rd ed. New York: Guildford.

Mills, H., Crone, D., James, D. V., and Johnston, L. H. (2012). Exploring the perceptions of success in an Exercise Referral Scheme: a mixed method investigation. *Evaluation review*, 36(6), 407–29.

Monti, P. M., Colby, S. M., Barnett, N. P., Spirito, A., Rohsenow, D. J., Myers, M., Woolard, R., and Lewander, W. (1999). Brief intervention for harm reduction with alcohol-positive older adolescents in a hospital emergency department. *Journal of Consulting and Clinical Psychology*, 67(6), 989.

Moore, G., Moore, L., and Murphy, S. (2011). Facilitating adherence to physical activity: exercise professionals' experiences of the National Exercise Referral Scheme in Wales. A qualitative study. *BMC Public Health*, 935(11), 935.

Morgan, O. (2005). Approaches to increase physical activity: reviewing the evidence for exercise-referral schemes. *Public Health*, 119(5), 361–70.

Müller-Riemenschneider, F., Reinhold, T., Nocon, M., and Willich, S. N. (2008). Long-term effectiveness of interventions promoting physical activity: a systematic review. *Preventive Medicine*, 47(4), 354–68. doi: http://dx.doi.org/10.1016/j.ypmed.2008.07.006.

Munro, J. F., Nicholl, J. P., Brazier, J. E., Davey, R., and Cochrane, T. (2004). Cost effectiveness of a community based exercise programme in over 65 year olds: cluster randomised trial. *Journal of Epidemiology and Community Health*, 58, 1004–10.

Murphy, S. M., Edwards, R. T., Williams, N., Raisanen, L., Moore, G., Linck, P., Hounsome, N., Din, N. U., and Moore, L. (2012). An evaluation of the effectiveness and cost effectiveness of the National Exercise Referral Scheme in Wales, UK: a randomised controlled trial of a public health policy initiative. *Journal of Epidemiology and Community Health*, 66(8), 745–53. doi: 10.1136/jech-2011-200689.

National Institute for Health and Care Excellence. (2013). *Physical activity: brief advice for adults in primary care. NICE public health guidance 44*. London: NICE.

National Institute for Health and Care Excellence. (2014). *Exercise referral schemes to promote physical activity*. London: NICE.

National Institute for Health and Clinical Excellence. (2006). *Four commonly used methods to increase physical activity: brief interventions in primary care, exercise referral schemes, pedometers and community-based exercise programmes for walking and cycling*. London: NICE.

National Institute for Health and Clinical Excellence. (2008a). *Occupational therapy interventions and physical activity to promote the mental wellbeing of older people in primary care and residential care*. London: NICE.

National Institute for Health and Clinical Excellence. (2008b). *Promoting and creating built or natural environments that encourage and support physical activity. NICE public health guidance 8*. London: NICE.

National Institute for Health and Clinical Excellence. (2008c). *Workplace health promotion: how to encourage employees to be physically active*. London: NICE.

National Institute for Health and Clinical Excellence. (2009). *Promoting physical actvity for children and young people. NICE public health guidance 17*. London: NICE.

National Institute for Health and Clinical Excellence. (2010). Measuring effectiveness and cost effectiveness: the QALY. Available at: http://www.nice.org.uk/newsroom/features/measur ingeffectivenessandcosteffectivenesstheqaly.jsp.

National Obesity Observatory. (2012). *Standard evaluation framework for physical activity interventions*. London: NOO.

Orrow, G., Kinmonth, A.-L., Sanderson, S., and Sutton, S. (2012). Effectiveness of physical activity promotion based in primary care: systematic review and meta-analysis of randomised controlled trials. *British Medical Journal*, 344. doi: 10.1136/bmj.e1389.

Pate, R. R., Pratt, M., Blair, S. N., Haskell, W. L., Macera, C. A., Bouchard, C., Buchner, D., Ettinger, W., Heath, G. W., King, A. C., Kriska, A., Leon, A. S. Marcus, B. H., Morris, J., Paffenbarger Jr, R. S., Patrick, K., Pollock, M. L., Rippe, J. M., Sallis, J., and Wilmore, J. H. (1996). Physical activity and public health: a recommendation from the Centers for Disease Control and Prevention and the American College of Sports Medicine, *JAMA.*, 273(5), 402–7.

Pavey, T. G., Anokye, N., Taylor, A. H., Trueman, P., Moxham, T., Fox, K. R., Hillsdon, M., Green, C., Campbell, J. L., Foster, C., Mutrie, N., Searle, J., and Taylor, R. S.. (2011a). The clinical effectiveness and cost-effectiveness of exercise referral schemes: a systematic review and economic evaluation. *Health Technol Assess*, 15(44).

Pavey, T. G., Taylor, A. H., Fox, K. R., Hillsdon, M., Anokye, N., Campbell, J. L., Foster, C., Green, C., Moxham, T., Mutrie, N., Searle, J., Trueman, P., and Taylor, R. S. (2011b). Effect of exercise referral schemes in primary care on physical activity and improving health outcomes: systematic review and meta-analysis. *British Medical Journal*, 343. doi: 10.1136/bmj.d6462.

Pavey, T., Taylor, A., Hillsdon, M., Fox, K., Campbell, J., Foster, C., Moxham, T., Mutrie, N., Searle, J., and Taylor, R. (2012). Levels and predictors of exercise referral scheme uptake and adherence: a systematic review. *Journal of Epidemiology and Community Health*, 66(8), 737–44. doi: 10.1136/jech-2011-200354.

Possidente, C. J., Bucci, K. K., and McClain, W. J. (2005). Motivational interviewing: a tool to improve medication adherence? *American Journal of Health-System Pharmacy*, 62(12), 1311.

Prince, S. A., Adamo, K. B., Hamel, M. E., Hardt, J., Gorber, S. C., and Tremblay, M. (2008). A comparison of direct versus self-report measures for assessing physical activity in adults: a systematic review. *International Journal of Behavioral Nutrition and Physical Activity*, 5(1), 56.

Rollnick, S., Butler, C. C., Kinnersley, P., Gregory, J. W., and Mash, B. (2010). Motivational Interviewing. *British Medical Journal*, 340, c1900.

Rollnick, S., Mason, P., and Butler, C. (1999). *Health behavior change: a guide for practitioners*. Elsevier Health Sciences.

Sharma, H., Bulley, C., and van Wijck, F. M. (2012). Experiences of an exercise referral scheme from the perspective of people with chronic stroke: a qualitative study. *Physiotherapy*, 98(4), 336–43.

Shephard, R. J., and Vuillemin, A. (2003). Limits to the measurement of habitual physical activity by questionnaires, *British Journal of Sports Medicine*, 37(3), 197–206. doi: 10.1136/bjsm.37.3.197.

Shircore, R. (2013). *Health trainers half year review 1st April – 30th September 2013. A critical assessment of health trainer activity, with particular reference to the most deprived social groupings, so as to assess the effectiveness and efficiency of the service in positively contributing to reducing health inequalities*. London: Royal Society for Public Health.

Sjöling, M., Lundberg, K., Englund, E., Westman, A., and Jong, M. C. (2011). Effectiveness of motivational interviewing and physical activity on prescription on leisure exercise time in subjects suffering from mild to moderate hypertension. *BMC research notes*, 4(1), 352.

Sørensen, J., Sørensen, J. B., Skovgaard, T., Bredahl, T., and Puggaard, L. (2011). Exercise on prescription: changes in physical activity and health-related quality of life in five Danish programmes. *The European Journal of Public Health*, 21(1), 56–62. doi: 10.1093/eurpub/ckq003.

South, J., Woodward, J., and Lowcock, D. (2007). New beginnings: stakeholder perspectives on the role of health trainers. *The Journal of the Royal Society for the Promotion of Health*, 127(5), 224–30. doi: 10.1177/1466424007081791.

Spanou, C., Simpson, S. A., Hood, K., Edwards, A., Cohen, D., Rollnick, S., Carter, B., McCambridge, J., Moore, L., Randell, E., Pickles, T., Smith, C., Lane, C., Wood, F., Thornton, H., and Butler, C. C. (2010). Preventing disease through opportunistic, rapid engagement by primary care teams using behaviour change counselling (PRE-EMPT): protocol for a general practice-based cluster randomised trial. *BMC Family Practice*, 11(1), 69.

Stevens, W., Hillsdon, M., Thorogood, M., and McArdle, D. (1998). Cost-effectiveness of a primary care based physical activity intervention in 45–74 year old men and women: a randomized controlled trial. *British Journal of Sports Medicine*, 32, 236–41.

Stokols, D. (1992). Establishing and maintaining health environments: toward a social ecology of health promotion. *American Psychologist*, 47(1), 6–22.

Tobi, P., Estacio, E., Renton, A., Yu, G., and Foster, N. (2012). Who stays, who drops out? Biosocial predictors of longer term adherence in participants attending an exercise referral scheme in the UK. *BMC Public Health*, 12(1), 347.

van Limpt, P. M., Harting, J., van Assema, P., Ruland, E., Kester, A., Gorgels, T., Knottnerus, J. A., van Ree, J. W., and Stoffers, H. E. (2011). Effects of a brief cardiovascular prevention program by a health advisor in primary care; the 'Hartslag Limburg' project, a cluster randomized trial. *Preventive Medicine*, 53(6), 395-401. doi: 10.1016/j.ypmed.2011.08.031.

Van Buskirk, K. A., and Wetherell, J. L. (2013). Motivational interviewing with primary care populations: a systematic review and meta-analysis. *Journal of Behavioral Medicine*, 37(4), 1–13. doi: 10.1007/s10865-013-9527-4.

Vinson, D., and Parker, A. (2012). Exercise, service and support: client experiences of physical activity referral schemes (PARS). *Qualitative Research in Sport, Exercise and Health*, 4(1), 15–31.

Williams, N. H. (2011). Promoting physical activity in primary care. *British Medical Journal*, 343. doi: 10.1136/bmj.d6615.

Williams, N. H., Hendry, M., France, B., Lewis, R., and Wilkinson, C. (2007). Effectiveness of exercise-referral schemes to promote physical activity in adults: systematic review. *British Journal of General Practice*, 57, 979–86.

World Health Organization. (2011). *mHealth: New horizons for health through mobile technologies: second global survey on eHealth*. Geneva: WHO.

Wormald, H., and Ingle, L. (2004). GP exercise referral schemes: improving the patient's experience. *Health Education Journal*, 63(4), 362–73.

Chapter 14

Evaluating stealth motivation interventions to promote Exercise Referral Scheme engagement and adherence

Samantha Meredith and Chris Wagstaff

Concerns for the uptake and maintenance of physical activity behaviours

Physical activity has long been considered a key behaviour for improving health, fitness, and wellbeing (for a review, see Penedo and Dahn, 2005). Indeed, the promotion of physical activity and structured exercise is a central concern for public health, both for the prevention and management of chronic disease, such as cardiovascular diseases, obesity, diabetes, cancer, and chronic respiratory diseases (e.g. World Health Organisation, 2010). In the current obesogenic society dominated by sedentary lifestyles (Swinburn et al., 2011), the government has launched various campaigns ('Moving More, Living More'; 'Change4Life') that aim to facilitate a more active society. Moreover, the benefits of regular physical activity, such as the regulation of body weight, improved insulin sensitivity, and reductions in hypertension (e.g. Bassuk and Manson, 2005) have led to the inclusion of structured exercise interventions within various rehabilitation settings to help effective management of chronic health conditions (e.g. cardiac rehabilitation, pulmonary rehabilitation, and GP referral schemes; Williams, 2011).

Current physical activity guidelines recommend that adults should achieve a total of at least 150 minutes over a week of at least moderate activity, in bouts of at least ten minutes duration (Department of Health, 2011). Despite national initiatives and agendas to enhance physical activity levels, the Health Survey for England (HSE) 2012 found that, according to self-reported physical activity data, 33 per cent of men and 45 per cent of women aged sixteen and over did not meet these guidelines (Health and Social Care Information Centre, 2015). Furthermore, beyond subjective self-report designs, results from an objective accelerometer study in 2008 (Health and Social Care Information Centre, 2015) found that only 6 per cent of men and 4 per cent of women achieved the government's recommended physical activity levels. These statistics highlight a growing health behaviour problem (Noar and Zimmerman, 2005).

Whilst the benefits of engaging, and risks of non-engagement, with physical activity are firmly entrenched within empirical and anecdotal accounts, there remains a dissonance between knowledge and action. That is, within society, individuals have reported a lack of motivation to initiate or sustain physical activity behaviour changes (see Health and Social Care Information Centre, 2015). Somewhat worryingly, even those patients with serious chronic health conditions who have been specifically prescribed exercise to manage disease are likely to fail to initiate or adhere to exercise referral schemes (see Pavey et al., 2012 for a systematic review and meta-analysis). Consequently, scholars pinpoint the need to identify factors that could create positive, effective exercise environments to foster engagement and adherence to exercise prescription (see Chapter 13). As such, psychologists have sought to examine the determinants of physical activity uptake and maintenance, revealing a range of influential factors affecting behaviour change, including self-efficacy, intentions, self-regulation, attitudes, perceived barriers, outcome expectations, and motivation (Amireault et al., 2013; Bauman et al., 2002; Michie et al., 2011). The reasons for altering or failing to modify behaviour are undoubtedly complex, and are likely influenced by myriad antecedents. However, a pivotal psychological construct for most behaviour-change theories is motivation (Biddle and Mutrie, 2007; Hagger and Chatzisarantis, 2007).

Motivation: self-determination theory

Motivation refers to an individual's drive or desire to approach or avoid a particular behaviour, and can alter the direction and intensity of one's effort towards a goal (Hollyforde and Whiddett, 2002). A comprehensive macro-theory of human motivation that has received substantial empirical attention and support is self-determination theory (Deci and Ryan, 1987, 2000). Self-determination theory focuses on types, rather than amounts, of motivation, delineating between autonomous motivation (i.e. acting through volition), controlled motivation (i.e. external pressures to act), and amotivation (i.e. no intentions to act). Deci and Ryan (1987) proposed that motivation is autonomous to the extent that behaviours are integrated into a sense of self, and individuals choose to act, feeling personal importance for a goal. Comparatively, controlled motivation comprises behaviours that have been driven by feelings of pressure, either internally (e.g. through a sense of guilt), or externally (e.g. through rewards, or being dictated by others). An array of research has found that the quality of an individual's motivation can have differing effects on behaviour (see Deci and Ryan, 2002). To elaborate, growing evidence suggests that controlled motivation undermines the impetus to change and harms well-being, whereas autonomous forms of motivation promote adherence to behaviours and allow people to flourish (Ryan and Deci, 2000). Therefore, it follows that the quality or orientation of an individual's motivation to be physically active is an important consideration when attempting to initiate and encourage sustained physical activity behaviour change.

The orientation of motivation concerns the underlying attitudes and goals that give rise to action (Deci and Ryan, 2000). That is, scholars need to be aware of the reasons that lead to the instigation of changes in physical activity and the essential motives that can help to maintain these changes. For instance, a coronary heart disease patient could be motivated to exercise by the social support and enjoyment of a rehabilitation group, or they could be motivated to exercise to gain approval from a significant other that is worried for their health. The amount of motivation does not necessarily vary in these examples, but the quality of it does. The former example refers to doing something because it is inherently interesting or enjoyable and is known as intrinsic motivation (i.e. an autonomous form of motivation), whereas the latter refers to enacting behaviour to achieve a separable outcome, labelled as extrinsic motivation (i.e. a more controlled form of motivation) (Deci and Ryan, 1987).

Ideally, exercise practitioners should aim to enhance an individual's intrinsic motivation to change, as this type of drive is far more powerful than any external motives to exercise (e.g. Sebire et al., 2009).

According to Deci and Ryan (2000), intrinsic motivation is defined as

> the doing of an activity for its inherent satisfactions rather than for some separable consequence. When intrinsically motivated a person is moved to act for the fun or challenge entailed rather than because of external prods, pressures, or rewards.
> (p. 56)

Comparatively, extrinsic motivation refers to external drivers of motivation that originate outside the individual. Self-determination theory (Deci and Ryan, 2000) proposes that there are four types of extrinsic motivation (Figure 14.1) that lie on a continuum from being very externally motivated to act, to being highly self-endorsed and volitional. That is, extrinsic motivation varies to the extent that it is self-determined or autonomous (Figure 14.1). Specifically, the most self-determined form of extrinsic motivation is 'integrated regulation', and refers to behaviours that are motivated by values and needs (Ryan and Connell, 1989). These behaviours are stable, highly-integrated (i.e. they are self-endorsed), and are enacted volitionally (e.g. exercise becomes incorporated into an individual's life goals and way of living). Next along the continuum of self-determined motivation is 'identified regulation', when an individual is motivated to behave because they identify with the given activity's purpose and value (e.g. a respiratory patient who exercises because they believe the activity will help to manage their condition). Moving further along the continuum to more controlling forms of extrinsic motivation, 'introjected regulation' involves enacting a behaviour in relation to internal contingencies for reward or punishment (e.g. an overweight man is motivated to exercise to avoid disapproval from his wife). Last, 'external regulation' refers to motivated behaviours for external rewards or punishment avoidance (e.g. exercising to complete the referral programme and receive a graduation certificate). It is important to note that all of the above examples represent intentional behaviour for an instrumental gain, but the types of extrinsic motivation vary in their relative autonomy (Deci and Ryan, 2000).

Self-determination theory and exercise

In a recent systematic review, Teixeira and colleagues (2012) found that identified regulation predicted short-term adoption of exercise more strongly than any other type of motivation. Identified regulation refers to being motivated by personal goals, outcomes, and product rather than enjoyment. By way of example, a large body of research suggests that individuals exercise to improve body shape and attractiveness (Prichard and Tiggemann, 2008; Vartanian et al., 2012). Although identified regulation is the most commonly employed motivation to initiate exercise, Teixeira et al. (2012) established that intrinsic motivation was more predictive of long-term exercise adherence. That is, intrinsic motives positively predict exercise participation across a range of samples (e.g. exercisers, healthy adults, students, office workers, cancer survivors, and exercise referral clients) and settings (e.g. cardiac rehabilitation, exercise referral schemes, schools, leisure centres). Thus, the experiential qualities

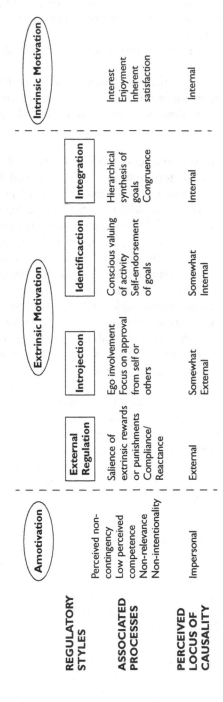

Figure 14.1 A continuum of self-determined motivation (adapted from Deci and Ryan, 2000).

of exercise are a critical factor mediating physical activity adherence (Rhodes and Pfaeffli, 2010).

Consequently, practitioners should seek to enhance an individual's intrinsic motivation to be physically active. However, it is unlikely that patients from a clinical population will be interested in, let alone intrinsically motivated to, changing their activity levels when they have been given an external prescription to participate in exercise (Markland and Tobin, 2010). Indeed, externally-regulated exercise behaviours might be perceived as controlling and undermining of an individual's self-determination (see Hagger and Chatzisarantis, 2008 for a review). Moreover, clinically-referred patients are more likely to have barriers to physical activity related to their medical condition (e.g. side-effects of medication; comorbidities; pain; fatigue). For instance, individuals with type 2 diabetes have reported exercise to be physically painful due to complications such as peripheral neuropathy, and comorbidities such as arthritic joint pain (e.g. Dutton et al., 2005). Moreover, clinical populations often report feelings of tiredness and anxiety, and fear the reoccurrence of symptoms (e.g. shortness of breath, chest pains) as common barriers to physical activity (e.g. Thomas et al., 2004; Thorpe et al., 2012; Yates et al., 2003). Perhaps not surprisingly, the effectiveness of promoting intrinsic motivation for increasing physical activity levels in this population group via prescription or exercise referral is not well evidenced, and might reflect a discord between theory and practice. Some practitioners might overcome some of these motivation-related barriers by using appropriately-tailored exercise prescription. However, physical activity interventions might benefit from more consistently and systematically incorporating self-determination theory intervention advice when attempting to enhance intrinsic motivation or psychical activity through transferring theory to practice (Michie et al., 2008).

Deci and Ryan (1987, 2008) suggest that intrinsic motivation can be enhanced through the creation of an environment that satisfies three innate psychological needs: the human desire for competence, relatedness, and autonomy. Feelings of competency can be gained from mastery experiences, such as the success of exercise experiences, or positive feedback from exercise practitioners. Competency is similar to self-efficacy, a concept introduced by Bandura (1977), who suggests that an individual's situation-specific self-confidence to perform a particular behaviour is an important facet of motivation. The psychological need of relatedness refers to one's personal connection with others and can be improved through facilitating positive social interactions. Autonomy refers to the self-endorsement of one's actions through the perception of choice and volition to engage in a given behaviour (Deci and Ryan, 2008). When an individual's environment supports these psychological needs, their motivation to engage in that behaviour is more self-determined and, thus, intrinsically motivated. Therefore, satisfying individuals' needs for autonomy, relatedness, and competency are the basis for developing and maintaining intrinsic motivation and promoting self-determined physical activity behaviours. Hence, practitioners might develop strategies that facilitate environments to support the satisfaction of patients' psychological needs. Indeed, the application of self-determination theory within a clinical setting to improve health behaviour change has been noted as an important approach to improve physical and mental health (Sheldon et al., 2003). Sheldon et al., (2003) also called for clinicians to advise patients regarding their need to understand how to attain health-related goals, and to feel that they can be effective in carrying out the necessary actions (competence); their need to feel a sense of choice and volition with respect to their health-related goals (autonomy); and their need to feel respected and cared for by practitioners and important others (relatedness).

In light of the research and theory described so far, there is a need for clinical exercise practitioners to better understand how interpersonal environments affect autonomous versus controlled motivation, by supporting psychological needs (see Table 14.1). Scholars have increasingly explored the predictive role of contextual factors (e.g. monetary rewards, an opportunity for choice) on an individual's motivation, and have intervened accordingly to improve the uptake and maintenance of physical activity behaviours (for a review see Hagger and Chatzisarantis, 2008). This is supported by some evidence showing that autonomous motivation is associated with exercise adherence (Chatzisarantis et al., 2003) and improved exercise intentions (Hagger and Chatzisarantis, 2007; Hagger et al., 2007; Wilson and Rodgers, 2004). Others have found that perceived autonomy support and higher self-determined motivation was associated with enhanced exercise behaviour in cardiac rehabilitation patients (Russel and Brady, 2010), increased physical activity levels in individuals with rheumatoid arthritis (Hurkmans et al., 2010), and improved engagement with exercise referral schemes (Markland and Tobin, 2010).

Therefore, nurturing psychological needs and self-determined motivation through providing supportive interpersonal relationships between the exercise instructor and the referred client is important to assist the maintenance of exercise within rehabilitation settings (Markland and Tobin, 2010). As a result, interventions to increase physical activity have focussed on including strategies to support these needs for autonomy, competence, and relatedness (Chatzisarantis and Hagger, 2009; Ryan et al., 2008; Silva et al., 2008). For instance, Silva et al. (2008) conducted a randomised, controlled trial examining the effect of a self-determination theory-informed behaviour change intervention on exercise adherence and weight control in overweight and moderately obese women, compared with a control group (no intervention). The intervention was designed to establish an autonomy-supportive climate for the participants. The overall goal was to bring each participant closer to making autonomous decisions about whether she wanted to change and how. Strategies to facilitate autonomy and intrinsic motivation included promoting competence by practicing the necessary skills (e.g. exercising at a given intensity), giving positive feedback, and providing participants with a menu of options and a variety of avenues for behaviour change (Silva et al., 2008). At twelve months, the intervention group showed greater weight loss (– 6.9 per cent ± 7.29 per cent) and higher levels of physical activity (300 ± 179 min/week of moderate plus vigorous exercise; 9902 ± 3331 steps/day), compared to controls (– 2.5 per cent ± 7.5 per cent weight loss; 162 ± 171 min/week of moderate plus vigorous exercise; and 7852 ± 3470 steps/day) (Silva et al., 2010). Moreover, individuals with higher autonomous motivation completed more physical activity after thirty six months, compared to those with lower autonomy (Figure 14.2). Hence, data from this trial suggested that providing environments that enhance self-determined motivation might facilitate uptake and adherence to physical activity programmes, thus helping to avoid the high attrition observed in programmes such as exercise referral schemes (Pavey et al., 2012; Williams et al., 2007).

Table 14.1 Strategies to support an exercise environment that fulfils autonomy, relatedness, and competence

Autonomy

Provide a choice of activities

Provide exercisers with a choice of activities that can suit their needs and preferences. Participants can be helped to identify appropriate activities based on instruction in public health guidelines and effective exercise parameters that fit their interests and lifestyles.

Offer a rationale for activities

Provide a clear rationale for activities, explaining the underlying purpose, to develop a positive perception of an activity.

Internalise behaviour by focussing on personal values

Facilitate internalisation by focusing on the value of exercise for a variety of outcomes, e.g. physical and mental health (i.e. autonomous motivation).

Utilise rewards sparingly and carefully

Rewards should be viewed primarily as a temporary motivating tool and should be used with caution by practitioners attempting to promote activity.

Competence

Give positive feedback

Give positive reinforcement and feedback to clients when they complete an appropriate action, and provide friendly corrective advice and instruction.

Set process goals

Individuals are more likely to engage in activity when their reference for success is based on the process of mastering a task rather than outperforming others.

Use SMART goals

Setting exercise goals that are specific, measurable, attainable, realistic, and timely can help to improve competence levels. Self-monitoring behaviour allows an individual to be aware of successful achievements. Setting goals that are realistic and achievable ensures client's experience successes to boost confidence levels.

Relatedness

Promote the development of social relationships

Provide an environment that promotes social connections between participants, such as introducing new clients and prompting conversation.

Create opportunities for social support

Encourage individuals to identify family and friends who could support their behaviour change.

Facilitators/instructors should be enthusiastic and supporting

Mix within the class and ensure availability during exercise training. Spend time chatting before the session, learn participant's name, and show enthusiasm. Present an attitude of caring, understanding, and listening in response to clients' needs regarding exercise and physical activity.

(Hsu et al., 2013; Kilpatrick et al., 2002)

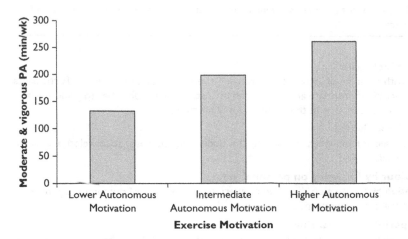

Figure 14.2 Self-reported minutes of moderate and vigorous exercise per week as a function of exercise autonomous motivation at thirty six months (i.e. two years following the intervention), adapted from Teixeira et al. (2012).

In summary, patients on exercise referral schemes are typically exercising for extrinsic means (e.g. to improve health outcomes; to adhere to a doctor's exercise prescription. For review see Hagger and Chatzisarantis, 2008). These reasons may be perceived as controlling, undermining participants' psychological needs and, thus, their self-determination, indirectly leading to a lack of motivation to persist with the behaviour (Markland and Tobin, 2010). This growing body of research suggests that clinical physical activity interventions would benefit from creating services that foster self-determination via the facilitation of psychological need satisfaction (increased variety of physical activity options; physical activity counselling; Edmunds et al., 2007).

However, sustaining an active lifestyle requires continued effort and repetition of activities. For many, health-related exercise is a behaviour that is seldom regulated or performed for intrinsic reasons alone (e.g. for the sake of the behaviour itself), but rather to attain an extrinsic outcome (Hagger and Chatzisarantis, 2008). The inherent enjoyment of exercise within the clinical domain might be unlikely given the relatively narrow choice of activities on offer in some exercise programmes. For instance, patients are often referred by health professionals to a community circuit programme or leisure centre facilities (e.g. gym, studio classes; Williams, 2011), which might not be enjoyable for some individuals. Whilst strategies can be developed to provide an autonomous exercise environment, scholars have proposed that regulation by identification with the outcomes of exercise might be more important than exercising for fun or enjoyment (Edmunds et al., 2006). For example, an obese individual with osteoarthritis, associated joint pain, and a lack of history of successful exercise experiences presents a challenging case study to enhance intrinsic motivation for physical activity. Therefore, when an individual does not enjoy exercise, it is important to make external reasons for change more internal to enhance their quality of motivation. Despite some evidence for the successful manipulation of contextual variables to create adaptive environments for exercise (for a review see Wilson et al., 2008) more innovative approaches to enhance the quality of motivation should be considered within exercise referral schemes. One such approach, and one that has recently gained growing acclaim for improving physical activity uptake and adherence, is the use of stealth interventions (BHFNC, 2014; Robinson, 2010).

Stealth interventions

In comparison to existing strategies that have tried to alter contextual variables to increase self-determined motivation to exercise (Kilpatrick et al., 2002), stealth interventions merge efforts to improve health with existing social movements that share behavioural goals (Robinson, 2010). That is, participants are intrinsically motivated to engage in an intervention that aims to achieve a social, more valued goal that might be unrelated to their health outcomes; healthy behaviours are a beneficial side effect. Robinson (2010) noticed that sizeable groups of the population readily change their attitudes, norms, and behaviours in line with social and ideological movements (e.g. anti-war, women's rights, animal rights, and anti-tobacco causes). Subsequently, he suggested that health projects could 'piggyback' on existing social movements to improve health-related behaviours. Physical activity by stealth refers to an intervention where the primary objective of the intervention, movement, or cause is unrelated to increasing physical activity levels. However, and most importantly, a supplementary outcome of the intervention is a sustainable change in physical activity behaviour. For instance, conservation volunteers (e.g. green gym projects) aim to develop green spaces for the wider public and engage in conservation work to improve the environment and help wildlife (see www.tcv.org.uk). Although the primary drive for such volunteering is related to engagement with, and the improvement of, the environment, the work involves moderate physical activity levels within a natural environment that can promote additional benefits for mood, and wellbeing (Pretty et al., 2007). Similarly, to achieve environmental sustainability (e.g. the cause, or movement), communities might design areas to improve the availability of walking and cycling paths, reduce mass transit, and decrease access to automobiles (e.g. the intervention). Consequently, opportunities for active travel to work and school improve, and enhanced physical activity levels become a by-product of the larger goal to improve climate change (see Table 14.2). This stealth approach is an appealing adjunct to current efforts of improving physical activity levels, as there is a focus on participants' intrinsic motivations and passions that might attract them to the projects, helping to sustain behaviour changes (Deci and Ryan, 2008).

According to Robinson (2010), stealth interventions enhance motivation through six key processes: identity formation; social interaction and membership; enhanced self-efficacy; collective responsibilities; beneficial emotional responses; and through influencing public policy. The incentive value of social movements allows the integration of beliefs to form strong identities that can align with individuals' deeper values and morals (Robinson, 2010). That is, an individual's drive to contribute towards a valued cause (e.g. preventing climate change) is more likely to be paralleled with their personal beliefs. This assimilation of values with idealised behaviours is a key step toward autonomous motivation (e.g. integrated regulation; intrinsic motivation), where an individual chooses to enact a behaviour that has been self-endorsed (Deci and Ryan, 2000). Moreover, the opportunities for social interaction, membership of a group, and the collective responsibilities available via stealth interventions might create strong social networks and interpersonal relationships that might subsequently satisfy one's need for relatedness (Deci and Ryan, 1987, 2000). Using the example of green gyms, an earlier evaluation of such a programme found that volunteers rated 'being a member of a social group' as a key motivator for taking part (Yerrell, 2008). Stealth interventions might also support the need for competency by providing vicarious and mastery experiences that are important for self-efficacy (Bandura, 1977). Indeed, Robinson (2010) recognised that the observation of influential models (e.g. observing group member successes) within social movements can enhance confidence levels, as well as the collective efficacy created by smaller successes achieved in the process of working as a group.

In adopting stealth approaches, previous interventions have utilised a valued cause, such as reducing youth crime (Hartmann and Depro, 2006), preventing climate change (Brockman and Fox, 2011), and reducing exposure to violent television programmes (Azevedo et al., 2013) to increase physical activity levels. By way of example, Brockman and Fox (2011) evaluated the effects of a workplace travel plan on levels of

Table 14.2 Social movements that are allied with physical activity behaviour change

Main valued outcome	Individual-level behaviours	Community/societal changes
Environmental sustainability/climate change e.g. preventing global warming and climate change, improving air quality	• Less automobile use • More walking • More cycling • Mass transit use (e.g. buses/trains)	Community design to increase ability to walk and cycle, improve mass transit and reduce access to automobiles
Anticonsumerism e.g. reducing consumer culture, or the influence of consumer culture	• Less television watching and other screen media use	School and community-based programmes and campaigns to reduce screen time and other exposures to marketing
Cause-related fundraising e.g. raising awareness and funding for charitable causes such as cancer research	• Walk-a-thons • Training and participation for endurance events • Long-distance bike rides	Greater use of physical activity-related fundraising organised by charities, increasing opportunities for physical activity in local communities.
Energy independence e.g. freeing nations from dependence on foreign oil	• Less automobile use • Increased walking • More cycling • Enhanced use of mass transit	Increased investment in, and availability of, public transportation and transportation infrastructure to promote non-motorised transportation to increase walking and cycling. Community design to increase walkability, bikability, and mass transit. Increased petrol taxes and consumer petrol prices.

Youth violence and crime prevention e.g. reducing youth involvement in gangs and crime	• Participating in after-school sports programmes for at-risk youths, or as mentors or coaches • Participating in community policing • Less screen time	Increased availability of after-school programmes, youth development programmes, including increased opportunities for physical activity and reduced screen time. Crime prevention policies for better street lighting, and greater police presence to reduce barriers to walking and outdoor recreation for community members.
Community safety, beautification, and traffic reduction e.g. improving safety and aesthetics to improve community quality of life and property values	• Gardening, clearing up, playground building, neighbourhood improvement, and repair projects • Spend more time participating in outdoor recreation and community social activities	Improved and increased pavements, bike lanes, walking paths, street lighting, lower speed limits, reduced availability, and increased costs of parking. Increased and improved parks and open spaces available for outdoor recreation in urban and suburban communities.

Adapted from Robinson, (2010).

active commuting. A travel survey conducted at the University of Bristol highlighted that staff who reported walking to work between 1998 and 2007 increased from 19 per cent to 30 per cent, and the percentage of regular cyclists increased from 7 per cent to 11.8 per cent (Figure 14.3). These changes were due to transport plans aimed at reducing car usage, such as restricting parking opportunities. Importantly, 70 per cent of staff who walked or cycled to work achieved a larger proportion of the recommended guidelines for physical activity through their active commuting (e.g. at least thirty minutes of moderate intensity activity on at least five days a week). Other stealth interventions that have successfully enhanced physical activity levels include projects aimed at reducing adolescent street crime and screen time by providing sports and dance clubs (Robinson et al., 2010). Indeed, the concern for the use of illegal recreational drugs and the associated elevations in youth crime rates has manifested in the development of initiatives designed to combat crime problems and promote social inclusion (Kelly, 2011). As such, sport now features in a range of youth programmes targeting deprived areas or 'at risk' groups/individuals, including 'Positive Futures – Catch 22', a national sport and physical activity-based social inclusion programme that works with young people in England and Wales (Home Office, 2013). For instance, mobile sports units providing opportunities to play various sports have been deployed in parks with reputations for anti-social behaviour and substance misuse by young people (Home Office, 2013).

Recently, the British Heart Foundation National Centre (BHFNC, 2014) hosted a conference, 'Creative partnerships: promoting physical activity by stealth', to share practice in the development and delivery of physical activity interventions. The focus

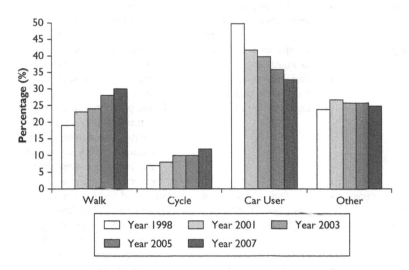

Figure 14.3 Percentage of individuals commuting through walking, cycling, car use, or by other modes of transport by year of survey (adapted from Brockman and Fox, 2011).

was on innovative stealth projects where the primary objective or end-goal of the intervention, movement, or cause was unrelated to increasing physical activity levels, but a supplementary outcome of the project was a change in physical activity behaviour, or projects that promoted people's intrinsic motivations and passions to attract them to physical activity. The conference highlighted a number of local stealth interventions, including real-world walking games (Box 14.1, Intelligent health, 2015), geocaching activities (e.g. a GPS treasure hunt game), projects to promote food foraging and outdoor activities, park regeneration projects, and parkour projects (BHFNC, 2014). The conference highlighted the potential public health importance of such interventions to contribute to through enhancing physical activity levels and sustaining adherence rates to these programmes through pursuit of a valued cause, or through engaging individuals through enhancing their intrinsic motivation.

Whilst the research discussed provides an indication of how stealth interventions might provide a means of promoting sustainable changes in physical activity levels, the majority of existing projects have targeted the general public and the prevention of chronic disease, rather than the management of disease *per se* (Brockman and Fox, 2011). Nevertheless, the stealth approach might be an attractive addition to traditional physical activity programmes, such as exercise referral schemes, to broaden patients' opportunities to be active. Given that externally-driven motivations could prevent sustained exercise changes (Teixeira et al., 2012), it might be fruitful to provide a range of activities and projects that harness self-determined physical activity behaviours. For example, the Welsh National Exercise Referral Scheme now offers gardening as an alternative activity to existing programmes (e.g. gym, circuits, and water-based classes) (BHFNC, 2014).

Moreover, empirical support for stealth interventions to cultivate intrinsic motivation and the ability to enjoy physical activity has since emerged, with an application to improving the uptake and adherence to health behaviours (Hunt et al., 2014a). Recent interventions in weight management have used innovative designs to maximise positive exercise atmospheres (e.g. satisfaction, intrinsic motivation, positive emotions, relatedness to group members, and mastery experiences; Hunt et al., 2014a). The intervention, known as Football Fans in Training (FFIT), was delivered to groups of Scottish men at top professional football clubs, targeting high-risk individuals to improve health behaviours (e.g. physical activity and healthy eating). Notably, the intervention attracted participants through focusing on enhancing their intrinsic motivation to change by involving their passions to be involved in a professional football club environment. The twelve-week scheme consisted of a pedometer-based walking programme, coach-led training at club stadia, portion size and healthy eating education, and behaviour change techniques such as self-monitoring of weight and physical activity, and goal-setting. Results from a randomised controlled trial demonstrate the effectiveness of FFIT in achieving clinically significant weight loss (4.36 per cent) at twelve months (Hunt et al., 2014b). Moreover, attendance throughout the programme was high, with 90 per cent retention at twelve weeks and twelve months follow-up (Hunt et al., 2014b). Importantly, qualitative interviews with participants revealed that the enjoyment and involvement with the football club improved engagement with the programme and enhanced adherence (Hunt et al, 2014b). Thus, the participants were not necessarily attracted to the programme through their motivations to alter their health behaviours, rather to enjoy membership and experiences within their admired sports club. Indeed, satisfaction with the content, context (the football club), and style of delivery (participative, peer-supported learning) likely predicted behavioural maintenance (Rothman et al., 2011). Therefore, nurturing positive subjective experiences (e.g. through enjoyment, and autonomy) might provide a successful means by which to captivate individuals in health behaviour interventions, and to enhance physical activity levels through stealth.

Box 14.1 Case study: physical activity stealth intervention

Beat the Street, Reading

Organisation: Intelligent Health

Aims and objectives: Beat the Street aims to reduce traffic congestion by promoting a community-wide walking competition. The main objectives were to raise awareness on the overdependence on cars for short journeys, and to build community cohesion through a fun real-world walking game.

Overview: Beat the Street took place in the local community of Reading on the streets and in the parks for five weeks beginning May 2014. Beat the Street turns an area into a real-life walking game where players register their movement by tapping RFID cards on 'beat boxes' placed around the town. The boxes flash and beep to register the activity. Tapping two or more walk tracking units records a journey. By using RFID technology, the competition is simple, engaging, and

(continued)

inclusive for the player, and measurable for the funder. As part of the challenge, schools and businesses can be invited to compete against each other to see who can accumulate the most points. The teams compete to walk the furthest, which is incentivised by prizes and raising money for charity. The intervention aims to act as a catalyst for longer-term behaviour change, encouraging individuals to explore walks and parks in the local area.

Evaluation/research methodology: The evaluation sought to measure any changes in physical activity. Baseline data were collected at registration via a registration website. This data included demographics (e.g. age, gender), the participant's post code, and completion of the single-item physical activity question (e.g. 'In the past week how many days have you done thirty minutes or more of physical activity, which was enough to raise your heart rate? This may include sport, exercise, and brisk walking or cycling, but not things that are part of your job.'). Moreover, participants were asked to complete a travel diary. A follow-up survey was then conducted on completion of the intervention, which repeated the single-item physical activity question and travel diaries. In addition, participants were asked to provide information about their attitudes, perceptions, and experiences of Beat the Street.

Results: Fifty teams competed in the competition, including thirty primary schools. In total, 15074 people took part, including 8416 children and 6658 adults. Results highlighted that the community walked a total distance of 244,537 miles. The majority of the journeys were through commuting to and from work or school. Individuals reported that the main reason they participated was for fun. Importantly, results showed a 10 per cent increase in the number of people meeting the governments' physical activity guidelines from 35 per cent at baseline to 45 per cent at the end of the intervention. At three months follow-up, 53 per cent of participants reported meeting these physical activity recommendations, indicating successfully-maintained behaviour changes. Notably, 12 per cent of participants had long-term health conditions, such as COPD, osteoarthritis, and diabetes. This suggests that this community scheme can improve physical activity levels and health, as both a tool for prevention and management of chronic disease.

Chapter summary

This chapter has focussed on the importance of self-determined motivation to enhance physical activity uptake and adherence, using stealth approaches as an example of how this can be applied. A large body of research acknowledges the importance of being intrinsically motivated to sustain physical activity changes. However, traditional programmes, such as exercise referral schemes, often seem to depend on participants' extrinsic motivation, such as advice from the health professional, so sustainable behaviour change may be unlikely. Current strategies to enhance intrinsic motivation have utilised tenets from self-determination theory to support an exercise environment that facilitates an individuals' psychological needs. Whilst these techniques have been shown to improve the integration of extrinsic motivation, innovative approaches might be required to elicit and develop intrinsic motivation to exercise within primary and secondary care. A burgeoning area of research and practice highlights the potential effectiveness of stealth interventions as a way of maintaining health-related behaviour change. Utilising an alternative cause that is highly valued, and which is allied to changes in physical activity behaviour, might be a useful adjunct to exercise referral approaches.

Study tasks

1 Review self-determination theory and list physical activity examples for each type of motivation detailed in the model.
2 Find a recent article that has researched the effectiveness of a physical activity intervention based upon self-determination theory. How did they transfer theory into practice? What specific intervention did they use and how was this outlined by self-determination theory?
3 Make a list of stealth intervention programmes that have increased physical activity in your local area. What are the specific components of the programmes? Who do the interventions target? What are the main goals of the interventions? How have these programmes been evaluated?
4 Create your own stealth physical activity intervention to incorporate into a GP exercise referral scheme.

Further reading

Hagger, M. S., and Chatzisarantis, N. (2008). Self-determination theory and the psychology of exercise. *International Review of Sport and Exercise Psychology*, 1(1), 79–103.
Robinson, T. N. (2010). Save the world, prevent obesity: piggybacking on existing social and ideological movements. *Obesity*, 18(S1), 17–22.
Teixeira, P. J., Carraça, E. V., Markland, D., Silva, M. N., and Ryan, R. M. (2012). Exercise, physical activity, and self-determination theory: a systematic review. *International Journal of Behavioural Nutrition and Physical Activity*, 9(78), 1–30.

References

Amireault, S., Godin, G., and Vézina-Im, L. A. (2013). Determinants of physical activity maintenance: a systematic review and meta-analyses. *Health Psychology Review*, 7(1), 55–91.
Azevedo, K. J., Mendoza, S., Fernández, M., Haydel, F., Fujimoto, M., Tirumalai, E. C., and Robinson, T. N. (2013). Turn off the TV and dance! Participation in culturally tailored health interventions: implications for obesity prevention among Mexican American girls. *Ethnicity and Disease*, 23(4), 452–61.
Bandura, A. (1977). Self-efficacy: toward a unifying theory of behavioral change. *Psychological Review*, 84(2), 191–215.
Bassuk, S. S., and Manson, J. E. (2005). Epidemiological evidence for the role of physical activity in reducing risk of type 2 diabetes and cardiovascular disease. *Journal of Applied Physiology*, 99(3), 1193–1204.
Bauman, A. E., Sallis, J. F., Dzewaltowski, D. A., and Owen, N. (2002). Toward a better understanding of the influences on physical activity the role of determinants, correlates, causal variables, mediators, moderators, and confounders. *American Journal of Preventative Medicine*, 23(2 suppl.), 5–14.

BHFNC. (2014). BHFNC 14th annual conference, creative partnerships: promoting physical activity by stealth-sharing practice booklet. Retrieved from website: http://www.bhfactive. org.uk/conference2014/index.html.

Biddle, S. J. H., and Mutrie, N. (2007). *Psychology of physical activity: determinants, well-being and interventions.* New York: Routledge.

Brockman, R., and Fox, K. R. (2011). Physical activity by stealth? The potential health benefits of a workplace transport plan. *Public Health*, 125(4), 210–16.

Chatzisarantis, N.L.D., and Hagger, M.S. (2009). Effects of an intervention based on self-determination theory on self-reported leisure-time physical activity participation. *Psychology and Health*, 24(1), 29–48.

Chatzisarantis, N.L.D., Hagger, M.S., Biddle, S.J.H., Smith, B., and Wang, J.C.K. (2003). A meta-analysis of perceived locus of causality in exercise, sport, and physical education contexts. *Journal of Sport and Exercise Psychology*, 25(3), 284–306.

Deci, E.L., and Ryan, R.M. (1987). The support of autonomy and the control of behaviour. *Journal of Personality and Social Psychology*, 53(6), 1024–37.

Deci, E.L., and Ryan, R.M. (2000). The 'what' and 'why' of goal pursuits: human needs and the self-determination of behavior. *Psychological Inquiry*, 11(4), 227–68.

Deci, E.L., and Ryan, R.M. (2002). *Handbook of self-determination research.* Rochester, NY: University of Rochester Press.

Deci, E. L., and Ryan, R.M. (2008). Self-determination theory: a macrotheory of human motivation, development, and health. *Canadian Psychology*, 49(3), 182–5.

Department of Health (2011). Physical activity guidelines for adults (19–64): factsheet 4. Retrieved from website: http://www.dh.gov.uk/en/Publicationsandstatistics/Publications/PublicationsPolicyAndGui dance/DH_127931.

Dutton, D.R., Johnson, J., Whitehead, D., Bodenlos, J.S., and Brantley, P.J. (2005). Barriers to physical activity among predominantly low-income African-American patients with type 2 diabetes. *Diabetes Care*, 28(5), 1209–10.

Edmunds, J., Ntumanis, N., and Duda, J. L. (2006). A test of self-determination theory in the exercise domain. *Journal of Applied Social Psychology*, 36(9), 2240–65.

Edmunds, J., Ntumanis, N., and Duda, J. L. (2007). Adherence and well-being in overweight and obese patients referred to an exercise on prescription scheme: a self-determination theory perspective. *Psychology of Sport and Exercise*, 8(5), 722–40.

Hagger, M. S., and Chatzisarantis, N. (2007). *Intrinsic motivation and self-determination in exercise and sport.* Leeds: Human Kinetics.

Hagger, M. S., and Chatzisarantis, N. (2008). Self-determination theory and the psychology of exercise. *International Review of Sport and Exercise Psychology*, 1(1), 79–103.

Hagger, M.S. Chatzisarantis, N.L.D., Hein, V., Pihu, M., Soós, I., and Karsai, I. (2007). The perceived autonomy support scale for exercise settings (PASSES): development, validity, and cross-cultural invariance in young people. *Psychology of Sport and Exercise*, 8(5), 632–53.

Hartmann, D., and Depro, B. (2006). Rethinking sports-based community crime prevention: a preliminary analysis of the relationship between midnight basketball and urban crime rates. *Journal of Sport and Social Issues*, 30(2), 180–196.

Health and Social Care Information Centre. (2015). Statistics on obesity, physical activity and diet, England 2015. Retrieved from website: http://www.hscic.gov.uk/catalogue/PUB16988.

Hollyforde, S., and Whiddett, S. (2002). *The motivation handbook.* London: Chartered Institute of Personnel and Development.

Home Office. (2013). Positive futures impact report, 2013. Retrieved from website: http://www. catch-22.org.uk/wp-content/uploads/2013/11/Positive-Futures-Impact-Report-2013.pdf.

Hsu, Y-T., Buckworth, J., Focht, B. C., and O'Connell, A. A. (2013). Feasibility of a Self-Determination Theory-based exercise intervention promoting Healthy at Every Size with sedentary overweight women: Project CHANGE. *Psychology of Sport and Exercise*, 14, 283–292.

Hunt, K., Gray, C. M., Maclean, A., Smillie, S., Bunn, B., and Wyke, S. (2014a). Do weight management programmes delivered at professional football clubs attract and engage high risk men? A mixed-methods study. *BMC Public Health*, 14(50), 1–11.

Hunt, K., Wyke, S., Gray, C. M., Anderson, A. S., Brady, A., Bunn, C., Donnan, P. T., Fenwick, E., Grieve, E., Leishman, J., Miller, E., Mutrie, N., Rauchhaus, P., White, A., and Treweek, S. (2014b). A gender-sensitised weight loss and healthy living programme for overweight and obese men delivered by Scottish Premier League football clubs (FFIT): a pragmatic randomised controlled trial. *Lancet*, 383(9924), 1211–21.

Hurkmans, E. J., Maes, S., de Gucht, V., Knittle, K., Peeters, A. J., Ronday, H. K., and Vliet Vlieland, T. P. M. (2010). Motivation as a determinant of physical activity in patients with rheumatoid arthritis. *Arthritis Care and Research*, 62(3), 371–7.

Intelligent Health. (2015). Beat the street: the physical activity programme that works. Retrieved from website: http://www.intelligenthealth.co.uk/our-workcase-studies/.

Kelly, L. (2011). 'Social inclusion' through sports-based interventions? *Critical Social Policy*, 31(1), 126–50.

Kilpatrick, M., Hebert, E., and Jacobsen, D. (2002). Physical activity motivation: a practitioner's guide to self-determination theory. *Journal of Physical Education, Recreation and Dance*, 73(4), 36–41.

Markland, D., and Tobin, V. J. (2010). Need support and behavioural regulations for exercise among exercise referral scheme clients: The mediating role of psychological need satisfaction. *Psychology of Sport and Exercise*, 11(2), 91–9.

Michie, S., Johnston, M., Francis, J., Hardeman, W., and Eccles, M. (2008). From theory to intervention: mapping theoretically derived behavioural determinants to behaviour change techniques. *Applied Psychology*, 57(4), 660–80.

Michie, S., van Stralen, M. M., and West, R. (2011). The behaviour change wheel: a new method for characterising and designing behaviour change interventions. *Implementation Science*, 6, 42.

Noar, S. M., and Zimmerman, R. S. (2005). Health behavior theory and cumulative knowledge regarding health behaviors: are we moving in the right direction? *Health Education Research*, 20(3), 275–90.

Pavey, T., Taylor, A., Hillsdon, M., Fox, K., Campbell, J., Foster, C., Moxham, T., Mutrie, N., Searle, J., and Taylor, R. (2012). Levels and predictors of exercise referral scheme uptake and adherence: a systematic review. *Journal of Epidemiology and Community Health*, 66(8), 737–44.

Penedo, F. J., and Dahn, J. R. (2005). Exercise and well-being: a review of mental and physical health benefits associated with physical activity. *Current Opinion in Psychiatry*, 18(2), 189–93.

Pretty, J., Peacock, J., Hine, R., Sellens, M., South, N., and Griffin, M. (2007). Green exercise in the UK countryside: effects on health and psychological well-being, and implications for policy and planning. *Journal of Environmental Planning and Management*, 50(2), 211–31.

Prichard, I., and Tiggemann, M. (2008). Relations among exercise type, self-objectification, and body image in the fitness centre environment: the role of reasons for exercise. *Psychology of Sport and Exercise*, 9(6), 855–66.

Rhodes, R. E., and Pfaeffli, L. A. (2010). Mediators of physical activity behaviour change among adult non-clinical populations: a review update. *International Journal of Behavioural Nutrition and Physical Activity*, 7(37), 1–11.

Robinson, T. N. (2010). Save the world, prevent obesity: piggybacking on existing social and ideological movements. *Obesity*, 18(S1), 17–22.

Robinson, T. N., Matheson, D. M., Kraemer, H. C., Wilson, D. M., Obarzanek, E., Thompson, N. S., Alhassan, S., Spencer, T. R., Haydel, F., Fujimoto, M., Varady, A., Killen, J. D. (2010). A randomized controlled trial of culturally tailored dance and reducing screen time to prevent weight gain in low-income African American girls. *Archives of Paediatrics' and Adolescent Medicine*, 164(11), 995–1004.

Rothman, A. J., Baldwin, A. S., Hertel, A. W., and Fuglestad, P. T. (2011). Self-regulation and behaviour change: disentangling behavioural initiation and behavioural maintenance. In K. D. Vohs, and R. F. Baumeister (Eds.), *Handbook of self-regulation: research, theory, and applications* (pp. 106–22). New York: The Guilford Press.

Russel, K. L., and Brady, S. R. (2010). Promoting self-determined motivation for exercise in cardiac rehabilitation: the role of autonomy support. *Rehabilitation Psychology*, 55(1), 74–80.

Ryan, R. M., and Connell, J. P. (1989). Perceived locus of causality and internalization: examining reasons for acting in two domains. *Journal of Personality and Social Psychology*, 57(5), 749–61.

Ryan, R. M., and Deci, E. L. (2000). Self-determination theory and the facilitation of intrinsic motivation, social development and well-being. *American Psychologist*, 55(1), 68–78.

Ryan, R. M., Patrick, H., Deci, E. L., and Williams, G. C. (2008). Facilitating health behaviour change and its maintenance: interventions based on self-determination theory. *The European Health Psychologist*, 10(1), 2–5.

Sebire, S. J., Standage, M., and Vansteenkiste, M. (2009). Examining intrinsic versus extrinsic exercise goals: cognitive, affective, and behavioral outcomes. *Journal of Sport and Exercise Psychology*, 31(2), 189–210.

Sheldon, K. M., Williams, G., and Joiner, T. (2003). *Self-determination theory in the clinic: motivating physical and mental health*. New Haven, CT: Yale University Press.

Silva, M. N., Markland, D., Minderico, C. S., Vieira, P. N., Castro, M. M., Coutinho, S. R., Santos, T. C., Matos, M. G., Sardinha, L. B., and Teixeira, P. J. (2008). A randomized controlled trial to evaluate self-determination theory for exercise adherence and weight control: rationale and intervention description. *BMC Public Health*, 8, 234.

Swinburn, B. A., Sacks, G., Hall, K. D., McPherson, K., Finegood, D. T., Moodie, M. L., and Gortmaker, S. L. (2011). The global obesity pandemic: shaped by global drivers and local environments. *Lancet*, 378(9793), 804–14.

Teixeira, P. J., Carraça, E. V., Markland, D., Silva, M. N., and Ryan, R. M. (2012). Exercise, physical activity, and self-determination theory: a systematic review. *International Journal of Behavioural Nutrition and Physical Activity*, 9(78), 1–30.

Thomas, N., Alder, E., and Leese, G. P. (2004). Barriers to physical activity in patients with diabetes. *Postgrad Medical Journal*, 80(943), 287–91.

Thorpe, O., Johnston, K., and Kumar, S. (2012). Barriers and enablers to physical activity participation in patients with COPD: a systematic review. *Journal of Cardiopulmonary Rehabilitation and Prevention*, 32(6), 359–69.

Vartanian, L. R., Wharton, C. M., and Green, E. B. (2012). Appearance vs. health motives for exercise and for weight loss. *Psychology of Sport and Exercise*, 13(3), 251–6.

Williams, N. H. (2011). Promoting physical activity in primary care. *British Medical Journal*, 343, d6615.

Williams, N. H., Hendry, M., France, B., Lewis, R., and Wilkinson, C. (2007). Effectiveness of exercise-referral schemes to promote physical activity in adults: systematic review. *British Journal of General Practice*, 57(545), 979–86.

Wilson, P. M., Mack, D. E., and Grattan, K. P. (2008). Understanding motivation for exercise: A self-determination theory perspective. *Canadian Psychology*, 49(3), 250–6.

Wilson, P.M., and Rodgers, W.M. (2004). The relationship between perceived autonomy support, exercise regulations and behavioural intentions in women. *Psychology of Sport and Exercise*, 5(3), 229–42.

World Health Organisation (2010). *Global status report on noncommunicable diseases.* Retrieved from website: http://www.who.int/nmh/publications/ncd_report2010/en/.

Yates, B. C., Price-Fowlkes, T., and Agrawal, S. (2003). Barriers and facilitators of self-reported physical activity in cardiac patients. *Research in Nursing and Health*, 26(6), 459–69.

Yerrell, P. (2008). National evaluation of TCV's green gym. Oxford: School of Health and Social Care, Oxford Brookes University. Retrieved from website: http://www.tcv.org.uk/sites/default/files/green-gym-evaluation-full.pdf.

Index